Certified Nurse Educator (CNE®) *and*
Certified Nurse Educator Novice (CNE®n)

EXAM PREP

Certified Nurse Educator (CNE®) *and*
Certified Nurse Educator Novice (CNE®n)

EXAM PREP

DONNA D. IGNATAVICIUS
MS, RN, CNE, CNEcl, ANEF, FAADN
President
DI Associates, Inc.
Littleton, Colorado

ELSEVIER

Elsevier
3251 Riverport Lane
St. Louis, Missouri 63043

Executive Content Strategist: Lee Henderson
Content Development Specialists: Dominque McPherson/Laura Goodrich
Publishing Services Manager: Julie Eddy
Senior Project Manager: Jodi Willard
Design Direction: Amy Buxton

Printed in India

Last digit is the print number: 9 8 7 6 5 4 3 2

Working together
to grow libraries in
developing countries

www.elsevier.com • www.bookaid.org

Contributors

SUSAN ANDERSEN, MS, RN, CNE
Director of Nursing Education
Kansas City Kansas Community College
Kansas City, Missouri

DEANNE A. BLACH, MSN, RN, CNE, NPD-BC
President
DB Productions
Green Forest, Arkansas

KAILEE BURDICK, DNP, RN, CNE
Clinical Simulation Specialist
Rural Health Innovation Collaborative Simulation Center
Terre Haute, Indiana

SOMER NOURSE, DNP, RN, CNE
Assistant Professor
School of Nursing
College of Health and Human Services
Indiana State University
Terre Haute, Indiana

ANGELA SILVESTRI-ELMORE, PhD, APRN,
  FNP-BC, CNE
Associate Dean for Entry and Prelicensure Education
University of Nevada, Las Vegas
Henderson, Nevada

LINDA KAYE WALTERS, PhD, RN, CNE
Professor/Undergraduate Coordinator
School of Nursing
College of Health and Human Services
Indiana State University
Rockville, Indiana

Preface

The Certified Nurse Educator® credential is a mark of professionalism that distinguishes the academic nurse educator's expertise within an advanced practice specialty role. The National League for Nursing (NLN) offers three different certification examinations for academic nurse educators:

- Certified Nurse Educator (CNE®)
- Certified Academic Clinical Nurse Educator (CNE®cl)
- Certified Novice Educator (CNE®n)

This excellent review and preparation book provides what you need to be successful on the CNE® and CNE®n examinations and consists of two parts: content review and practice questions.

Content Review

The content of this book is organized within 10 chapters written by expert academic nurse educators across nursing program types. Each chapter specifies learning outcomes, CNE®/CNE®n Key Points, current end-of-chapter references, and a summary of content you will need to know to pass the exams. Chapters 1 and 10 focus on tips for exam preparation and success; Chapters 2 through 9 highlight the essential knowledge you need for each academic nurse educator core competency. Each of these chapters presents a robust content review aligned with the test plans for each core competency, followed by multiple practice questions that simulate CNE®/CNE®n test items.

The specific emphasis for each chapter content review is summarized here:

- Chapter 1, entitled "Getting Ready for the Certified Nurse Educator (CNE®) and Certified Nurse Educator® Novice (CNE®n) Exams," introduces the educator to the Certified Nurse Educator® credential and differentiates the design and content of the CNE® and CNE®n exams.
- Chapter 2, entitled "Facilitating Learning," describes selected teaching-learning activities based on commonly used educational theories. Strategies for creating a safe, evidence-based learning environment are also discussed.
- Chapter 3, entitled "Facilitating Learner Development and Socialization," identifies evidence-based strategies to assist learners to develop as professional nurses and become socialized into the nursing profession.

- Chapter 4, entitled "Using Assessment and Evaluation Strategies," focuses on using valid and reliable strategies to assess and evaluate learning in the cognitive, psychomotor, and affective domains.
- Chapter 5, entitled "Participating in Curricular Design and Evaluation of Program Outcomes," describes the major components of a nursing curriculum and program assessment, including how to develop an effective systematic evaluation plan.
- Chapter 6, entitled "Functioning as a Change Agent and a Leader," discusses the role of the nurse educator in creating and sustaining change as a leader within the program and organization.
- Chapter 7, entitled "Pursuing Continuous Quality Improvement in the Nurse Educator Role," describes the process for socialization to the academic nurse educator role, including scholarship.
- Chapter 8, entitled "Engaging in Scholarship of Teaching," describes the development of an academic nurse educator as a nursing scholar with an emphasis on the scholarship of teaching.
- Chapter 9, entitled "Functioning Within the Educational Environment," explains the role of the nurse educator in program and institutional governance and ways to build a supportive organizational climate.
- Chapter 10, entitled "Planning for Success on the Certified Nurse Educator (CNE®) and Certified Nurse Educator Novice (CNE®n) Exams," explains how to develop an individualized study plan, manage cognitive test anxiety, and approach questions on the certification exams.

Practice Questions

Unlike most other CNE®/CNE®n review books, this comprehensive resource provides an abundance of valid practice questions that simulate today's certification exams. Eight chapters (Chapters 2 through 9) end with multiple test items that assess knowledge of the core competency reviewed in each chapter. All test items are presented as multiple-choice questions with a situation in the item stem and four answer options from which to choose. Correct answers with rationales and current references are provided at the end of this book.

In addition, following Chapter 10, a 150-item comprehensive test that simulates the certification examination is provided. All test items are presented as multiple-choice questions with a situation in the item stem and four answer options from which to choose. Similar to what is provided for the chapter practice questions, correct answers for the comprehensive test with rationales and current references are found at the end of this book.

It is my hope that you enjoy this review and preparation resource and obtain the CNE® or CNE®n credential soon!

Donna "Iggy" Ignatavicius

*To the nurse educators who are passionate about
shaping students into new roles, I applaud you.*

*To my husband of 45 years, who continues to
support my work with love and patience, I thank you.*

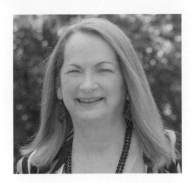

DONNA D. "IGGY" IGNATAVICIUS,
MS, RN, CNE, CNEcl, ANEF, FAADN
President, DI Associates, Inc.

Nationally recognized as an expert in nursing education and medical-surgical/gerontologic nursing, Iggy has a wealth of experience in education, clinical nursing, and administration. She has taught in AD and BSN programs for many years. Currently, Iggy speaks at national and state conferences and provides program consultation on such topics as curriculum development and program assessment through her company, DI Associates, Inc. She has conducted over 2000 presentations in all 50 states and Canada during the past 20 years. Additionally, Iggy is the author of a number of articles, chapters, and books, including her leading textbook, *Medical-Surgical Nursing: Concepts for Clinical Judgment and Collaborative Care,* 11th edition (in press), and *Developing Clinical Judgment for Practical/Vocational Nursing Practice and Next-Generation NCLEX-PN® Success* and *Developing Clinical Judgment for Professional Nursing Practice and NGN Readiness,* 2nd edition (in press). In 2007 Iggy was inducted as a fellow into the very prestigious Academy of Nursing Education (ANEF) for her national contributions to nursing education. She obtained her Certified Nurse Educator credential in 2016 and the Certified Academic Clinical Educator credential in 2020. In 2021 she recertified as a CNE® and was accepted as a fellow in the Academy of Associate Degree Nursing (FAADN).

Acknowledgments

Developing and producing a first edition book requires the talents of many people, starting with Lee Henderson, Elsevier Executive Content Strategist, Nursing Content, who encouraged me to coordinate this project. My contributor team were certified expert academic nurse educators who submitted high-quality manuscripts to produce an excellent resource.

Laura Goodrich and Dominque McPherson, Content Development Strategists, helped guide me during the development of the book to prepare for production and publication. I was especially fortunate to work with Jodi Willard, Senior Project Manager for Elsevier's Global Book Production, who mastered the many details of this book and kept me on schedule. Julie Eddy, Publishing Services Manager; Amy Buxton, Senior Book Designer; and Gregory Wade, Print Specialist, were also instrumental in helping to get this book published.

Publishing a book takes many experts, but equally important are the people who ensure that the book is appropriately marketed to the right customers. David Peery, Assistant Marketing Manager, made sure that this book would reach our audience of academic nurse educators. Many thanks to all of these Elsevier team members who helped make this book such a valuable resource!

Contents

Certified Nurse Educator (CNE®) *and*
Certified Nurse Educator Novice (CNE®n)

EXAM PREP

PART I

Preparing for the CNE® and CNE®n Exams for the Academic Nurse Educator

Getting Ready for the Certified Nurse Educator (CNE®) and Certified Nurse Educator Novice (CNE®n) Exams

DEANNE A. BLACH

LEARNING OUTCOMES

1. Identify the purpose of the Certified Nurse Educator (CNE®) and Certified Nurse Educator Novice (CNE®n) credentials.
2. Describe the design and content of the CNE® and CNE®n examinations.
3. Delineate the eight core competencies for the academic nurse educator.
4. Summarize how to prepare for certification and recertification as an academic nurse educator.

An *academic nurse educator* is an individual who functions as a faculty member in an academic nursing program that prepares learners to become practical/vocational nurses (PNs/VNs), registered nurses (RNs), or advanced practice registered nurses (APRNs) (Christensen & Simmons, 2020). The National League for Nursing (NLN) developed *The Scope of Practice for Academic Nurse Educators* in 2005 and revised that document slightly in 2012 as a result of their 2011 practice analysis.

Purpose of the Certified Nurse Educator® Credential

Graduate study and certification are common ways to develop specialized knowledge and skills for advanced practice nurses. As nurses with an advanced practice specialty, academic nurse educators gradually develop mastery skills over time with mentorship, experience, knowledge acquisition, and continuing professional development.

To demonstrate this specialized knowledge, the NLN developed the first Certified Nurse Educator® examination based on *The Scope of Practice for Academic Nurse Educators'* eight core competencies. The Certified Nurse Educator® (CNE®) credential is a mark of professionalism that distinguishes the academic nurse educator's expertise within an advanced practice specialty role. Passing a standardized exam allows the educator to use the CNE® designation for a 5-year period, at which time the educator may apply for recertification.

According to the NLN (2022), an academic nurse educator may qualify to take the CNE® exam in two ways. The criteria for the first option to qualify include licensure, education, and experience requirements. These requirements have remained the same since the CNE® exam was developed:

- Documentation of valid licensure/certificate or other documentation of unencumbered practice in the country of residence
- A master's or doctoral degree in nursing (with a major emphasis in a role other than nursing education)

- At least 2 years of employment in a nursing program in an academic institution within the past 5 years

The second option to qualify to take the CNE® exam includes licensure and education requirements and was added within the past 10 years to allow educators to take the exam without meeting the experience requirement. This option has enabled consultants, including those employed by state boards of nursing, and new educators to qualify for the exam and obtain the CNE® credential:

- Documentation of valid licensure/certificate or other documentation of unencumbered practice in the country of residence
- A master's or doctoral degree in nursing with a major emphasis in nursing education *or*
- A master's or doctoral degree in nursing plus a post-master's certificate in nursing education *or*
- A master's or doctoral degree in nursing and nine or more credit hours of graduate-level education courses (e.g., curriculum development, evaluation, and testing)

The first CNE® exam was offered in 2005. The first-time CNE® pass rate has decreased dramatically since 2005. One likely explanation for this decrease is that experienced nurse educators initially took the exam with success compared with less experienced educators more recently taking the exam with little or no teaching experience. The second possible reason for decreasing pass rates is that the NLN expanded the eligibility for new graduates of master's and doctoral nursing programs to take the exam with no required educator experience. Even though nurse educators coming out of graduate school meet the eligibility criteria, the exam was not developed to measure graduate program outcomes. A recent study by Fitzgerald et al. (2020) found that graduate programs offering a focus on or degrees in nursing education typically only address four of the eight core competencies of the academic nurse educator used as the basis for the CNE® exam.

As a result of the decline in CNE® exam pass rate and the desire of new educators to become certified, the NLN piloted a new Certified Nurse Educator Novice (CNE®n) examination in 2022. This exam is based on seven of the eight core competencies for academic nurse educators but has a larger percentage of questions on those competencies that new educators have likely achieved in 3 or fewer years of experience.

As a distinct specialty of advanced nursing practice, academic nursing education certification brings professional credibility and shows a commitment to lifelong learning. Many educators indicate there is a personal level of satisfaction in being certified in an advanced practice role. Nurse educators who have achieved the CNE® credential are role models for other faculty colleagues and learners. Poindexter et al. (2019) reported that academic nurse educators ranked professional accomplishments, such as obtaining the CNE® credential, more important than professional recognition or rank.

Obstacles that educators often face in becoming certified include the cost of the exam, a lack of time to study for the exam, inadequate support for the credentialing process, and lack of employer recognition of certification significance. Research is needed to correlate certification to the ability to better prepare nursing learners and demonstrate a relationship between certification and improved learner and patient outcomes.

Description of the CNE® and CNE®n Exams

The CNE® exam is designed to evaluate the nurse educator's knowledge about the role of the academic nurse educator in the full scope of practice. As of 2021 about 8000 academic nurse educators were CNE® certified (L. Simmons, personal communication, 5/3/21). The new CNE®n exam is primarily designed to evaluate the novice nurse educator's knowledge and expertise in facilitating learning, but most other competencies are measured.

Both exams consist of 150 multiple-choice items; 130 are scored, and 20 pretest items are not scored. The items are not distinguished separately on the exam, so candidates do not know which ones are scored. Pretest items are analyzed, and those that meet the statistical criteria are approved and placed into the test bank.

Exam pass rates may vary based on difficulty level of the test items. Several versions of the exams are used concurrently. The pass score may be different on each, depending on what information is being collected from the exams. The pass score for all versions is psychometrically reviewed by NLN and Scantron. After determining the mean scores for each exam version, the passing score is set at the low end of the confidence range. Many of the questions on both certified nurse educator exams are at the application and analysis cognitive levels to measure the critical thinking ability of the nurse educator in a variety of situations.

Overview of the Scope of Practice for Academic Nurse Educators

The Scope of Practice for Academic Nurse Educators provides a framework for what nurse educators are expected to perform at a competent level. The standards of practice outlined in the *Scope of Practice* publication organize the roles and functions of the academic nurse educator into eight core competencies (Fig. 1.1).

Several theories and models are used as the foundation of this document and are summarized briefly in Table 1.1. As a specialty of advanced nursing practice, academic nurse educators have a distinct set of values and beliefs. These values and beliefs of the academic nurse educator are outlined in the *Scope of Practice* document and are summarized in Table 1.2.

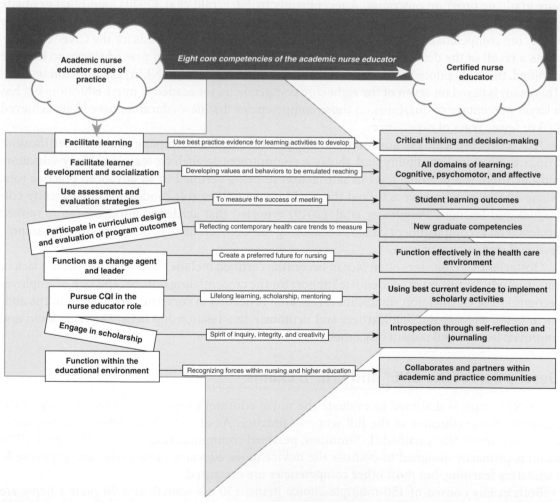

FIG. 1.1 Core Competencies of the Academic Nursing Educator and the Certified Nurse Educator® Credential. *CQI,* Continuous quality improvement. *(Courtesy Deanne A. Blach.)*

TABLE 1.1	Foundational Theories and Models Used in the Scope and Standards of Practice for the Academic Nurse Educator
Boyer's Model of Scholarship	The academic nurse educator should be prepared to embody the role of the nurse educator in scholarship, service, leadership, and self-improvement. Boyer's Model of Scholarship is often used by nurse educators to document portfolio development in career advancement.
Kolb's Experiential Learning Theory	Learning style preferences are used to collect (sensing/thinking) and process (watching/doing) information. There are diverse learning style preferences based on how information is processed (Kolb & Kolb, 2005): • Convergers (abstract, hands-on) • Divergers (concrete, reflective) • Assimilators (abstract, use inductive reasoning) • Accommodators (concrete, hands-on) The nurse educator uses this cycle of learning to facilitate the most appropriate learning activities for successful student learning outcomes.
Bloom's Revised Taxonomy	Bloom's revised taxonomy is used to develop measurable learning outcomes, usually developed as a result of analysis and identification of gaps in knowledge, skills, and practice. **Lower-Order Cognitive Levels (Not Thinking)** • Remembering (Knowledge) • Understanding (Comprehension) **Higher-Order Cognitive Levels (Thinking)** The higher cognitive levels require the learner to recall and use two or more pieces of knowledge and connect them to a new situation to make the best decisions. • Applying (Application) • Analyzing (Analysis) • Evaluating (Evaluation) • Creating (Synthesis)
Knowles' Adult Learning Principles	Based on real-life experience, adults are self-directed, problem-centered, and want direct involvement in planning their own learning. They prefer a relaxed space and "hands-on" learning.
Community and Academic Partnerships	Nursing programs collaborate with community and clinical agencies to provide rich clinical experiences for learners. Measuring program outcomes is important to determine if external stakeholders are satisfied with the new graduate. Although the response rate can be a struggle, it is essential to gather this information to ensure the program outcomes are being measured and the program is effective.

The major component of the *Scope of Practice* document is the delineation of eight Core Competencies of Nurse Educators with Task Statements. These competencies outline the specific responsibilities and functions of the academic nurse educator and serve as the framework for the CNE® exam. Table 1.3 lists each core competency with a brief description of each. Specific task statements for each competency can be found in the *Scope of Practice* document.

Use of Core Competencies as the CNE® and CNE®n Exam Framework

To ensure validity of the CNE® examination, the NLN periodically conducts a practice analysis of the roles, functions, and responsibilities of academic nurse educators. The most recent analysis resulted in the identification of eight core competencies that demonstrate the specialized knowledge and abilities of the academic nurse educator. The new CNE®n examination measures all of these competencies except for one. Each of these competencies is briefly summarized next.

TABLE **1.2**	NLN Hallmarks of Excellence in Academic Nursing Education

1. Student Engagement

2. Diverse, Well-Prepared Faculty

3. A Culture of Continuous Quality Improvement

4. Innovative, Evidence-Based Curriculum

5. Innovative, Evidence-Based Approaches to Facilitate and Evaluate Learning

6. Resources to Support Goal Attainment

7. Commitment to Pedagogical Scholarship

8. Effective Institutional and Professional Leadership

Data from National League for Nursing. (2012). *The scope of practice for academic nurse educators.* New York: Author.

TABLE **1.3**	Academic Nurse Educator Core Competencies and Description	
Competency Number	**Core Competency**	**Description of Competency**
1	Facilitate Learning	Create an environment in classroom, laboratory, and clinical settings that facilitates student learning and the achievement of desired cognitive, affective, and psychomotor outcomes.
2	Facilitate Learner Development and Socialization	Assist learners' development as nurses, and integrate the values and behaviors expected of those who fulfill that role.
3	Use Assessment and Evaluation Strategies	Use a variety of strategies to assess and evaluate student learning in classroom, laboratory, and clinical settings, as well as in all domains of learning.
4	Participate in Curriculum Design and Evaluation of Program Outcomes	Formulate program outcomes and design curricula that reflect contemporary health care trends; prepare graduates to function effectively in the health care environment.
5	Function as a Change Agent and Leader	Function as change agents and leaders to create a preferred future for nursing education and nursing practice.
6	Pursue Continuous Quality Improvement in the Nurse Educator Role	Recognize that the role of the academic nurse educator is multidimensional, requiring an ongoing commitment to develop and maintain competence in the role.
7	Engage in Scholarship	Recognize that scholarship is an integral component of the faculty role and that teaching itself is a scholarly activity.
8	Function Effectively Within the Institutional Environment and the Academic Community	Be knowledgeable about the educational practice environment and recognition of how political, institutional, social, and economic forces affect the nurse educator role.

Data from National League for Nursing. (2012). *The scope of practice for academic nurse educators.* New York: Author.

Competency 1: Facilitate Learning

This competency represents the largest percentage of content on both the CNE® and CNE®n examinations. The nurse educator uses evidence-based teaching learning strategies to foster clinical reasoning in multigenerational, multicultural learners. Developing a trusting, respectful relationship is foundational to facilitate learning. To effectively facilitate learning, the educator is mindful of the characteristics of today's learners to individualize their learning progression. Communicating effectively using a variety of platforms and recognizing how one's personal behavior is perceived by others are necessary for positive relationship building with learners, faculty, and clinical agency partners. Nurse educators plan learning activities that help develop critical thinking and decision making. Educators show enthusiasm in their role and model professional behaviors to inspire learners to be their best.

Competency 2: Facilitate Learner Development and Socialization

This competency focuses on developing values and behaviors in the learner that are expected in the role of a new nurse generalist or APRN. Emphasis is placed on meeting the learning needs of learners from diverse backgrounds and integrating cultural and diversity concepts in all learning environments. Educators reach learners most effectively when providing experiences that include the cognitive, affective, and psychomotor domains of learning. The educator implements a variety of teaching styles to foster interpersonal relationships and meet student learning outcomes. The nurse educator provides opportunities for learners to use self-reflection and personal goal setting, which promote socialization into the role of the lifelong learner.

Competency 3: Use Assessment and Evaluation Strategies

A major responsibility of the academic nurse educator is developing or selecting evidence-based assessment tools to evaluate achievement of learning in the cognitive, psychomotor, and affective domains. Assessment of student learning should be appropriate to each learner and learning outcome and needs to be constructive and timely. Examples of common assessment methods used for formative and summative evaluation include tests, clinical evaluation tools, clinical paperwork, discussion forums, projects, papers, and presentations.

Competency 4: Participate in Curricular Design and Evaluation of Program Outcomes

Designing or revising a curriculum is one of the most time-consuming responsibilities of the academic nurse educator. The nurse educator needs to have the knowledge of how to design or revise all components of a curriculum, including philosophy, program learning outcomes, competency statements, and lesson plans. As a change agent in the revision process, the educator uses the principles of change theory to identify strengths, weaknesses, opportunities, and threats. In addition to considering societal and local health and nursing trends, feedback from internal and external stakeholders, program data, and learner surveys is essential to help develop a contemporary curriculum that best prepares learners for generalist or advanced practice. Program data and analysis documented on the systematic plan for evaluation (SPE) ensures continuous program quality improvement.

Competency 5: Function as a Change Agent and Leader

The academic nurse educator uses leadership skills to create and implement change within the nursing program, the institution, and the community. To help manage the organizational culture, the nurse educator recognizes the need for participation from members of the organization, quality two-way communication, congruent structures with consistent policies and procedures, and resource allocation. As a leader, the nurse educator is actively involved in evaluating organizational effectiveness and implementing strategies for organization change. The nurse educator shows creativity, flexibility, and cultural sensitivity during the change and works to sustain the change. This competency is *not* measured on the CNE®n examination.

Competency 6: Pursue Continuous Quality Improvement in the Nurse Educator Role

Engaging in activities that promote socialization to the role includes lifelong learning, in part, by participating in professional nursing development opportunities and professional organizations. The nurse educator fulfills teaching, scholarship, and service requirements of the educational institution. Mentoring new educators and supporting other educators in their role development are additional ways to improve team performance. The nurse educator practices self-reflection and uses feedback from learners, peers, and administration to improve role effectiveness.

Competency 7: Engage in Scholarship

This competency includes demonstrating a spirit of inquiry in the teaching/learning process, participating in or conducting research, sharing teaching expertise with others, and demonstrating integrity and creativity as a scholar using best current evidence. The academic nurse educator designs and implements scholarly activities in an established area of expertise.

Competency 8: Function Within the Educational Environment

The academic nurse educator functions as a leader on committees within the nursing profession and educational environment and develops collaborations and partnerships within the academic community. To function in this role, the educator recognizes the influence of social, economic, political, and institutional forces on higher and nursing education.

Preparing to Take the CNE® or CNE®n Exam

Steps for Applying to Take the CNE® or CNE®n Exam

To prepare for taking the CNE® or CNE®n exam, the academic nurse educator needs to complete each of the following activities. Chapter 10 discusses specific strategies for being successful and passing these exams.

- To begin, enter the NLN website www.nln.org to access the Certification Page and the portal for CNE® or CNE®n examination registration.
- Review the latest version of the NLN *Certified Nurse Educator (CNE®) Candidate Handbook* or *Certified Nurse Educator Novice (CNE®n) Candidate Handbook* for eligibility criteria, a detailed test blueprint, and testing guidelines (www.nln.org/certification).
- Follow the application process described in the handbooks. The application is reviewed within 2 to 3 days after online submission and is either approved or additional data will be requested. New exam software has greatly reduced the wait time for notification of being accepted for the exam.
- After receiving the approval to test, schedule a date to take the exam within 90 days. The CNE® or CNE®n exam can be taken at a Scantron Testing Center during selected hours from Monday through Saturday. The Scantron website https://schedule.psiexams.com/ has specific information about the available testing centers. Due to the COVID-19 pandemic, nurse educators may also request online testing at home or at another location.

Basic Test Plans for the CNE® and CNE®n Exams

The content of the CNE® exam is based on the test plan developed from the Academic Nurse Educator Practice Analysis in 2011. To ensure the content is current and applicable to the nurse educator, the practice analysis is regularly updated.

The test plans in the handbooks outline the CNE® and CNE®n exam content areas, which are weighted with a percentage of questions that correspond to each area (Table 1.4). These content areas align with the eight core competencies described earlier in this chapter. The academic nurse educator should carefully review the relevant test blueprint to focus on essential content to be successful on the exam. Although each major content area is represented in every exam with the appropriate percentage of items and cognitive levels, not all content subareas are included on every form of the test.

Key Resources to Prepare for the CNE® and CNE®n Exams

The NLN *Certified Nurse Educator (CNE®) Candidate Handbook* and *Certified Nurse Educator Novice (CNE®n) Candidate Handbook* include a lengthy list of resources that can help the academic nurse educator prepare for the examination. In addition to *The Scope of Practice for Academic Nurse Educators,* examples of these resources include:

General Nursing Education and Role of the Educator
- Billings, D. M., & Halstead, J. A. (2020). *Teaching in nursing: A guide for faculty* (6th ed.). St. Louis: Elsevier.
- Halstead, J. A. (Ed.). (2019). *NLN core competencies for nurse educators: A decade of influence.* Philadelphia: Wolters Kluwer.

Facilitating Learning
- Bradshaw, M. J., Hultquist, B. L., & Hagler, D. (2021). *Innovative teaching strategies in nursing and related health professions* (8th ed.). Burlington, MA: Jones & Bartlett Learning.
- Cannon, S., & Boswell, C. (2016). *Evidence-based teaching in nursing: A foundation for educators* (2nd ed.). Burlington, MA: Jones & Bartlett Learning.

TABLE **1.4**	Test Blueprint for the CNE® and CNE®n Examinations		
Category	Major Content Area	Percentage of CNE® Exam	Percentage of CNE®n Exam
1	Facilitating learning	22%	39%
2	Facilitating learner development and socialization	15%	11%
3	Using assessment and evaluation strategies	19%	15%
4	Participating in curriculum design and evaluation of program outcomes	17%	5%
5	Pursuing continuous quality improvement in the academic nurse educator role	12%	8%
6	Engaging in scholarship, service, and leadership • Functioning as a change agent and leader • Engaging in scholarship • Functioning effectively within the institutional environment and the academic community	15%	15% N/A 4% 11%

Data from National League for Nursing. *Certified Nurse Educator (CNE®) 2022 candidate handbook and Certified Nurse Educator Novice (CNE®n) 2022 candidate handbook.* New York: Author.

- Oermann, M. H., DeGagne, J. C., & Phillips, B. C. (2022). *Teaching in nursing and role of the educator* (3rd ed.). New York: Springer Publishing.

Assessment and Evaluation of Learning

- Oermann, M. H. (Ed.). (2017). *A systematic approach to assessment and evaluation of nursing programs.* Philadelphia: Wolters Kluwer.
- Oermann, M. H., & Gaberson, K. B. (2021). *Evaluation and testing in nursing education* (6th ed.). New York: Springer Publishing.

Curriculum Development

- Iwasiw, C. L., Andrusyszyn, M., & Goldenberg, D. (2020). *Curriculum development in nursing education* (5th ed.). Burlington, MA: Jones & Bartlett Learning.
- DeBoor, S. S. (2023). *Keating's curriculum development and evaluation in nursing education* (5th ed.). New York: Springer Publishing.

CNE® Recertification Process

Because the CNE®n credential is the newest certification, the process for recertification has not been established at the time of this writing. The academic nurse educator who earned the CNE® credential, however, is responsible for managing all aspects of renewal. Two options are available for CNE® renewal—renewal by credits and renewal by examination. Either option must be completed by September 30 of the CNE® expiration year. Most nurse educators choose to renew by credits to avoid taking the CNE® exam again. To renew by credits, the following criteria must be met by the educator:

- Hold an active RN license in United States or in one of its territories
- Have the equivalent of 2 or more years of employment in the past 5 years functioning in the full scope of the academic faculty role
- Have Certified Nurse Educator Code of Ethics compliance
- Pay renewal fees by the certification expiration date
- Maintain a 5-year renewal cycle per the CNE® certificate expiration date
- Demonstrate continued maintenance or expansion of knowledge relevant to the role of academic nurse educator within the 5-year renewal cycle

Academic nurse educators who choose to renew by credits and meet the criteria noted earlier need to provide documentation of 50 renewal credits. Renewal credits are professional activities that demonstrate continued professional development of the nurse educator. Starting in 2026, 75 renewal credits will be required for recertification. These activities must be related to at least five of the eight core competencies and be spread across the previous 5-year period.

If choosing the renewal by credit option for recertification, most educators find it easier to track and organize activities as they occur rather than waiting until the end of the 5-year renewal cycle to locate their documentation. The process for the CNE® recertification process should be started soon after passing the exam. The renewal cycle begins the day the official passing score is received and continues until the last day of the fifth year. Retired CNEs have the option to retain their credentials. After approval, "CNE-Ret" may be used.

Beginning in 2021 the NLN recognizes an outstanding person or group who has championed the cause for CNE® certification. According to the website, this *Certification Star Award* recognizes outstanding individuals, programs, or organizations who have made a significant difference or substantial impact on nursing education, embraced nurse education through adoption and/or promotion of certification, and helped to sustain certifications and excellence in education. The award is presented each year at the NLN Education Summit.

References

Asterisk (*) indicates a classic or definitive work on this subject.

Christensen, L. S., & Simmons, L. E. (2020). *The scope of practice for academic nurse educators and academic clinical nurse educators*. Washington, DC: National League for Nursing.

Fitzgerald, A., McNelis, A. M., & Billings, D. (2020). NLN core competencies for academic nurse educators: Are they present in the course descriptions of academic nurse educator programs? *Nursing Education Perspectives, 41*(9), 4–9.

*Kolb, A. Y., & Kolb, D. A. (2005). Learning styles and learning spaces: Enhancing experiential learning in higher education. *Academy of Management Learning and Education, 4*(2), 193–212.

National League for Nursing. (2022). *Certified Nurse Educator (CNE®) 2022 Candidate Handbook*. http://www.nln.org/docs/default-source/default-document-library/cne-handbook-2022.pdf?sfvrsn=2.

Poindexter, K., Lindell, D., & Hagler, D. (2019). Measuring the value of academic nurse educator certification: Perceptions of administrators and educators. *Journal of Nursing Education, 58*(9), 502–509.

CHAPTER 2

Facilitating Learning

DEANNE A. BLACH | DONNA D. IGNATAVICIUS

LEARNING OUTCOMES

1. Identify selected teaching-learning strategies to engage and motivate learners in a variety of educational settings.
2. Apply common educational theories to select evidence-based teaching-learning strategies for diverse learners.
3. Identify effective communication skills to promote a positive, student-centered learning environment.
4. Describe effective methods for assisting learners to develop critical and reflective thinking.
5. Discuss personal attributes needed for nurse educators to create a safe, evidence-based learning environment.
6. Explain the need for nurse educators to function as a role model in the clinical practice environment.

The primary role of the academic nurse educator is to facilitate learning using a variety of approaches and strategies and is therefore the largest content area measured on the CNE® and CNE®n certification examinations. The nurse educator is responsible for creating an effective learning environment and facilitating learning for diverse students in all educational settings—classroom, online, laboratory, clinical agency, and simulation. As a role model, the nurse educator should implement evidence-based teaching-learning strategies and demonstrate effective relationship skills when communicating with learners, peers, and clinical agency personnel. Nurse educators should also engage in self-reflection and ongoing professional development to improve teaching practices that facilitate learning.

Implementing a Variety of Teaching Strategies

Teaching can be viewed as the instructional approach that academic nurse educators use to impart content knowledge. Using teaching as the approach is within the educator's control and may not consider the learners' needs. This approach is *teacher-centered* rather than learner-centered. *Learning* is an approach in which the nurse educator plans instructional experiences based on learners' needs. When learning occurs, the learner changes behavior by translating the new knowledge into practice (Oermann et al., 2022). This approach is *learner-centered* rather than teacher-centered.

Learning can be categorized as passive or active. In *passive learning*, learners use their senses to acquire knowledge through activities such as attending lectures, viewing video or audio resources, and reading assignments. However, passive learning fosters short-term knowledge memorization and minimal, if any, critical thinking development.

Nurse educators commonly use a passive learning approach because learners may prefer it based on previous educational experiences (Billings & Halstead, 2020). The most common strategy used for passive learning is lecture accompanied by a lengthy slide presentation. Although slides can be useful for visual learners, nurse educators should follow best practices when preparing slides, which include (Billings & Halstead, 2020):

- Use a large-size font with a contrasting (but light) background.
- Do not include more than two to three summary points on each slide.
- Include graphic images as appropriate instead of massive amounts of text.
- Present slides in a landscape format.

Active learning allows learners to be more involved in the learning process. Depending on the teaching-learning strategy, benefits of active learning include (Billings & Halstead, 2020):

- Increased knowledge retention, understanding, and retrieval
- Increased critical thinking development
- Increased interest in learning
- Improved ability to meet learning outcomes

> ### CNE®/CNE®n Key Point
>
> **Remember:** Passive learning fosters short-term knowledge, memorization, and minimal, if any, critical thinking development. Active learning allows learners to be more involved in the learning process and increases critical thinking.

Learning can be also differentiated as surface learning and deep learning. *Surface (superficial) learning* is short-term and occurs when learners try to memorize and recall knowledge; it does not contribute to brain development. As a result, learners are unable to retrieve knowledge when needed at a later time. Surface learning tends to be extrinsically motivated, meaning that learners usually memorize knowledge for taking tests (Billings & Halstead, 2020).

By contrast, *deep learning* allows learners to understand new knowledge, connect new knowledge with previously learned knowledge, and create meaning through continued brain development. Learners are usually able to retrieve knowledge when needed to solve problems or make decisions. Deep learning is typically intrinsically motivated by a desire to learn to meet personal goals (Billings & Halstead, 2020).

Learning can be either synchronous or asynchronous. In a *synchronous learning* environment, all students are scheduled for the experience at the same time. *Asynchronous learning* allows students to learn at different times. For example, online or remote learning provides an opportunity for students to learn asynchronously. This teaching method is also referred to as distance learning because the educator and learners are separated by geography and possibly time.

Teaching strategies, often referred to as *teaching-learning strategies,* are specific active and passive activities, methods, and approaches that are purposefully planned by the nurse educator to facilitate learning. Although nurse educators have the academic freedom to select how to teach, all teaching-learning strategies should be evidence-based (Cannon & Boswell, 2016).

Most educators use strategies with which they feel most comfortable and experienced; however, several other factors should influence the selection of teaching-learning methodologies. The nurse educator plans meaningful learning by selecting a variety of evidence-based teaching strategies that are appropriate for the:

- Course content and educational setting
- Learning outcomes
- Students' learning needs and style preferences
- Instructional delivery method

Implementing Teaching Strategies Based on Course Content, Course Context, and Educational Setting

The content and context of a course and where it is taught direct the type of teaching-learning strategies the nurse educator selects. For example, some courses are entirely didactic, meaning that the course is taught in a classroom or online. Other courses have a clinical focus and require that the nurse educator determine how to help learners translate knowledge into practice. For both didactic and clinical settings, nurse educators need to explore recent advances in technology that support education and practice. The use of educational technology is discussed later in this chapter.

Didactic Learning Environments

Using a variety of teaching-learning approaches in didactic settings (either classroom or online) is essential for developing critical thinking, engaging and motivating learners, and making content knowledge more interesting (Cannon & Boswell, 2016). However, for many years nurse educators have relied on the traditional *lecture* combined with a slide presentation as the primary method for didactic teaching. This method is what many educators experienced during their own basic nursing education programs.

The traditional lecture format with slides remains the most commonly used passive teaching-learning strategy today. This method has the advantage of providing a large amount of content in a short period (Oermann et al., 2022). Characteristics of an effective lecture include:

- Planning the lecture based on course objectives (content learning outcomes)
- Organizing the lecture in a logical manner, building on learners' previous knowledge
- Allowing time for discussion, questions, and answers to clarify content knowledge
- Summarizing and highlighting content key points for learners

The purpose of lecture is to help learners acquire and remember knowledge, but it does not guarantee the learners' ability to retrieve knowledge, critically think, or actively engage in the learning process. Several newer models for teaching lend themselves to more active learning when students are in classroom settings.

Cooperative learning encourages peer interaction and collaboration in groups while maintaining individual learner accountability in the classroom or online environment. The nurse educator facilitates group formation, ensuring that each group is a mix of two to four diverse learners. Cooperative learning engages learners, promotes deep learning, and helps develop critical thinking skills (Oermann et al., 2022).

Best practice for forming groups includes knowing the characteristics of the learners. Based on this information and purpose of the learning activity, the nurse educator selects group members with either similar or different attributes. It is often helpful to group learners together based on similar attributes so they can bond as a team. However, working with diverse learners enhances learning about various aspects of diversity. Group make-up should be based on and reflect the learning outcomes and purpose of the learning activity. As an icebreaker, the nurse educator could ask each group to select a team name based on something they have in common. This method of selecting groups can be used for both face-to-face and online instruction.

Two structured cooperative learning approaches are team-based and problem-based learning. *Team-based learning* consists of three phases: preparation by learners, assessments of readiness (both individual and group through testing), and application of concepts in case-based scenarios that promote thinking (Oermann et al., 2022). The teams then share their responses to the application activities for discussion and learning. *Problem-based learning* is also a student-centered cooperative learning experience in which discovery of learning occurs through self-direction. Both approaches require the nurse educator to facilitate group learning rather than present information in a lecture format.

One of the newest approaches for teaching-learning in the face-to-face setting is the *flipped classroom*. Using this pedagogical model, learners are required to engage in significant preclass learning activities that prepare them for class (Billings & Halstead, 2020). Then, in class they work individually and/or collaboratively in groups to apply and expand what they learned in meaningful critical thinking activities. Many nursing faculty and learners do not prefer this learning methodology because:

- The traditional lecture format is more commonly used and familiar.
- Nurse educators and learners are socialized to passive learning, like the lecture format.
- Preparing for a flipped classroom experience requires more work for both the educator and learners.

Instead of a pure flipped classroom approach, some learners prefer a mix of active learning strategies interspersed with mini-lectures ("lecturettes") in which the nurse educator shares information to clarify, highlight, and update what is gleaned from the learning activity. This mix of activities engages learners and promotes learning and thinking. Like the flipped classroom approach, learners complete significant preclass learning activities that prepare them for class. Barnett (2014) named this approach the *scrambled classroom.*

Regardless of educational approach, nurse educators determine which learning activities are most appropriate for the content of a course. For instance, a support course like pathophysiology requires knowledge of medical terminology, which must be memorized. Games such as *Jeopardy* can help learners acquire and recall medical terminology as part of the didactic learning experience. By contrast, a core course focusing on nursing care requires use of those terms and application to make appropriate clinical judgments. Case studies are commonly used in this type of course to allow learners the opportunity to develop cognitive skills to make appropriate clinical decisions. These learning activities and others are described in detail later in this chapter.

Clinical Learning Environments

Practice settings for clinical learning may include the campus laboratory to practice nursing skills or health assessment techniques, clinical simulation, and clinical agency experiences. The nurse educator selects a variety of learning strategies that are appropriate for each learning practice setting.

Sometimes referred to as the learning laboratory or learning resource center, the campus *skills laboratory* is designed to simulate a clinical setting to provide a safe environment for learners to practice clinical nursing skills on peers, standardized patients, mannequins, and/or task trainers. Exposure to the skills laboratory begins in the first nursing semester of a prelicensure program in which learners practice basic clinical skills. Integrated throughout the program and as part of graduate education, learners progress to practicing more complex and advanced skills. The learner's performance of selected skills is evaluated by the educator or peer learner to demonstrate competence, typically before the learner performs those skills in a clinical agency.

Clinical simulation is a scenario-based active learning experience that brings the learner into the center of the experience to foster critical thinking and clinical reasoning. Based on experiential learning theory, clinical simulation engages learners with diverse perspectives to reflect and better understand practice, connecting the "thinking like a nurse" to the "doing like a nurse" (Billings & Halstead, 2020).

Clinical simulation is typically provided in a campus laboratory equipped with a combination of mid- and high-fidelity (most humanlike) mannequins to provide learners with a nonthreatening opportunity to provide complex nursing care in a variety of clinical scenarios (see Table 5.7 in Chapter 5 for mannequin fidelity levels). These learning environments are usually managed by a credentialed simulation coordinator who is a master's-prepared registered nurse. Like all educational experiences, the coordinator or nurse educator develops learning outcomes for each scenario and provides debriefing as an essential component of learning.

Debriefing is an interactive reflective learning activity after a simulation experience that is usually led by the nurse educator facilitator. During the debriefing process, learners reflect on what they did well and what they could have done differently and focus on how clinical decisions were made during their experience. The learning facilitator requires special debriefing training to learn how to best provide detailed and constructive feedback to learners. Research shows this learning strategy helps students improve clinical competence, gain self-confidence, develop deep learning, and have a perception of being prepared for nursing practice (Bradshaw et al., 2021).

Clinical learning also occurs in health care agencies in the local community with which the educational institution has a contractual agreement. Like clinical simulation, the *clinical practicum* allows learners the opportunity to experience what practicing generalists or advanced practice nurses do each day. The nurse educator plans activities that help learners meet course outcomes, including direct care activities and focused learning (thinking) activities. Debriefing occurs in a postclinical conference either immediately or soon after the clinical learning experience. The clinical experience is discussed later in this chapter in more detail.

Implementing Teaching Strategies Based on Desired Learning Outcomes

The nurse educator develops learning outcomes to delineate desired learner expectations in a variety of educational settings. Outcomes that measure learning at the content level are often referred to as *course objectives*. These objectives are placed in the syllabus or topical outline to communicate to learners the expectations they will need to achieve in a course for each content topic. The objectives operationalize the curriculum and direct all learning activities (Billings & Halstead, 2020). Chapter 5 describes learning outcomes and course objectives in detail.

Course objectives represent learning in the cognitive, affective, and psychomotor domains and are briefly described here (Oermann et al., 2022):

- *Cognitive domain:* Learning involves acquiring knowledge and developing thinking, which cannot be directly observed.
- *Affective domain:* Learning involves attitudes, values, and beliefs, which cannot be directly observed.
- *Psychomotor domain:* Learning involves hands-on performance of technical skills, which can be directly observed.

Table 2.1 provides examples of evidence-based teaching-learning strategies to develop learning in each domain.

TABLE **2.1**	**Examples of Teaching-Learning Strategies by Learning Domain**	
Learning Domain	**Teaching-Learning Strategy Example**	**Description of Teaching-Learning Strategy**
Cognitive domain	Lecture	Educator led to provide information; effective for large classes.
	Focused group discussion	Learners form groups (either random or volunteer) and discuss assigned topic.
	Case studies	Individual learners or groups of learners answer questions about a clinical scenario to promote thinking and to make clinical judgments.
Affective domain	Reflection activity based on a video or video clip	Learners watch a video clip or full video and answer reflection questions to improve awareness of values.
	Focused reflective journaling	Learners write a journal entry about values and feelings related to clinical experience; educator directs focus of journal entry.
Psychomotor domain	Technical skill practice	Learners practice skills in laboratory setting to gain confidence and competence.
	Simulation experience	High-fidelity mannequins used to simulate actual clinical experiences for learners to practice psychomotor and critical thinking skills.

> **CNE®/CNE®n Key Point**
>
> *Remember:* Learning occurs in the cognitive, affective, and psychomotor domains.
> - *Cognitive domain:* Learning involves acquiring knowledge and thinking, which cannot be directly observed.
> - *Affective domain:* Learning involves attitudes, values, and beliefs, which cannot be directly observed.
> - *Psychomotor domain:* Learning involves hands-on performance of technical skills, which can be directly observed.

Nurse educators develop course objectives based on the educational setting. For example, learning in didactic environments focuses primarily on the cognitive domain, but affective learning may also occur. In clinical environments, learners have the opportunity for cognitive, affective, and psychomotor learning as they provide patient care.

When developing course objectives, the nurse educator considers the level of learners based on their prerequisite knowledge and thinking level. For example, a beginning prelicensure learner has minimal nursing knowledge or skills. Therefore the educator would create basic-level objectives, such as "Identify common physiologic changes of aging." The verb "identify" informs the nurse educator that the learning strategy to meet this objective would need to help learners acquire and recall knowledge. Games are appropriate learning activities to help learners meet this objective.

By contrast, course objectives written for learners in a last-semester prelicensure nursing program would require more thinking and be more complex. An example is "Prioritize collaborative care for the mechanically ventilated patient." This objective could be used for didactic learning using a case study as the learning strategy or for clinical learning in a critical care setting. Table 2.2 provides examples of learning outcome verbs that can be used for each domain and common verbs for each taxonomic level of the cognitive learning domain.

Implementing Teaching Strategies Based on Learning Needs and Learning Style Preferences

Students are diverse learners who have varying needs and preferences for how they learn best. As mentioned earlier, the nurse educator should be *learner-centered* rather than teacher-centered. Being learner-centered means that the educator focuses on meeting the needs of learners. For example, some students learn best in groups and others learn best on their own as individuals. The educator assesses which learning method the class prefers or uses both methods to meet the needs of diverse learners (Billings & Halstead, 2020).

TABLE 2.2	Examples of Verbs Appropriate for Learning Domains	
Learning Domain	**Learning Domain (Lowest Level to Highest Level)**	**Verb Examples**
Cognitive domain	• Remembering • Understanding • Applying • Analyzing • Evaluating • Creating	• Identify, define • Explain, describe • Apply, demonstrate • Analyze, differentiate • Evaluate, interpret • Develop, plan
Affective domain	• Awareness • Values development	• Reflect, recognize • Challenge, promote
Psychomotor domain	• Basic • Complex	• Obtain, set up • Perform, demonstrate

Learners have differing learning style preferences. An evidence-based way of differentiating learning styles is using the *VARK model*:

- V = Visual learner
- A = Aural (Auditory) learner
- R = Read/Write learner
- K = Kinesthetic learner

A visual learner prefers information in a graphic format, but an auditory learner prefers information that can be heard or spoken. A read/write learner prefers to learn information in text format, and a kinesthetic learner prefers to learn information using "hands-on" or experiential activities. The VARK learning style inventory can be accessed at http://vark-learn.com/the-vark-questionnaire/. Table 2.3 provides examples of teaching-learning strategies that are appropriate for each type of learner based on the VARK model.

Implementing Teaching Strategies Based on Instructional Delivery Method

Instructional delivery methods vary depending on the type of nursing program in which the educator teaches. However, unexpected societal or health events can change the planned delivery method. Nurse educators must be able to respond effectively to unexpected events that affect instruction. For example, at the beginning of the COVID-19 pandemic in 2020, educational institutions had to rapidly convert face-to-face programs to completely online. Many nurse educators had never previously engaged in online learning but had to plan and implement their courses, often without formal professional development. Some learners did not have access to high-speed Internet or appropriate electronic devices, which presented challenges to successful online education. A number of nursing programs continue to provide more online learning opportunities than those offered before the pandemic.

Online learning can be classified by the percentage of time that a learner is engaged in distance education. Each university, college, or school has definitions of how online learning is classified. Most graduate programs in nursing are completely online except for the clinical practicum. Some courses in undergraduate are *hybrid* or *blended,* meaning that part of the course is face-to-face and part is online. For example, didactic learning may be offered online, but clinical learning is usually in person. Any type of nursing program may offer *web-enhanced courses* that are usually provided in a classroom setting; learners use their learning management system (LMS) to engage in selected teaching-learning activities before or after class. Often part of the preclass activities is viewing the voice-over lecture/slide presentation.

The most important role of the nurse educator who teaches in an online environment is to facilitate communication and use presence to connect with learners (Oermann et al., 2022). Establishing social, cognitive, and teaching presence is especially challenging, but is an important best practice for creating the learning community (Ignatavicius, 2019). As in any educational

TABLE **2.3**	Examples of Teaching-Learning Strategies by Learning Style Preference
Learning Style Preference	**Teaching-Learning Strategy Example**
Visual	• Graphic organizers, such as concept maps • Videos and video clips • Graphic images
Auditory	• Lecture • Face-to-face or online group/peer discussion
Read/write	• Textbook reading assignment • Taking notes in class
Kinesthetic	• Psychomotor skill practice • Patient care in practice setting • Virtual or high-fidelity clinical simulation • Digital tools

setting, the educator needs to use active learning techniques and provide prompt feedback to learners while addressing their diverse needs.

Peer interaction is an effective online educational strategy that reduces the feeling of learner isolation and reinforces lifelong collegial learning. The nurse educator plans activities that require online peer interaction, including case studies, concept maps, and group work. Online *discussion forums* allow learners to interact asynchronously in a meaningful way and promote critical thinking. The educator provides challenging questions on course topics for learner response with supporting literature citations. The educator may also participate to provide feedback to learner comments or to challenge learners to consider other aspects of the discussion.

CNE®/CNE®n Key Point

Remember: The most important role of the nurse educator who teaches in an online environment is to facilitate communication and use presence to connect with learners (Oermann et al., 2022).

Using Teaching Strategies Based on Educational Theories and Current Evidence

The nurse educator facilitates learning by linking how learners process information with how the information is delivered. Learning theories, also referred to as educational theories, describe the processes used to change student thinking and behavior (performance) or how students understand or organize the learning environment.

Nurse educators use general principles of learning theories as a guide when planning teaching-learning approaches and activities. For example, *adult learning theory* posits that adults are motivated to learn and are accountable for their own learning and decision making. The nurse educator might consider a flipped or scrambled classroom approach in which adults could work collaboratively in groups. *Constructivism* is a group of theories in which learners build new knowledge based on previous knowledge, often through real-life experiences. Clinical simulation provides an opportunity for learners to discover and build new knowledge. Table 2.4 lists examples of teaching-learning approaches and activities that are based on common learning theories.

In addition to using one or more educational theories as a guide for planning instructional methods, nurse educators need to select teaching-learning strategies and approaches that are based on sound evidence. For example, *concept mapping* is a commonly used evidence-based teaching-learning method that promotes critical thinking as learners make connections among concepts. Each concept map is unique because learners construct knowledge based on their previous knowledge (Oermann et al., 2022). Some nurse educators are resistant to having learners use this instructional tool because they prefer more traditional tools that are more uniform, structured, and easy to grade.

Modifying Teaching-Learning Strategies Based on Learner Diversity and Clinical Experience

Chapter 3 includes a detailed discussion regarding the unique learning needs of diverse learners and resources that can help meet those needs. The nurse educator respects the needs of diverse learners and considers them when planning evidence-based teaching-learning strategies.

Generational Groups

Many nursing classes include a multiple-age range of learners, each with their uniqueness, styles of communication, and learning needs. Some nursing programs tend to attract more *traditional learners* who are recent high school graduates, and other programs attract a large number of nontraditional learners. *Nontraditional learners* tend to be older than traditional learners with

TABLE 2.4	Examples of Teaching-Learning Strategies by Learning Theory	
Learning Theory	**Characteristics of Learning Theory**	**Teaching-Learning Strategy Example**
Behaviorism	Learning is a change in behavior that occurs between a stimulus and response, using immediate feedback and positive reinforcement for the behavior change. There is a reward for a change in behavior. Controlling the external environment is key to managing what people learn.	Memorizing steps of a procedure Quiz after content delivery Completing assignments
Cognitive psychology	Cognitive psychology is an internal mental/cognitive process that focuses on thinking, understanding, organizing, and consciousness.	Active learning Case studies
Adult learning theory	Adults are responsible for their own learning and decision making; prefer active learning and building on life experiences.	Reflective journaling Group work
Constructivism	Knowledge is constructed through real-life experiences. New information is built upon the foundation of preexisting knowledge, then rearranged and reordered until it makes sense to the learner in the learner's own unique way. Learning is active and outcome-oriented; focus on meaningful learning rather than rote memorization.	Concept mapping Clinical simulation
Social learning theory	Learning occurs through observation of others, imitation, and modeling that behavior. The goal is self-efficacy, which reflects confidence in the ability to control one's motivation, behavior, and environment. Learners who believe they can perform at a high level will have the confidence to do well.	Role modeling Mentoring Clinical learning
Humanism	Process of learning involves learning with and through others. Learners are self-directed and can choose how they want to learn. Internal motivation and experiential learning are keys.	Icebreakers Workshops Affective learning
Multiple intelligences	Learners have their own unique profile of eight preferences for learning (intelligences): verbal, mathematical, visual, kinesthetic, musical, interpersonal, intrapersonal, and naturalistic. A learner's unique profile of intelligences is used for problem-solving and interacting with the environment. A learner's problem solving is influenced by learning and experiences of life.	Group interaction using different intelligences (music, movement, critical thinking)
Experiential learning	A continuous experiential (mind and feelings) learning process includes transforming the experience (concrete), reflecting on the experience (reflective observation), gaining meaning from the experience (abstract conceptualization), and applying the meaning (active experimentation). There are two types of perceptions (sensing/thinking) and two types of information processing (watching/doing): • Converger—thinking/doing • Diverger—feeling/observing • Assimilator—thinking/observing • Accommodator—thinking/feeling	*Converger*—Clinical learning activities *Diverger*—Role-playing, brainstorming, seminars, and experience *Assimilator*—Content experts, reading, independent learning, and online learning *Accommodator*—Group work, case studies, precepted clinicals, and online learning
Brain-based learning	A mind–body (holistic) approach to learning, which creates deep learning. Left brain is the analytical, logical side; right brain is the holistic, artistic side.	Cooperative learning Clinical learning

varying work and/or life experiences. Most nontraditional learners have family and work responsibilities while completing their education, which can increase stress and affect learner success. However, nontraditional learners are generally very intrinsically motivated to learn and achieve their career goals.

Chapter 3 details generational differences among the *Baby Boomers* (1945–1964), *Generation X (1965–1979)*, *Millennials (Generation Y) (1980–1994)*, *and Generation Z (i-Generation)* (born after 1995). Each learner generation has unique values the educator must recognize to promote a positive and collaborative learning environment. Understanding generational differences encourages open-mindedness and brings an awareness of life differences from others of a different generation. Any one generational group has some of the same characteristics, but consideration of an individual's learning characteristics is essential. Table 2.5 lists examples of generational considerations when selecting teaching-learning strategies for learner success.

TABLE 2.5	Examples of Teaching-Learning Strategies by Generational Groups	
Generational Group	**Common Characteristics**	**Teaching-Learning Strategy Example**
Baby Boomers (born 1945–1964) Nurse educators in this age-group are nearing retirement, contributing to the crisis of the faculty shortage.	• Optimistic with a strong work ethic and value career over personal life • Love–hate relationship with authority • Prefer live communication over email or texting • Prefer face-to-face instruction • Work as a team with cooperation and competition • Need recognition and praise for hard work • Feeling valued and needed are motivators	• Explain the purpose of learning strategy. • Be aware that they prefer cooperative learning for problem-solving. • Include lecture and small-group discussion to allow for discovery and experimentation. • Assign reflective journaling, critical incidents, and portfolios to incorporate life experiences into learning.
Generation X (born 1965–1979) This is the dominant age-group in the work force for the next 20 years.	• More informal, self-directed, creative, flexible, and self-reliant • Prefer to be rewarded based on individual performance • Work well in teams • Do not want public acknowledgment, prefer privacy • Value work–life balance • Adaptable to changes, including technology, using email, and texting as primary tools for communication • Motivated by freedom, removal of rules, and time off • Want clear information with practicality	• Be aware that they prefer active learning strategies, on-the-job training, and e-learning. • Facilitate learning by giving learners the opportunity to do things their own way. • Make learning fun. • Assign reading assignments with guided lecture. • Provide ongoing, regular feedback.
The *Millennials/ Generation Y* (born 1980–1994) This is the first generation of digital natives.	• Digital natives; expect technology and Internet resources to be available • Confident multitaskers who are high achievers • Want immediate access to learning opportunities • Team player • Communicate through social media, email, and texting • Value personal life over careers • Motivated by time off and to work with skilled people	• Use technology in class and clinical simulation. • Provide short bursts of information. • Establish assignments with clear outcomes. • Provide opportunities for cooperative learning. • Encourage mentorship. • Provide frequent feedback.
Generation Z (born after 1995) Traditional learners are members of this generation.	• Ethically diverse, globally aware, environmentally aware • Digital natives • Have decreased attention spans • Social media is a primary means to communicate • Prefer combining their use of technology with real-world experiences	• Similar to *Gen Y;* use active learning instead of lecture. • Foster learner engagement (establish learner community using blogs, online interactions, and group projects). • Stimulate intellectual development (e.g., storytelling with engagement). • Build rapport with learners (e.g., immediate and useful feedback).

Cultural Background

The learning process is also significantly affected by each person's cultural background, especially influencing how information is interpreted and used. A learner's response to culture is primarily unconscious and has intellectual and emotional components. Academic nurse educators should advocate to improve efforts in increasing diversity and inclusion, providing learning experiences that reach both intellectual and emotional responses to different cultures. By incorporating cultural humility into teaching-learning processes, nurse educators may be able to reduce bias and promote the inclusive learning environment necessary to retain diverse nursing learners.

Nurse educators must recognize the strength that a multicultural educational approach has on the success of minority and underrepresented learners. Learners need mentors and role models to foster role development from a variety of cultural backgrounds.

Nurse educators must integrate cultural diversity into the curriculum and evaluate its effectiveness in producing culturally competent graduates. As a role model for learners, the nurse educator disseminates best practices by providing meaningful learning that incorporates inclusion, equity, diversity, and the social determinants of health on patients' experiences within the health care system.

Nurse educators need to use a variety of engaging teaching-learning strategies to improve cultural competence and minority learner retention, including role-playing, games, vignettes, case studies, media, books, interviews, storytelling, experiential immersion, exchange experiences, service learning, ethnographies, and workshops. Critical thinking activities should be developed to promote learning in the affective domain by using self-reflection as learners continue to develop cultural competence.

Past Life, Educational, and Clinical Experiences

Nontraditional learners enter a nursing program with a variety of life, educational, and clinical experiences, which should be considered by nurse educators as they plan teaching-learning approaches and activities. The nurse educator should explore what experiences learners have had and build on them as appropriate. For example, a number of young and middle-aged *veterans* are returning to school to achieve a new career. Veterans are part of a unique culture and share a common bond to protect the country. Other common characteristics are that veterans:

- Are committed and loyal
- Are stoic and able to endure hardship
- Have strong moral values
- Strive for excellence
- Prefer group work and interactions

The nurse educator could modify teaching-learning strategies for these learners by planning more group work to solve problems and make decisions. For example, veteran experiences and training regarding moral values could be used as a basis for discussions about professional nursing ethics.

In addition to life and educational experiences, some learners have had clinical experience in nursing or other health care role. The nurse educator asks learners about details of their experience, especially in clinical learning experiences. Depending on the time and depth of the clinical experience, the nurse educator might ask the learner to assist in learning or skill demonstration. For example, if a learner is a licensed practical nurse (LPN) who works in an outpatient surgical center as the "IV nurse," the nurse educator might ask the LPN to share personal experience about performing the procedure. A paramedic could share experiences about prehospital care and collaboration with the emergency department health care team.

> ### CNE®/CNE®n Key Point
>
> *Remember:* Nurse educators must integrate cultural concepts into the curriculum and evaluate its effectiveness in producing culturally competent graduates. In addition, nurse educators need to recognize that nontraditional learners have a variety of life, educational, and clinical experiences, which must be considered as they plan teaching-learning approaches and activities.

Using Technologies to Support the Teaching-Learning Process

Today's academic nurse educator must know how to implement technology to support the teaching-learning process in any setting and understand generational traits that affect its use. The nurse educator recognizes learners have different abilities when using technology. *Digital natives,* such as Generations Y and Z, have been immersed in technology since early childhood and are naturally fluent in digital language. They function best when networked and do best with engaging in instant feedback, rewards, and gaming as learning strategies. Digital immigrants had little or no exposure to information technology during formative years. Some still prefer print to reading from a computer screen and can struggle with online or web-based learning. Many educators are members of Generation X or Baby Boomers and are considered digital immigrants because they were digitally naïve.

Because many nurse educators are not familiar with the use of educational technology, professional development is essential to learn best practices for online learning. Continuing education regarding the technology is often offered through the university, college, or school. However, additional development is needed to assist educators with how to customize this technology for nursing education.

Technology can be incorporated into any learning environment, including the classroom, laboratory, and clinical learning environment. In the classroom, one of the most commonly used educational technology tools is *audience response systems,* usually applied through electronic mobile devices. Audience response apps allow the educator to formatively assess learners by asking polling questions for their responses. Polling can also occur as part of online instruction.

One of the most common areas for technology in nursing education is the use of clinical simulation. The academic nurse educator creates active, experiential learning for learners integrating knowledge and psychomotor skills into realistic patient scenarios using problem-solving to make clinical decisions. Low-, medium-, and high-fidelity mannequins and other equipment assist learners for hands-on skills development that addresses all domains of learning. One advantage of clinical simulation is that it provides real-time performance feedback and can be used in both formative and summative assessment. It is also a way to facilitate interprofessional communication and collaboration.

One of the newest types of computer-based technology is *virtual reality.* Used most commonly for clinical learning, learners participate in virtual simulation, which creates opportunities to practice clinical reasoning to make appropriate patient care decisions with members of the interprofessional health care team. This virtual reality world enables learners to interact with each other through patient avatars. Virtual technology is also being used for clinical skills practice, such as inserting a urinary catheter. The learner may wear headgear to practice and master the clinical skill using game-based technology (Billings & Halstead, 2020).

Using Effective Communication Skills to Foster Positive Educator–Learner Relationships

The nurse educator is expected to clearly and respectfully communicate with learners using professional interpersonal skills to foster the faculty–learner relationship and create a positive learning environment. Nurse educators must be genuine, showing feelings of caring, patience, and integrity to establish trust. One behavior to develop trust is for the educator to follow through on commitments to learners. For example, if the educator informs learners that a paper will be graded and returned to them by a certain date, the educator should be sure to meet that expectation.

Essential educator behaviors that can foster positive educator–learner relationships include:

- Use active listening skills.
- Be truthful in all communication.
- Be respectful and inclusive of all learners.
- Maintain professional boundaries.
- Strive for cultural humility in every learner encounter.
- Convey empathy.
- Avoid condescending language.
- Avoid negative nonverbal behaviors, such as eye-rolling.
- Serve as a role model for civil behavior and communication.

The majority of communication is nonverbal. Nurse educators seeking to improve communication skills need to understand how body language and other nonverbal communication affects others and what techniques encourage engagement, manage challenging learners, and show enthusiasm. Using body language to promote communication between educators and learners can help build a positive learning environment. For instance, the academic nurse educator should not stand or sit behind a classroom podium, but rather should be moving around the room to engage learners and refocus attention. Facing learners is an effective way to observe understanding and reactions.

Personal attributes of the academic nurse educator not only promote positive interpersonal relationships with learners but can also facilitate learning. For example, in the classroom, the educator can encourage thinking and problem-solving by briefly pausing before asking a question. Pausing several seconds allows learners to reflect and produce an answer to share. The educator cautions learners not to immediately shout out an answer to allow all learners time to think. When asking a question, anxiety and embarrassment can be avoided by not calling learners out by name or pointing to them to provide a response. Additional information about the impact of personal attributes of nurse educators is provided later in this chapter.

Using Effective Oral and Written Communication Skills

Nurse educators need to know how to effectively communicate with learners, peers, administrators, and external stakeholders. The nurse educator applies best practices in oral, written, and electronic communication that reflects an awareness of self and others and the ability to convey ideas in a variety of ways.

In addition to promoting positive educator–learner relationships as described earlier, nurse educators must provide learner feedback and document learner performance in a variety of educational environments. Verbal feedback to learners should be timely, meaningful, and constructive. Feedback can be provided in a private setting either during an educator's office hours or at another time that is mutually agreed upon. Frequent feedback provides information to the learner about academic progress and allows the learner to improve as needed. The nurse educator should document all learner meeting discussions in case the information is needed for reference at a later time (Billings & Halstead, 2020).

Providing written feedback on learner performance is also part of the nurse educator's role. For example, graded assignments should include educator comments to inform learners about the strengths of the assignment and areas that need improvement. Written comments should be specific, constructive, and related to the grading rubric. In some cases, educators may allow an opportunity for learners to use written feedback to resubmit the assignment to help master the learning.

Written feedback is also important when documenting learner clinical performance. The nurse educator maintains ongoing notes during the clinical experience regarding each learner's performance to assist in determining if the learner met clinical expectations on the summative tool. Specific, constructive written feedback related to these clinical criteria assists learners in identifying areas for improvement.

Nurse educators have multiple opportunities to communicate with peers in committee meetings, task groups, and faculty organization meetings. The educator should actively participate in meetings as part of program, departmental, and institutional governance. If the educator has a concern, the educator would meet with the course coordinator, lead instructor, or program administrator, depending on the nature of the concern, to verbalize the information. In some cases, written proposals for change may be requested.

Electronic communication via email is another important communication method for nurse educators. Although this method of communication is often appropriate for learners and peers, it is best used for brief informational purposes only. Email should not be used for sensitive, confidential, or lengthy communication that could be misinterpreted or cause an unexpected emotional response. Sensitive, confidential, and lengthy information should be communicated in a face-to-face format, including virtual video formats such as Zoom.

Educators also contribute to creating documents for continuing program approval and accreditation. The nurse educator needs to be proficient in electronic documentation, including the use of basic computer programs such as Word and Excel. These computer skills are also important for the nurse educator to create a portfolio or dossier to document professional scholarship activities for tenure and promotion.

CNE®/CNE®n Key Point

Remember: Written feedback is important when documenting learner clinical performance. Specific, constructive written feedback related to these clinical criteria assists learners in identifying areas for improvement.

Modeling Reflective Thinking Practices

Reflection is an example of critical thinking about values, beliefs, and attitudes in the affective learning domain. For learners, reflection is necessary to help develop critical thinking and clinical reasoning. Reflection can be used to evaluate the learner's level of understanding and fosters development of personal awareness. The nurse educator assigns reflective thinking activities like clinical journaling, debriefing after simulation, reaction papers, and debates to promote professional and personal growth.

The nurse educator models reflective thinking by engaging in self-reflection about teaching-learning ability as an essential component of professional development and growth. Like any skill, it must be practiced and refined. *Critical reflection* is the intentional process of identifying and checking the validity of the teaching assumptions educators work from (Bradshaw et al., 2021). These actions are based on the assumptions of how students learn best. Assumptions come from a variety of sources and may or may not be accurate.

As part of the reflection process, the academic nurse educator considers different viewpoints. The self-view is used for self-assessment to reflect on current teaching practices. Considering the learner view includes using feedback from course evaluations, assessments, journals, focus groups, and/or interviews. Colleagues can offer different ideas, views, understanding, and support through peer observation or coaching.

Creating Opportunities for Learners to Develop Critical Thinking

In the process of developing clinical judgment skills for safe, competent patient care, nurse educators have a responsibility to help learners develop critical thinking and clinical reasoning in preparation for the generalist or advanced practice role. The nurse educator purposefully engages learners in active learning strategies to help acquire, retain, and retrieve knowledge that is needed to make appropriate clinical judgments (Ignatavicius, 2019). Clinical judgment requires the use of knowledge for application in patient care.

Educational games or games that can be adapted for education are appropriate for didactic course content. Sometimes called *gaming* or *gamification,* these activities allow the learner to acquire, retain, and retrieve knowledge needed for thinking and making clinical decisions. Examples of commonly used games in nursing education are *Jeopardy* and *Who Wants to Be a Millionaire?* Kahoot is a digital game app that is also popular for knowledge retrieval. A major advantage of gaming is that learners can receive immediate feedback. However, games can be very time-consuming, and a designated period should be allocated for each game (Billings & Halstead, 2020).

Other active learning strategies that help to acquire, retain, or retrieve knowledge include:

- *Numbered Heads Together*: Learners count off to form groups of three or four and look up information as requested by the educator. This activity can be used in the classroom or online.
- *Directed or Guided Reading*: Learners are provided a list of questions to answer while reading to narrow their reading focus. This activity is used by individual learners either before or after class.

The nurse educator provides opportunities for learners to engage in active learning strategies that foster critical thinking and clinical decision making. For each strategy, the educator provides a *reflection* time to reflect on the activity focus, summarize key points, and correct any misperceptions. Examples of these active learning and thinking activities include:

- *Think-Pair-Share Activity*: After posing a question to the group, each learner writes down the answer; in pairs, learners share and compare their answers, which may then be shared with the entire learner group. This activity can be used in the classroom, online, or postclinical conference.
- *Venn Diagram*: Learners work individually or in pairs to create this compare-and-contrast *graphic organizer* (Fig. 2.1). This activity can be used in the classroom, online, or postclinical conference.
- *Concept Maps*: Learners construct a unique concept map, making connections regarding different components of patient care as a plan of care or different components of a concept. This *graphic organizer* activity can be created individually or in groups of learners in the classroom, online, or clinical learning environments.
- *Socratic Questioning*: The educator asks learners questions about clinical or policy situations, which promote and expand critical thinking. Examples are "What else?" "Why?" "Can you explain?" "What does that mean?" This activity can be used for individual learners or in groups in the classroom, online, or clinical learning environments.

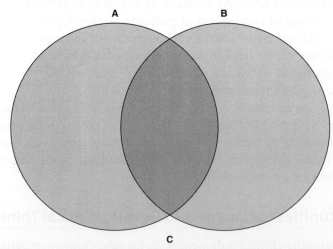

FIG. 2.1 Venn Diagram Used for Compare-and-Contrast Thinking Activities. A and B are overlapping circles, which represent two concepts or topics. Similarities of the two concepts or topics are placed in the overlapped area (C). Differences are placed in the remaining portions of the circles (A and B).

- *Send-a-Problem*: Learners, in groups or individually, develop test questions and pass them to another individual or group to answer; answers are reviewed after all learners have answered all of the questions.
- *Structured Controversy*: Learners get into pairs and discuss a selected ethical issue or dilemma by defending both sides of the issue to each other for 1 minute each. The educator then facilitates a group discussion about both sides of the issue.
- *Case Studies*: Learners analyze a clinical scenario and answer critical thinking questions about patient care or a professional nursing issue. This activity can be used individually or in groups in the classroom, online, or in clinical learning environments, including postclinical conference. Four types of case activities that the educator can assign include (Oermann et al., 2022):
  - *Case method,* which presents one short clinical or professional issue scenario followed by two to three thinking questions.
  - *Case study,* which presents more information in one clinical or professional issue scenario followed by multiple thinking questions.
  - *Unfolding case,* which presents an initial clinical or professional issue scenario followed by one or more additional phases of the scenario demonstrating change over time. Multiple questions are presented for each phase of the scenario.
  - *Reverse case study,* which allows learners to develop a case study in small groups after the educator provides partial patient information, such as health problem(s) and medications, if any.

Creating a Positive Learning Environment

A positive learning environment can be fostered when nurse educators demonstrate an interest in and respect for all learners. Learning environments should be welcoming and encourage collaboration between the educator and learners. One way to present a welcoming environment is to present a "warm" syllabus that is learner-centered. Characteristics of a warm and welcoming course syllabus include (Billings & Halstead, 2020):
- Positive and friendly language that demonstrates educator flexibility
- Self-disclosure to provide insight into the educator's teaching-learning or interpersonal style
- Enthusiasm about the course
- Compassion that demonstrates educator flexibility and caring
- Rationales for course assignments to show how learning can be achieved

The nurse educator and learner need to examine attitudes and beliefs that each bring to the learning environment. Learners may lack confidence in their abilities, especially if they are first-generation college learners. The nurse educator recognizes the presence of a power dynamic between educators and learners because of the inherent power role of the educator. Learners can become empowered when the nurse educator demonstrates an attitude of caring and commitment by being courteous and respectful. When learners recognize they have a role to play in developing their own learning experience, it can prove to be an empowering experience for them.

In the clinical setting, the academic nurse educator creates a positive learning environment using teaching strategies to support the learner's needs, the learning outcomes, and course outcomes. Opportunities are sought to develop critical thinking and clinical reasoning skills in the learner. Teaching-learning strategies are grounded in theory, and evidence-based teaching practices are employed and often supported by technology.

Debriefing and *reflection* are essential critical thinking activities and should be part of any active learning strategy. For example, after learners complete a case study, the nurse educator reviews the correct answers and provides rationales to support them. Discussion about learner responses help learners determine what they did well and what areas need review and improvement. Postclinical conference should be used as a debriefing time after every clinical learning experience to ensure that learners gained the appropriate knowledge and understand how to use it to make appropriate care decisions.

Demonstrating Enthusiasm for Teaching, Learning, and the Nursing Profession

When nurse educators show a passion for teaching, learning, and the nursing profession, they inspire learners and provide motivation for success. Presented by the nurse educator with enthusiasm, the topic becomes much more interesting and pertinent and helps create a positive learning environment. Some students struggle with learning difficult or uninteresting content.

Showing enthusiasm and passion for the content by using body language, speech patterns, and eye contact are approaches to get students inspired to learn (Nelson, 2020). Providing upbeat music that communicates to the learners before class begins and appropriate use of humor can help provide an enthusiastic learning environment. Including learner engagement strategies, such as games, YouTube videos, and group discussions about the course content can promote a positive environment for learning. Soliciting learner feedback can improve the learning environment. For example, the educator can ask "What's working for you?" or "What do you need to help promote learning?"

The nurse educator demonstrates genuine caring about learners' success. One strategy is to offer a short informal assessment of the class after the first few weeks of a course. Based on learner feedback, the educator can make adjustments in the teaching-learning process. If requested changes are addressed, learners may be more enthusiastic because they recognize their suggestions are taken seriously.

Demonstrating Personal Attributes That Facilitate Learning

The most effective nurse educators are respectful of others, evidence-based, confident, fair, approachable, creative, and enthusiastic. They are able to communicate, promote critical thinking, and have realistic expectations. The educator's personal attributes of caring, confidence, patience, integrity, and flexibility facilitate learning.

Academic and clinical integrity in the academic nurse educator is exhibited through professionalism based on a foundation of using values, morals, and ethical principles to guide teaching practice. The academic nurse educator facilitates the development of integrity in learners through role modeling and providing a learning environment with trust and the free exchange of ideas.

Establishing Professional Boundaries

Just as nurses in practice must maintain professional behaviors and establish professional boundaries with patients, academic nurse educators are obligated to establish professional boundaries with learners as part of personal integrity. The caring nature of educators may be misconstrued by some learners as friendship, especially when learners are about the same age or older than educators. To help prevent any misperception, some nursing programs require that educators be addressed by their last name, such as Dr. Brown or Miss Sanchez. In other programs, learners and educators are addressed by their last names as a symbol of mutual respect.

Orientation for new nurse educators should include information about establishing professional boundaries. Ongoing continuing education through webinars and group discussions help to remind educators about the need for professional behaviors at all times in all learning environments. Role-playing may help novice faculty learn how to respond to specific situations between learners and educators.

At times, educators may feel it is acceptable to attend social gatherings such as going to lunch at a local restaurant with learners at the end of a course or clinical learning experience. However, this behavior is not professional and does not respect boundaries. If learners request for the educator to attend such an event, the educator should politely decline the invitation and explain that attendance would violate professional boundaries. Instead, if learners desire to celebrate the end of a term, they might plan a luncheon during a class break.

Responding Effectively to Unexpected Events Affecting Instruction

Natural disasters, snow storms, and other unexpected external events often close the educational institution for 1 or more days. Internal events like heating and cooling mechanical failures may also result in school closure. These events usually occur unexpectedly and quickly, preventing educators from preplanning alternative learning experiences. However, educators must be proactive and be prepared for these events at any time.

As discussed earlier in this chapter, the COVID-19 pandemic was an unexpected event that affected the lives of nurse educators and learners across the globe. National and local regulatory agencies provided direction on adapting classes based on social distancing recommendations. The pandemic presented unique challenges and put the nurse educator in a situation of quickly adapting traditional instructional delivery methods for new ones.

The pandemic also emphasized the importance of preparing nurses to adequately respond and care for a large number of very ill and infected patients. Learner and educator safety was key in making the transition to a remote learning environment. Many nurse educators were in a new environment and out of their "comfort zone." Changing to online learning required the willingness for educators to adapt and be flexible in learning educational methodologies without formal training. Nurse educators were empowered to work remotely when possible. Just-in-time learning was essential during the pandemic to ensure all students were aware of the frequently changing practices surrounding the pandemic.

In addition to global pandemics and natural disasters, other unexpected events occur and require adaptation by the nurse educator. For example, clinical sites (in nonpandemic times) often decrease census at certain times of the year or make major institutional changes that require intensive staff development. When these events occur, the educator may need to consider options for clinical learning, such as clinical simulation, virtual simulation, and/or skills laboratory practice. Missed class or clinical hours need to be made up through appropriate alternative learning activities to meet regulatory approval and accreditation standards. Being able to seek these alternative experiences demonstrates educator flexibility and integrity.

Developing Collegial Working Relationships With Clinical Agency Personnel

The ability to establish and maintain effective working relationships with clinical agencies is based on a shared mission, values, and trust. A collegial working relationship is developed through effective, clear communication and commitment to addressing conflicts. Opportunities for developing a collaborative partnership from a contractual agreement is a complex and time-consuming process with early planned discussions. However, developing collegial working relationships with clinical agency personnel is essential because agencies continue to be more difficult to acquire for learner practice.

The nurse educator develops strong relationships with clinical agency partners to maximize student learning opportunities and help learners navigate the clinical experience. The ability of the clinical faculty to facilitate students' learning can be enhanced when an effective working relationship is established with the clinical agency. Successful relationships begin with effective communication, which must be practiced in an ongoing way to maintain relationships and facilitate learning outcomes. To help maintain positive collegial relationships, the educator may request unit nurses recommend the best patient assignments to meet clinical learning outcomes. Soliciting staff assistance may help unit nurses feel their expertise is valued by the nurse educator.

The successful nurse educator understands the clinical environment and the roles individuals have within the environment, has flexibility to modify teaching activities to fit the situation, and establishes effective relationships to improve the learning experience. The nurse educator must clearly communicate the expected learning outcomes, level and ability of learners, clinical practice expectations, and clinical schedule to relevant agency staff. When expert nurses foster learning, especially in the clinical setting, learners feel welcomed and supported, which improves communication and ultimately improves patient safety (Billings & Halstead, 2020).

Developing a Safe Learning Environment

Research on the clinical practicum indicates that learners experience a variety of stressors in the clinical learning environment (Oermann et al., 2022). These concerns can be categorized as physical, psychological, and emotional and should be addressed as part of clinical orientation to assure learners that the educator is responsible for creating a safe learning environment.

One major physical stressor for learners is the fear of contracting a disease or getting sick from caring for patients, especially during the recent pandemic. During the pandemic, most nursing programs did not allow learners to go to community clinical sites to prevent them from becoming infected. When learners returned to the clinical agency, educators assessed whether the agency had adequate personal protective equipment (PPE) and learners knew when and how to use it properly. If adequate PPE was not available in an agency or unit, the educator did not assign learners to the site.

The daily stressors and frustrations of nurses (especially during the pandemic), for example, frequently leads to negative behaviors that may be directed towards learners and/or the educator. Staff incivility can cause learners to have psychological and emotional responses that include emotional exhaustion and burnout. The nurse educator is responsible for functioning as a gatekeeper to prevent these outcomes (Oermann et al., 2022).

Learners may also fear making mistakes during patient care and causing harm. Nurse educators must reassure learners that they will supervise key aspects of care provided by learners. This reassurance should begin in clinical agency orientation and be reinforced frequently during every clinical learning experience.

Using Knowledge of Evidence-Based Practice for Instruction

Nurse educators have the dual responsibility of modeling evidence-based clinical practice and utilizing evidence-based instructional methods in any learning environment. Educators first need to gain knowledge about the evidence that supports instructional methods and approaches, including evidence-based teaching-learning strategies for a variety of environments. Then educators need to select those instructional methods that meet the needs of diverse learners and are appropriate for the type of program. For example, app-driven audience response activities in the classroom would be most appropriate for learners who are *digital natives,* such as Generations Y and Z.

Effective clinical teaching involves the ability of clinical nurse educators to optimize the learning environment by providing meaningful experiences grounded in current evidence. For example, nurse educators facilitate cooperative learning strategies such as peer teaching and pairing learners as they provide care and participate in postclinical conferences.

Ongoing professional development through journals, webinars, workshops, and conferences assists nurse educators in keeping current and up to date with the latest nursing education research. Educators may desire to conduct their own studies on instructional methods or approaches as part of the Scholarship of Discovery. Findings should be published in a peer-reviewed nursing education journal to help advance the science of nursing education.

Demonstrating the Ability to Teach Clinical Skills

The most important attribute of an academic nurse educator who teaches in the clinical learning environment is clinical competence. Educators must keep current in their area of clinical expertise through professional development activities and maintain competence in clinical nursing skills to serve as role models for learners. They may need to teach and demonstrate a new skill that learners have not learned or practiced. If educators have not practiced selected clinical skills recently or are not current with skills, they should seek opportunities to update and practice in the clinical agency or simulation laboratory.

> **CNE®/CNE®n Key Point**
>
> *Remember:* The most important attribute of an academic nurse educator who teaches in the clinical learning environment is clinical competence. Educators must keep current in their area of clinical expertise through professional development activities and maintain competence in clinical nursing skills to serve as role models for learners.

Nurse educators may teach clinical skills in the campus laboratory, clinical simulation laboratory, or community clinical agency. The campus skills and clinical simulation laboratories usually have more educational tools for teaching the skill, such as video and audio resources, task trainers, mannequins, and multiple supplies, when compared with clinical agencies. Depending on the skill, the nurse educator in the campus laboratory:

- Assigns learners to read about how to perform the skills before the lab is conducted
- May assign learners to view a video skill demonstration
- Gives a reading quiz to learners before skill practice in the lab
- Demonstrates the skill using role-play, standardized patient, equipment, supplies, and/or mannequin, and explains each skill performance step
- Provides opportunities for learners to practice the skill with constructive feedback by the educator

If the skill is taught in the clinical agency, often with a patient, the educator performs the demonstration with explanation and permission of the patient.

As discussed earlier, nurse educators must also serve as role models for reflective and critical thinking and be able to help learners develop critical thinking. Critical thinking and clinical reasoning are needed to make safe and appropriate clinical decisions or clinical judgments, especially when a patient's condition deteriorates or changes significantly.

Acting as a Role Model in Practice Settings

In the clinical practice setting, the nurse educator acts as a professional role model for learners and staff. Role modeling is an active, dynamic process involving observational learning, and it aims to explore the process involved. Role models are important for learners to socialize into the role of a nurse, but they are especially essential for the success of minority learners who must overcome additional barriers and benefit the most from positive learner–educator relationships. Mentoring and coaching by the nurse educator is the single most important strategy that successfully helps in retention of learners. Being available as a nurse educator to learners when needed and providing timely, frequent, and meaningful feedback on learner clinical performance can also help learners to be successful (Billings & Halstead, 2020).

Role modeling is also important for clinical practice nurses and other staff to demonstrate professional behaviors and develop positive collaborative relationships. Clinical practice nurses, learners, and educators should have the opportunity to evaluate their experience and the clinical learning site after the clinical practicum is completed.

References

Barnett, P. E. (2014). *Let's scramble, not flip, the classroom.* Inside Higher (Ed). https://www.insidehigh-ered.com/views/2014/02/14/flipping-classroom-isnt-answer-lets-scramble-it-essay.

Billings, D. M., & Halstead, J. A. (2020). *Teaching in nursing: A guide for faculty* (6th ed.). St. Louis: Elsevier.

Bradshaw, M. J., Hultquist, B. L., & Hagler, D. (2021). *Innovative teaching strategies in nursing and related health professions.* Burlington, MA: Jones & Bartlett Learning.

Cannon, S., & Boswell, C. (2016). *Evidence-based teaching in nursing: A foundation for educators* (2nd ed.). Burlington, MA: Jones & Bartlett Learning.

Ignatavicius, D. (2019). *Teaching and learning in a concept-based nursing curriculum: A how-to best practice approach.* Burlington, MA: Jones & Bartlett Learning.

Nelson, Y. M. (2020). Strategies to maintaining enthusiasm in the classroom. *Nurse Educator, 45*(6), E61.

Oermann, M. H., DeGagne, J. C., & Phillips, B. C. (2022). *Teaching in nursing and role of the educator* (3rd ed.). New York: Springer Publishing.

CHAPTER 2 Practice Questions

1. The nurse educator is planning a skills laboratory practice experience for learners. In which learning domain will the educator plan this teaching strategy?
   A. Cognitive domain
   B. Affective domain
   C. Visual domain
   D. Psychomotor domain

2. The nurse educator is planning a teaching-learning strategy that would help visual learners best understand the course content. Which strategy would the nurse educator most likely select?
   A. Case study
   B. Lecture
   C. Concept map
   D. Discussion forum

3. Which statement by the novice nurse educator about online learning requires follow-up by the mentor?
   A. "I can let students learn on their own for online learning."
   B. "I think my students are very motivated to use online learning."
   C. "I will give learners prompt feedback about their online assignments."
   D. "I plan to participate in the discussion forums to respond to learners."

4. Which of these teaching strategies would be the best for the nurse educator to select to help students achieve learning in the cognitive domain?
   A. Practicing listening to breath sounds
   B. Taking a quiz on medical terminology
   C. Taking a final course examination
   D. Working on a case study during class

5. Which teaching strategy would the nurse educator select to help learners acquire or recall knowledge?
   A. Case study
   B. *Jeopardy*
   C. Reflective journaling
   D. Simulation

6. Which teaching-learning strategy would the nurse educator employ to help learners achieve deep learning?
   A. Watching online videos
   B. Taking notes in live lecture format
   C. Completing preassigned worksheets
   D. Developing a concept map

7. Which statement by the nurse educator indicates the use of a constructivism-based teaching-learning strategy?
   A. "I will be using concept mapping for clinical assignments."
   B. "I'm going to assign each learner a topic to research and present."
   C. "I'm going to co-teach this course with another faculty member."
   D. "I'm going to post a discussion forum online."

8. Which teaching-learning activity would most likely help learners achieve deep learning about care of patients experiencing diabetic ketoacidosis (DKA)?
   A. Compare and contrast DKA and hypoglycemia.
   B. Create a teaching plan for a diabetic who becomes ill.
   C. Read selected materials on metabolic acidosis.
   D. Write a reflective postclinical paper about the assigned client in DKA crisis.

9. Which of the following factors does the nurse educator recognize as most important in creating a learning environment conducive to the nontraditional learner?
   A. Encourage a competitive environment.
   B. Avoid "busywork" assignments.
   C. Minimize technology.
   D. Decrease the use of collaborative learning.

10. Which statement by the novice nurse educator would indicate a need for the mentor to follow up about how to teach the i-Generation learners?
    A. "I'll have learners collaborate in small groups."
    B. "I'm going to post a discussion forum online."
    C. "I'm going to assign projects to research and present on a YouTube video."
    D. "I'm going to reduce electronic assignments this semester."

11. Which outcome requires learning in the psychomotor domain?
    A. Define medical terminology related to care of the cardiac patient.
    B. Explain where to place a stethoscope when listening to heart sounds.
    C. Write a personal plan for physical fitness.
    D. Locate S_1 and S_2 as a part of cardiac assessment.

12. Which statement by the novice nurse educator about creating case studies indicates best practice?
    A. "I ask learners to create the case on the topic we are studying."
    B. "I may need to grade the case study questions."
    C. "I include minimal data so learners can interpret from their own perspective."
    D. "I include psychosocial data and the family situation to make it realistic."

13. Which of the following verbs would assess learning in the affective domain?
    A. Reflect
    B. Explain
    C. Develop
    D. Plan

14. Which of the following teaching-learning approaches is the best for the nurse educator to use for cooperative learning?
    A. Flipped classroom
    B. Team-based learning
    C. Scrambled classroom
    D. Structured learning

15. The nurse educator reviews a course objective that states "Apply knowledge of pathophysiology to determine common assessment findings for patients who have multiple sclerosis." Which learning domain does this objective assess?
    A. Affective
    B. Psychomotor
    C. Cognitive
    D. Behavioral

16. Which of the following teaching-learning approaches is an example of asynchronous learning?
    A. Concept map
    B. Discussion board
    C. Structured controversy
    D. Reverse case study

17. Which statement about using educational games in class by the novice nurse educator would require follow-up by the mentor?
    A. "Games are good for engaging learners in the classroom."
    B. "Games help promote critical thinking and clinical reasoning."
    C. "Games help learners acquire and recall knowledge."
    D. "Games tend to take a lot of time to implement."

18. Which of the following active learning strategies is considered a graphic organizer?
    A. Unfolding case study
    B. Concept map
    C. Send-a-Problem
    D. Virtual reality

19. Which outcome requires learning in the affective domain?
    A. Compare and contrast affective disorders and schizophrenia.
    B. Distinguish between primary, secondary, and tertiary mental health care.
    C. Become self-aware using exploration of personal mental health practices.
    D. Demonstrate a neurologic assessment on a client with a history of a stroke.

20. Which learning activity demonstrates the divergent role in Kolb's learning theory?
    A. Group work on a case study
    B. Role-playing communication techniques
    C. Completing a concept map
    D. Inserting a urinary catheter

21. The nurse educator is developing objectives for a new course. Which would be the best example to include as a psychomotor objective?
    A. Discuss the proper use of body mechanics for lifting.
    B. Develop a case study for simulation.
    C. Reflect on the case study implemented in clinical simulation.
    D. Demonstrate how to insert an intravenous catheter.

22. The nurse educator is planning an activity in the classroom for visual learners. What activity would be the best to create?
    A. Listen to a podcast and summarize in a report.
    B. Read the textbook assignment and review in small groups.
    C. Watch a film clip and discuss in a think-pair-share activity.
    D. Demonstrate a skill as part of a competency assessment.

23. How does the nurse educator provide the best learning environment for learners from different generations?
    A. Use think-pair-share as a primary cooperative learning strategy.
    B. Arrange study sessions for different times of the day.
    C. Provide learning opportunities for learners to work online in small groups.
    D. Find commonalities among the groups and connect with technology.

24. A learner develops a concept map for patient teaching regarding a new medication regimen and explains how the medications work to decrease symptoms. What type of learning has the learner demonstrated?
    A. Knowledge retention
    B. Deep learning
    C. Memorization
    D. Superficial learning

25. The nurse educator modifies teaching strategies and learning experiences based on which of the following?
    A. Enthusiasm for learning
    B. Ability to teach others
    C. Clinical sites
    D. Cultural background

26. What learning strategy would be best for the nurse educator to use to improve diversity and inclusion in the learning environment?
    A. Revise the curriculum to increase cultural awareness.
    B. Include cultural content on each exam.

C. Assign learners to participate in cultural activities on campus.
D. Create a self-study unit on cultural humility.

27. The novice nurse educator asks the mentor how the nursing program has broken down barriers for learners with diverse backgrounds. What is the mentor's best response?
    A. "We include content regarding diversity on our exams."
    B. "We discourage social activities among nursing students."
    C. "We do a personal inventory of our own feelings and beliefs.
    D. "We have modified our curriculum to include LGBT content."

28. In the skills lab the nurse educator demonstrates how to do a neurologic assessment for learners. After the demonstration, a few learners state they are unsure about the assessment. What would be the best strategy to ensure a clear understanding of the information?
    A. Have learners practice neurologic assessment in pairs.
    B. Repeat the demonstration for the class.
    C. Provide a film on assessment of the client with neurologic deficits.
    D. Have learners listen to an audiotape on neurologic assessment.

29. What is the nurse educator's first step in fostering a sense of community in the online environment?
    A. Use feedback from learners.
    B. Use a discussion board to establish presence.
    C. Schedule an initial face-to-face meeting with the class.
    D. Develop a culture of academic integrity.

30. High-fidelity clinical simulation experiences are influenced by which theory?
    A. Kolb's Learning Theory
    B. Constructivism
    C. Boyer's Scholarship
    D. Deep Learning Theory

31. The novice nurse educator asks the mentor what elements are included in structuring the debriefing process for clinical simulation. What is the best response?
    A. "Select one model of a debriefing design."
    B. "Use a teacher-centered approach for learning."
    C. "Special debriefing training is necessary."
    D. "Use a guide for cognitive retraining."

32. What type of teaching-learning activity would be most preferred by visual learners?
    A. Case study
    B. Journaling
    C. Concept maps
    D. Debriefing

33. Which statement by the novice nurse educator regarding unfolding case studies would require follow-up by the mentor?
    A. "Using case studies supports student-centered learning."
    B. "New faculty would benefit from professional development on how to develop case studies."
    C. "Case studies are not a form of experiential learning."
    D. "Case studies are most effective with complex patient situations."

34. The nurse educator uses which teaching-learning methodologies for learners who prefer auditory learning?
    A. Notetaking and print resources
    B. Case studies and examples
    C. Guest speakers and debates
    D. Maps and charts

35. Which question in a case study best stimulates critical thinking?
    A. What are the risk factors for hypertension?
    B. What happens to the blood vessels in chronic hypertension?
    C. What focused assessment will be performed?
    D. What medications are most likely to be prescribed?

36. Which learner activity is consistent with the theory of behaviorism?
    A. Writing a scholarly paper for publication
    B. Participating in cooperative learning activities
    C. Completing a physical assessment on a child, adult, and older adult
    D. Practicing test questions until scoring is consistently above 80%

37. What question would the nurse educator ask to assess how well the learner performed in the affective domain in the clinical learning environment?
    A. "Is the learner able to adapt clinical skills to different patient situations?"
    B. "Does the learner interact well with the patients and health care team?"
    C. "Has the learner shown accurate relationships on concept maps?"
    D. "Does the learner demonstrate improved critical thinking abilities?"

38. Which teaching-learning activity is an example of constructivism?
    A. Developing an unfolding case study
    B. Taking a dosage calculation test
    C. Learning the steps of a clinical procedure
    D. Practicing frequently in the simulation lab

39. The nurse educator develops a clinical experience for learners to work alongside the charge nurse to analyze how communication promotes safe patient care. What domains of learning does this experience represent?
    A. Psychomotor and cognitive
    B. Communicative and affective
    C. Cognitive and communicative
    D. Behavioral and cognitive

40. A learner asks the clinical nurse educator to help insert a urinary catheter for the first time. What is the best response by the clinical educator?
    A. "Ask the nurse to help you because I'm busy right now."
    B. "I'll let you know when I am available."
    C. "When do you need me to help you?"
    D. "Ask the nurse to insert the catheter this time and you can watch."

41. Which learner assignment by the nurse educator best develops critical thinking skills?
    A. Developing a slide show
    B. Watching a film clip
    C. Reading an article
    D. Journaling after a clinical experience

42. Learners beginning a clinical learning experience express that they are concerned they will accidently make a mistake that could harm a patient. What is the nurse educator's best response?
    A. "The staff nurses will be watching you carefully, so you don't need to worry."
    B. "You should not make any mistakes because you all passed your skills check-offs."
    C. "I will be observing every invasive skill that you perform for patients."
    D. "The staff nurses are accountable for patient care, but I will be available if you need me."

43. Which of the following communication methods would be the best for the educator to use to provide feedback to a learner who is failing a course?
    A. Email
    B. Texting
    C. Face-to-face
    D. Social media

44. Which teaching-learning activity would be the most appropriate when helping learners reflect on ethical dilemmas?
    A. Concept map
    B. Think-pair-share
    C. Send-a-Problem
    D. Structured controversy

45. Which teaching-learning activity would the nurse educator select for a group of Generation Z learners?
    A. Lecture
    B. Voice-over slide presentation
    C. Virtual simulation
    D. Reading assignment

46. Which teaching-learning strategy would the nurse educator select for a group of learners with varying learning style preferences?
    A. Concept map
    B. Lecture
    C. Slide presentation
    D. Final examination

47. Which communication method is preferred by Generation Z learners?
    A. Social media
    B. Email
    C. Texting
    D. Face-to-face

48. Which learning domain is represented by this learning outcome: "Demonstrate how to perform wound care"?
    A. Affective domain
    B. Cognitive domain
    C. Psychomotor domain
    D. Behavioral domain

49. Which verb would best measure learning at the remembering/cognitive level?
    A. Differentiate
    B. Perform
    C. Reflect
    D. Identify

50. Which active teaching-learning activity would the nurse educator select to help gain learning in the cognitive domain?
    A. Case study
    B. Journaling
    C. Skills practice
    D. Role-playing

51. The novice nurse educator is planning strategies to help learners use therapeutic communication techniques. What is the best teaching-learning activity to meet this goal?
    A. Provide handouts on communication.
    B. Assign a reading about communication.
    C. Plan a role-play demonstration on communication.
    D. Provide a reverse case study focused on communication.

52. Which statement by the novice nurse educator demonstrates understanding of the purpose of lecture?
    A. "It can include a large amount of content for a large group of learners."
    B. "It provides an opportunity for in-depth discussion and understanding."
    C. "It promotes critical thinking needed to make appropriate clinical judgments."
    D. "It is difficult to plan and organize, given my group of diverse learners."

53. Which teaching-learning activity would be best for the nurse educator to use to help learners make appropriate clinical judgments?
    A. Unfolding case study
    B. Socratic questioning
    C. Think-pair-share
    D. Discussion board

54. What is the primary domain of learning used in the classroom or online learning environment?
    A. Affective domain
    B. Cognitive domain
    C. Psychomotor domain
    D. Behavioral domain

55. What is the primary domain of learning used in the skills laboratory?
    A. Affective domain
    B. Cognitive domain
    C. Psychomotor domain
    D. Behavioral domain

56. Which of the following is included in best practices for creating slides for a presentation?
    A. Use a small-size font to be able to include more information per slide.
    B. Avoid using multiple pictures or graphic organizers.
    C. Provide slides for every class that learners can use as study guides.
    D. Place two to three points of information as summary or key points for each slide.

Facilitating Learner Development and Socialization

SOMER NOURSE | KAILEE BURDICK

LEARNING OUTCOMES

1. Discuss the implications of student learning styles, unique learner needs, and learner characteristics on role socialization.
2. Identify advisement strategies for promoting learner development.
3. Describe selected resources for diverse student learning.
4. Differentiate learning activities that assist the learner to develop within the cognitive, psychomotor, and affective domains.
5. Describe methods to assist learners to develop skills in reflection, self-evaluation, and peer evaluation.
6. Explain the role of professional development in the lifelong learning of the nurse.

Academic nurse educators have a responsibility to help learners develop not only as nurses but in the broader concept of global citizens. Educators assist learners in developing nursing knowledge and skills but are also tasked with ensuring that learners develop the moral and ethical code required of nurses. The American Nurses Association (ANA) Code of Ethics (2015) calls for nurses to demonstrate compassion, advocacy, competence, and accountability. Nurses are charged with consistently demonstrating not only personal ethical practices but also with improving the ethical environment of the health care setting (ANA, 2015). The academic nurse educator is accountable for modeling the values and behaviors of the profession and promoting growth in learners.

Identifying Unique Learning Styles and Needs of Learners

Facilitating learner development requires that nurse educators are knowledgeable about learning styles, motivational factors, and characteristics of diverse learners. Faculty must create an environment where a variety of learning styles can be accommodated and where learner values and needs are respected. Effective teaching involves assessing student learning styles and adapting teaching to individual learners to promote learner development. Nurse educators must be aware of their own learning styles because many tend to teach in the manner they best learn. Understanding the characteristics of diverse learners can also help educators identify motivational factors and readiness to learn.

Learner Motivation

Understanding what motivates students to learn is equally as important as understanding the different methods of how they learn. *Motivation* may be *intrinsic* (arising from internal factors) or *extrinsic* (arising from external forces). Learners may have intrinsic motivation to achieve a nursing degree because they have a genuine desire to help others, feel accomplished, or serve a higher purpose. Extrinsic factors affecting learners' motivation to do well in nursing courses may include getting good grades, graduating with honors, maintaining a scholarship, getting a good job, or parental and societal pressures. According to Keller's (2009) ARCS model of motivational design, there are four factors to consider when promoting motivation in learners:

- *Attention:* Gain the learner's attention through perceptual or visual arousal. Play games, pose questions, use humor, use a visual stimulus, or encourage brainstorming.
- *Relevance:* Establish relevance by using concrete language and examples familiar to the learners. Identify how this learning will help achieve current and future goals and allow learners to choose different methods for completing the learning.
- *Confidence:* Promote learner confidence by providing objectives and prerequisites. Make sure learners are aware of performance requirements and evaluation criteria. Provide feedback for success. Allow for small successes to build confidence.
- *Satisfaction:* Learning must be rewarding and satisfying. Provide opportunities for learners to use their knowledge in useful ways in real or simulated settings. Provide positive feedback and reinforcement.

Educators can use these motivational strategies to keep learners interested and actively engaged. Faculty should evaluate motivational strategies based on the generational and learner characteristics of each cohort of learners. Educators can incorporate many of the ARCS principles by using active learning strategies such as role-playing, case studies, simulation, or problem-solving activities (Cannon & Boswell, 2016).

> **CNE®/CNE®n Key Point**
>
> *Remember:* Encourage learner motivation through active learning strategies, such as role-playing, simulation, and case studies.

Academic nurse educators also need to be aware that motivation is needed for learners to be successful for *online learning*. A systematic review of the literature by Cadet (2021) found that the necessary characteristics for online learners include:

- Motivation
- Readiness to learn
- Self-efficacy
- Self-persistence
- Autonomy

The researcher concluded that nurse educators should assess online learners to determine what needs they may have to be successful with this mode of instructional delivery.

Readiness to Learn

The learning theories and approaches described in Chapter 2 provide insight into how learners acquire new information and what motivates them. Learners must also be assessed to determine if they are ready and willing to process new information. An assessment of readiness to learn helps learners and educators discover if the learner is physically and mentally prepared to take on a new challenge. One method for assessing readiness is use of Lichtenthal's (1990, as cited in Bastable, 2016) *PEEK model for learner readiness*. Before deciding on an appropriate learning activity, the educator must first "take a PEEK" into the four major types of learner readiness: physical readiness, emotional readiness, experiential readiness, and knowledge readiness. The four types of readiness may act as barriers or facilitators of learning. Specific attributes of each type of readiness must be considered when determining the level of readiness to learn.

- P—Physical Readiness: Measure of ability, complexity of task, environmental effects, health status, and gender
- E—Emotional Readiness: Anxiety level, support systems, motivation, risk-taking behavior, frame of mind, developmental stage
- E—Experiential Readiness: Level of aspiration, past coping mechanisms, cultural background, locus of control, orientation
- K—Knowledge Readiness: Present knowledge base, cognitive ability, learning disabilities, learning styles (Bastable, 2016)

Nurse educators can use their skills of assessment to determine if learners are ready and willing to take on a new challenge. If readiness-to-learn barriers are present, nurse educators may attempt to modify certain attributes or wait to provide the teaching when the learner is more amenable to accepting new information.

Learning Styles and Theories

A *learning style* is a unique approach in which an individual receives, processes, and reacts to information and new opportunities. Individuals can learn using all modalities of learning, but most people prefer one style over others, and that preferred style remains relatively stable over time. Understanding one's own style can help the learner identify specific learning needs and how to approach new learning. Additionally, educators must understand the various styles of learning to maximize learning in the educational setting. Chapter 2 provides information about selected educational theories. Several commonly used theories related to adult learning are briefly summarized here.

As described in Chapter 2, Fleming and Mills (1992) describe the four most common classic learning styles using the acronym VARK: visual, aural/auditory, read/write, and kinesthetic. *Visual* (spatial) learners prefer to learn through seeing, such as viewing pictures, charts, and demonstrations. The use of computers and graphics is helpful for visual learners. *Aural* learners learn best through listening and speaking. An aural learner prefers to have information presented through discussions, debates, lectures, and tutorials. *Read/write* learners learn best through text-based materials and prefer slide show presentations and reading. *Kinesthetic* learners are active learners who prefer movement and sense of touch. They like to actively experiment, role-play, play games, and use simulation. Learners can obtain knowledge of their own learning styles by completing a 16-item VARK tool. Learners are encouraged to identify their own learning styles to understand and take responsibility for meeting their own learning needs.

Kolb's experiential learning theory suggests that learning is cyclical in nature and occurs during a combination of watching, doing, feeling, and thinking. New learning takes place when old ideas are replaced with new ones. Kolb's learning style inventory differentiates between four main learning style preferences based on how the learner perceives information (concrete versus abstract) and processes information (active experimentation versus reflective observation) (McLeod, 2017). Table 3.1 delineates how these learning preferences align with the perception and processing of information.

Howard Gardner's (1999) multiple intelligences theory proposes that rather than a single type of intelligence that generally focuses on cognitive abilities, there are instead multiple types of "intelligences" that individuals may possess. The different types of intelligences influence how

TABLE 3.1 Kolb's Learning Style Inventory Preferences		
	Active Experimentation (AE) (Doing)	**Reflective Observation (RO) (Watching)**
Concrete Experience (CE) (Feeling)	Accommodating (CE/AE)	Diverging (CE/RO)
Abstract Conceptualization (AC) (Thinking)	Converging (AC/AE)	Assimilating (AC/RO)

TABLE **3.2**   Gardner's Learning Styles/Intelligences

Type of Learning Style/Intelligences	Description of Learners by Learning Style/Intelligences
Linguistic intelligence	Are sensitive to spoken and written languages and prefer to read, write, speak, and discuss
Logical/mathematical intelligence	Prefer experimentation, problem-solving, and working with numbers; like to find logical solutions to problems
Spatial intelligence	Have the ability to recognize and manipulate patterns and tend to "think in pictures"; may prefer to draw, read, view pictures, or create designs
Bodily/kinesthetic intelligence	Are able to use their bodies to perform skills, create products, or solve problems; prefer to manipulate things, use tools, move around, and use many senses to learn
Musical intelligence	Have the ability to recognize rhythms and patterns; may create songs to help them learn and listen to music
Interpersonal intelligence	Are able to recognize and understand the moods, emotions, and intentions of others; enjoy working with groups, sharing knowledge, and collaborating with others
Intrapersonal intelligence	Have the ability to recognize one's own mood, desires, and intentions; prefer to work alone; are deeply reflective, independent, and understand how to achieve their goals
Naturalistic intelligence	Are able to differentiate the types of plants, animals, and other parts of the natural world; these learners prefer to explore nature and are interested in the lived experiences of other humans

Data from Gardner, H. (1999). *Intelligence reframed: Multiple intelligences for the 21st century*. New York: Basic Books.

people learn. These eight learning styles or "intelligences" include linguistic, logical/mathematical, spatial, bodily/kinesthetic, musical, interpersonal, intrapersonal, and naturalistic (Table 3.2).

Other types of learners may include:

- *Tactile learners*: These learners require movement and manipulation of objects for optimal learning. They prefer to draw, write, or conduct experiments. They enjoy playing Scrabble.
- *Global learners*: These learners tap into emotion and intuition when making decisions. They prefer creative projects, group work, and storytelling.
- *Intuitive learners*: These individuals are fast, innovative learners but do not like work that requires memorization or repetition because they will easily become bored. At times they may make careless mistakes on tasks because of a lack of attention to details.
- *Digital (online) learners*: These learners are typically individuals from the Millennial or younger generations who enjoy collaborative learning that involves technology, specifically smart phones or other handheld devices.

Learner Development and Socialization

Although many learners have a preferred learning style, most learners are *multimodal*, meaning that they learn using multiple styles and methods. Learning styles are influenced by cultural background, age, and experience and may change over time as the learner adapts to new learning environments. It is important that educators help learners identify their own preferences for learning; however, educators should design learning experiences that encompass a variety of methods so that students may learn through a variety of experiences and be challenged in new ways.

> **CNE®/CNE®n Key Point**
>
> *Remember:* Although many learners have a preferred learning style, most learners are *multimodal,* meaning that they learn using multiple styles and methods.

Learner development and socialization can be facilitated using a set of guiding principles for higher education. After reviewing decades of pedagogical research, Chickering and Gamson (1987) created a set of seven principles for good practice in undergraduate education. These principles were designed for faculty, learners, and administrators to improve teaching and learning in higher education. Although these principles were initially created for undergraduate education, they are directly applicable to all levels and settings of education:

1. Encourage contact between learners and faculty: Frequent contact is essential for maintaining learner motivation and involvement.
2. Encourage cooperation among learners: Team learning increases involvement in learning and deepens understanding. Good learning should be collaborative and social, not isolated.
3. Encourage active learning: Students do not learn well by just listening to teachers. They need to be discussing what they are learning, relating it to past experiences, and using it in their daily lives.
4. Give prompt feedback: Learners need frequent opportunities to perform and receive suggestions for improvement. Learners need appropriate feedback in order to benefit from learning.
5. Emphasize time on task: Allocating realistic amounts of time is critical to effective learning, and some students may need help learning time management skills.
6. Communicate high expectations: Expecting learners to perform well is a self-fulfilling prophecy, and all types of learners will benefit from being held to high expectations.
7. Respect diverse talents and ways of learning: Students may have different styles of learning, and they need opportunities to demonstrate their talents in a manner that works for them. They also can be encouraged to learn in new ways.

Meeting the Needs of Diverse Learners

As the demographic composition of the student body has continued to evolve, so too must academic nurse educators continue to modify their teaching practices and role model positive relationships to create a healthy diverse classroom (Frazer et al., 2021). The National League for Nursing (NLN, 2016) describes *diversity* as the uniqueness of and differences among people, including their physical characteristics (e.g., race and ethnicity), beliefs (e.g., religious and political), and other attributes. These differences must be recognized and respected by nurse educators and all learners such that everyone feels included, a concept referred to as *inclusivity.*

As institutions of higher education continue to modify their admissions practices, more opportunities become available for a diverse student body. Educators are tasked with improving success for learners whose backgrounds may vary according to culture, ethnicity, gender, age, use of technology, previous education, sexual orientation, gender identity, and personal and financial challenges. Meeting the needs of these learners requires knowledge of their characteristics, challenges of each group, and provision of available resources.

Generational Diversity and Characteristics of Learners

The learners and faculty in a classroom may include multiple generations of learners, each with its own characteristics, preferred modes of communication, and learning needs. Each generation has its own set of unique values that must be understood by the educator in order to promote a positive and collaborative learning environment. Each group will display many of the same characteristics, but individuals vary and have their own characteristics. Regardless of generation, some students are group learners and benefit from the knowledge and characteristics of others. Other students prefer to learn as individuals and do not like group work. Table 3.3 describes key attributes of each generation of learners with whom the academic nurse educator may interact.

Cultural Diversity

Creating an environment of *inclusivity* involves intentionally using strategies to promote a sense of belonging among diverse individuals or groups with differing traits, perceptions, and experiences (Metzger et al., 2020). Having a diverse nursing workforce that is representative of the diverse patient population is essential to providing quality health care. Having minority faculty role models is important for minority learner success. The total number of minority graduates in baccalaureate and graduate nursing education has continued to rise over the past decade (American Association of Colleges of Nursing [AACN], 2021), but attrition rates remain higher for minority learners than for members of the majority. Promoting an environment of inclusivity to increase success for culturally diverse and minority learners requires commitment from faculty and the larger institution.

Common barriers for culturally diverse learners may include:
- Episodes of discrimination
- Financial difficulties
- Lack of academic support or preparation
- Lack of peer support
- Lack of family support
- Lack of diverse faculty role models

Creating an environment of inclusivity can help improve learning outcomes for diverse learners. All aspects of a student's *learning community,* which includes the learner, the learner's peers, faculty, staff in the clinical setting, overall institutional culture, and family and friends outside of school, act as facilitators or barriers to inclusivity and diversity (Metzger et al., 2020). A lack of belongingness, which may result from discrimination, is associated with adverse learning outcomes.

TABLE 3.3	General Characteristics of Generational Learners
Generational Learner Group	**General Characteristics**
Baby Boomer generation (born 1945–1964)	• Have strong work ethic and value career over their personal life • In-person communication preferred over email or texting (technology naïve) • Prefer face-to-face classroom learning • Motivated by being praised, recognized, and feeling valued
Generation X (born 1965–1979)	• Value work–life balance • Adapt well to change, including the use of technology • Use email and texting as primary communication • Motivated by freedom, removal of rules, and time off from work
Generation Y (Millennials) (born 1980–1995)	• Are digital natives and technologically savvy • Like to multitask • Are more team-oriented than other generations • Use social media, email, and texting as primary communication • Value personal life over career/work but can be high achievers • Need frequent feedback from educators
Generation Z (born after 1995)	• Are technology natives and almost always digitally connected • Use social media as primary communication • Prefer combining technology with real-world experiences • Embrace education and work

Strategies for faculty to foster a sense of belonging may include:

- Learning student names
- Organizing diverse clinical and study groups
- Modifying case studies and learning materials to be more inclusive
- Intervening in episodes of discrimination
- Showing interest in other cultures
- Exhibiting supportive, encouraging, and accepting behaviors

Faculty strategies to foster a sense of belonging and institutions devoted to appreciating diversity and inclusivity can increase learning and self-confidence and improve the academic outcomes of learners from diverse backgrounds.

English as an Additional Language

Multilingual learners for whom English is an additional language (EAL) may experience challenges in nursing school related to language difficulties. Medical terminology, colloquialisms, and communicating with patients and staff may be difficult for some EAL learners, also sometimes referred to as *English language learners* (ELL). The Test of English as a Foreign Language (TOEFL) can be used to assess a learner's ability to communicate in English and identify at-risk learners who may need additional support services. Other tests are also available. Educators should work to create an environment that values and respects cultural diversity and be aware that EAL learners may need additional time to complete activities and exams because of language comprehension. The English language is the most difficult to learn, and many words have different meanings depending on their context.

Providing the following accommodations may help increase success for EAL learners:

- Use TOEFL or similar examination to identify at-risk learners.
- Allow EAL learners to audiotape class sessions.
- Use small groups so that EAL learners may benefit from working with native English speakers.
- Practice communication with patients and staff using role-playing exercises.
- Use role-playing to help with improved understanding as appropriate.
- Use simple, common vocabulary during class sessions and on examinations.
- Provide copies of class handouts.
- Use multiple methods of learning assessment.
- Allow additional time for examinations and class activities.
- Highlight key words on assignments and examinations.

CNE®/CNE®n Key Point

Remember: Implement learning strategies that help promote success of EAL learners, including allowing audiotaping of class sessions, using common vocabulary terms, and small-group activities.

Traditional Versus Nontraditional Learners

Traditional learners are those who enter college immediately after completing high school and begin a prelicensure program. Nontraditional learners may include individuals who are first-generation college learners, older learners, individuals who entered the workforce before entering higher education, learners with current employment, learners with family responsibilities, and adult learners with previous college degrees. Traditional and nontraditional learners each have unique characteristics, stressors, and life experiences that may affect their educational experience.

Traditional learners may be experiencing their first time away from home in a new and challenging environment. Traditional learners may find the initial college transition overwhelming and need additional assistance learning to navigate campus and classroom locations, study habits, time management, and test-taking skills. These transitional challenges are further compounded for first-generation college learners who are the first in their families to attend higher education. First-generation learners may not have a family role model to help them navigate the challenges of college life, so these learners may need to be referred to campus resources to help ensure their success.

Adult learners' motivation to learn is generally centered on making a life change. Adult learners may display a variety of learner characteristics but are typically self-directed learners who draw on past experiences when learning new material. They prefer learning that is problem-centered and has direct application. Adults tend to be active participants in the learning process and like immediate feedback. Adult learners, however, present with their own unique set of challenges. The demands of home, family, and job responsibilities may mean that adult learners lack sufficient time to complete assignments and may have scheduling conflicts. They may also experience lack of confidence and anxiety related to fear of academic failure. These competing demands should cause educators to consider creating learning experiences for adult learners that are relevant and practical. Adult learners do not want to waste time on activities that they consider to be irrelevant to achieving their goal.

Strategies for facilitating development of adult learners include:

- Actively involve adult learners in the learning process.
- Create a relaxed environment that fosters a climate of trust and mutual respect.
- Create a climate that promotes a sense of responsibility for one's own learning.
- Design learning activities that encourage reflection on past and present experiences.
- Use collaborative learning contracts with clearly detailed evaluation criteria.
- Design learning activities that are relevant and meaningful.
- Avoid "busywork" assignments.
- Be respectful and considerate of learners' personal needs and concerns.
- Encourage collaboration with others to achieve learning objectives.
- Allow for self-directed and self-controlled learning.

Learners With Disabilities

The Rehabilitation Act of 1973 was instrumental in antidiscrimination efforts for persons living with disabilities. This act states that any program or activity that receives federal funding cannot deny access or participation to persons with disabilities. The Americans with Disabilities Act (ADA) of 1990 and the updated Americans with Disabilities Act Amendments Act (ADAAA) of 2008 led to additional protections for individuals with disabilities and require that learners with mental or physical illnesses or disabilities be offered reasonable accommodations for learning. Learners may have physical, emotional, and cognitive disabilities that affect their learning. Learners with disabilities may include but are not limited to:

- *Physical disabilities*: musculoskeletal or nervous system disorders
- *Sensory disabilities*: vision, hearing, smell, and touch deficits
- *Cognitive/learning disabilities*: dyslexia, attention-deficit/hyperactivity disorder (ADHD)
- *Mental illness*: anxiety disorder, depression, schizophrenia, chemical dependency problems
- *Other chronic diseases*: diabetes mellitus, systemic lupus

It is the learner's responsibility to seek out the institution's disability services in order to receive reasonable accommodations for learning. The institution and faculty have a legal and ethical obligation to provide reasonable accommodations for learners with a reported, documented disability. Faculty should collaborate with disability services at the institution to provide appropriate accommodations for learners and make every effort to provide reasonable accommodations for learners with disabilities. The academic nurse educator must maintain confidentiality of the student's learning disability, as it is up to the learner to decide when and with whom to disclose the nature or presence of a disability and accommodations.

A *learning disability* is one of the most common disabilities among college learners. Many learners may enter college unaware that they have a learning disability. Faculty may recognize that a student may have a learning disability when there is a discrepancy between clinical and classroom performance. For example, the learner may perform well in the clinical setting but struggle in the classroom with test taking.

Common characteristics of learners with learning disabilities include:

- Reading and spelling difficulties
- Difficulty with basic reading skills
- Mathematical difficulties
- Difficulty following instructions
- Difficulty organizing ideas verbally or into written text
- Inability to prioritize
- Time management difficulties
- Anxiety and self-confidence issues

If a nurse educator believes a learner may have a learning disability, the learner may be referred to the institution's disability services. The disability officer makes decisions about the accommodations needed for the learner. These accommodations may include taking examinations at a different secure location, extended time for completing examinations, a qualified proctor to read the test to the learner, assistance of an in-class note-taker, and use of audio-recorded classroom sessions while still holding the learner to the same standards as those without learning disabilities.

> **CNE®/CNE®n Key Point**
>
> *Remember:* Faculty must make every effort to provide reasonable accommodations for learners with disabilities while ensuring students can meet learning outcomes.

Veterans and LGBTQ Learners

Veterans in the post-9/11 era present with similar characteristics as many other adult learners, but may also have physical or psychological injuries that affect their learning. Returning to civilian life after deployment may be challenging for some veterans. They may experience challenges related to balancing school with job and family responsibilities. Veterans also have many strengths that contribute to their success in nursing school. If they were medics in the military, they possess skills valuable for clinical practice. Veterans have valuable life experiences to draw from; they are good at working in teams and skilled at focusing on tasks. Nurse educators, however, should be sensitive to classroom or clinical situations that may trigger previous traumas. Veterans may benefit from assistance from the veteran support office or disabilities services office on campus.

Nursing students who identify as *lesbian, gay, bisexual, transgender, or queer/questioning (LGBTQ)* are more likely than others to experience episodes of harassment and discrimination that may affect their ability to learn. LGBTQ learners are often at greater risk for mental health and suicidal issues as a result of discrimination. Faculty should continue to learn more about the unique needs of this learning group. Increasing awareness of diverse sexual orientations in the nursing curricula, use of preferred pronouns, and discouraging discrimination are a few methods that can be used by nurse educators to create an environment of inclusivity. Academic nurse educators can also promote development of this group of learners by using inclusive language on assignments, in class, and on examinations.

Providing Resources for Diverse Learners

Increasing success of learners from diverse backgrounds requires a concerted effort from academic institutions and individual faculty members. Learners from diverse backgrounds may experience a number of barriers that can affect their academic success. Being a first-generation college learner means that there may be a lack of family role models to help prepare for and succeed during college. Financial insecurity; lack of academic preparation; lack of family support; socioeconomic disparities; lack of English skills; and a lack of racial, ethnic, and gender diversity among faculty can all affect learner success. Learners from diverse backgrounds may require additional academic and peer support in addition to having faculty role models. Faculty members are expected to know about learner resources on the institution's campus and how learners may access those resources. Creating a culture that appreciates diversity and inclusivity can help improve the outcomes of learners from diverse backgrounds.

Campus Resources

When identifying learners who are struggling in class, the educator may want to refer them for tutoring services. Tutoring may take the form of formal tutoring services provided by campus tutoring services, peer tutoring, or the faculty member may provide tutoring. Tutoring may be one-on-one or in a group setting. Some institutions have dedicated tutors for nursing courses. Learners who are struggling to be successful on writing assignments may be referred to the campus writing center for additional assistance. Campus writing centers provide strategies for writing assignments and assist learners with mechanics, formatting, and spelling and grammar. Learners who struggle with medication calculations may be referred to the campus math center for additional assistance. Many nursing programs also have a learning resource center where students can use equipment in the skills laboratories to practice, refine, or remediate clinical skills. Educators may also suggest that learners engage in peer groups. Peer support, especially within nursing programs, can help improve learner success.

Learners may be doing well academically but struggling with a sense of belonging. Different campus cultural groups may help learners find support from others from a similar cultural background to help foster a sense of belonging. Living-learning communities are dormitories on campus that group individuals who share an academic major. Nursing students who reside in living-learning communities live together, can have study groups, may have dedicated nursing tutors, and can provide emotional support to others who are experiencing the same challenges. Living-learning communities allow for socialization into the role of nursing student, mentoring, peer interaction, and peer support through common learning. There is evidence that living-learning communities contribute to higher academic self-confidence, mentoring, and civic engagement (Brower & Inkelas, 2010).

Campus resources for learners may include but are not limited to:
- Referral services
- Writing center
- Math center
- Tutoring
- Learning resource center (including library and health sciences librarian)
- Peer tutoring and mentoring groups
- Campus wellness services/health center
- Campus mental health services
- Campus cultural centers
- Career center
- Disability services
- Veteran services
- Living-learning communities

A common barrier for diverse learners is a lack of diverse faculty role models. Minority backgrounds are underrepresented in nursing education, with approximately 16% of full-time nursing faculty coming from a minority background (AACN, 2019). Faculty can help support diverse nursing students by identifying and offering access to role models or mentors among practicing minority nurses. Educators can help minority learners feel connected by helping them access campus support services and promoting an environment of inclusivity.

High-Impact Educational Practices

Knowledge of learning styles, characteristics, and needs of learners and knowledge of resources to support diverse learners are essential for nurse educators to meet the needs of today's learners. The use of high-impact educational practices can further support diverse learning needs and result in positive learning outcomes. *High-impact educational practices* are active learning strategies that can contribute to an increase in learner engagement and retention. The following high-impact educational practices can help foster deep learning and contribute to positive learning outcomes (American Association of Colleges and Universities [AACU], 2008):

- First-year seminars: Programs that bring in small groups of learners and faculty together regularly during the first year to help learners develop intellectual and practical skills for success.
- Common intellectual experiences: A set of common courses that include integrative studies or participation in a learning community.
- Learning communities: Two or more linked courses taken together as a group to encourage integration of learning across courses.
- Writing-intensive courses: Courses with an emphasis on writing to improve quantitative reasoning, oral communication, information literacy, and ethical inquiry.
- Collaborative assignments and projects: Courses that require learning and collaborating with others to solve problems.
- Undergraduate research: Encouraging research early on in the learner's college experience to actively involve learners in systematic investigation and empirical observation.
- Diversity/global learning: Courses that help learners explore different cultures and worldviews to broaden their thinking, which may include experiential learning and study abroad opportunities.
- ePortfolios: Maintaining an electronic collection of learners' work for self-reflection on their achievements and goals.
- Service learning/community-based learning: Experiential learning strategies that allow learners to work with community partners to solve real-world problems and develop citizenship.
- Internships: Connecting learners with real-world experiences in work settings in their field of study.
- Capstone courses and projects: Culminating experiences near the end of college to integrate and apply what they have learned during a program of study.

CNE®/CNE®n Key Point

Remember: Knowledge of learning styles, characteristics, and needs of learners and knowledge of resources to support diverse learners are essential for nurse educators to meet the needs of today's learners.

Advising Learners to Meet Professional Goals

Academic advisement is important for academic success and learner retention. Some nursing programs may utilize staff as academic advisors, but many institutions consider academic advising a responsibility of the faculty. The primary role of an academic advisor is to ensure that learners enroll in the correct courses and complete the curriculum required for graduation. The role of faculty as academic advisor may also include providing general program and course information, creating a plan of study for sequencing of courses, ensuring that learners enroll in the proper courses, providing study strategies, ensuring learners have applied for graduation, and discussing career options and future goals. Advisors may provide resources for learners planning to continue their education. It is common for academic advisors to serve as a reference and provide letters of recommendation for learners who are applying for internships, employment, scholarships, or advanced degrees. Learners typically remain with the same academic advisor during completion of a program, so there is potential for meaningful relationships to develop over time. The advisor may also provide counseling or resources for learners struggling with a variety of academic, social, and economic issues.

Faculty need knowledge of tutoring services, supplemental instruction, and services such as the writing and math centers to refer learners who may be struggling academically. For learners who are experiencing financial difficulties, faculty may need to refer them to the offices of financial aid and scholarships. Many campuses may also have additional support programs for learners with food insecurity. Learners may experience significant life events during their time in college and may have difficulty coping with these life events and significant changes.

Advisors may need to refer the learner to the campus mental health resources office for additional support.

Academic advising can benefit both learner and advisor, and implementation of sufficient advisor training, time management, and use of multiple modes of communication can increase the efficacy of advisement (Chan et al., 2019). Advisement may be delivered one-on-one in person, through videoconferencing, or to a group of learners. Specific characteristics of advisors are needed for an effective advisor relationship, such as being knowledgeable about the advising role, program curriculum policies, and procedures; having good communication and interpersonal skills; being organized and good at problem-solving; and having a friendly demeanor (National Academic Advising Association [NACADA], 2017a). The most common barrier to effective advising for learners and faculty is lack of time, but providing support for faculty as academic advisors and using advisement technology tools may offer a possible solution (Chan et al., 2019). Many institutions provide software to make scheduling academic advisement appointments easier. Services such as Zoom or Skype can make it easier for faculty to meet with learners remotely, yet still provide the same face-to-face communication during advisement appointments. Faculty commitment to advising and a balance of the values of caring, commitment, empowerment, inclusivity, integrity, and professionalism will positively influence the relationship between the learners and faculty member (NACADA, 2017b). See Table 3.4 for more information on desirable advisor values and behaviors.

Theoretical approaches to advising vary based on the needs of the learner and the desired outcomes. The two most common approaches to advisement are prescriptive and developmental advising (He & Hutson, 2016) (Table 3.5). *Prescriptive advising* is authoritarian and informational in nature, with the faculty member providing the expert advice and ensuring that the learner registers for the correct courses. Prescriptive advising sessions may be limited to academic matters, and faculty may choose to provide group sessions when providing prescriptive advisement. *Developmental advising* involves a shared responsibility between the advisor and advisee to help the learner explore career and life goals and resources, in addition to creating a plan of study and registering for the correct courses. During developmental advising, the faculty member will spend time talking to and getting to know the learner. Developmental advising may be a bit more time-consuming, but the learner and faculty are able to develop a more meaningful relationship and make short-term and

TABLE **3.4**	Desirable Advisor Core Values and Behaviors
Core Value	**Advisor Behaviors**
Caring	• Nurtures and supports the learners • Is compassionate and empathetic
Commitment	• Is dedicated to learner success • Is committed to learners and the institution through continued learning and professional development
Empowerment	• Motivates and encourages learners to achieve their potential
Inclusivity	• Values a culturally diverse environment • Fosters an environment that supports the needs and perspectives of all learners
Integrity	• Values honesty, transparency, and accountability • Acts ethically and professionally
Professionalism	• Acts according to a set of values that benefits learners, colleagues, the institution, and higher education
Respect	• Builds positive relationships through a learner-centered approach of appreciating learner views and values

Data from National Academic Advising Association (NACADA). (2017b). *NACADA core values of academic advising.* https://nacada.ksu.edu/Resources/Pillars/CoreValues.aspx.

long-term goals. Prescriptive advising may be more appropriate for first-year learners who need specific information about which courses to take, whereas the developmental approach may be more suitable for junior and senior students who are beginning to think beyond graduation.

Creating Learning Environments to Facilitate Goal Setting and Role Socialization

Socialization to the role of nursing is an important aspect of the educational process. Nursing is a profession, and socialization to its culture is imperative to lifelong success. Adopting the norms, values, and beliefs of the profession are all part of socialization that learners must go through to develop their identity (Cannon & Boswell, 2016). As new nurses, learners move into a novice role in organizations and bring with them the attitudes and beliefs that were modeled and experienced during their education. Modeling behaviors and educating about goals and outcomes encourages development among learners. Nurse educators have a responsibility to shape the experiences of learners as they move through their educational program.

Moving from learner to professional generalist or advanced practice nurse is a significant transition and can come with challenges. Role transition to these professional roles can be made more challenging without appropriate socialization during the education period. For example, a theory–practice gap can be one factor that ties into the shock that new entry-level graduates can experience when entering their first professional role (Murray et al., 2019). Changing the role from learner to novice professional can result in struggles to define oneself and balance the new expectations of professional life with personal life. Many changes are often occurring at one time, and the identity of the learner is shifting in multiple ways.

Benner (1984) developed a classic theory delineating the advancement from novice to expert in the nursing role. The five phases include:

- Novice
- Advanced beginner
- Competent
- Proficient
- Expert

Education on Benner's theory should be included in nursing curriculum to develop learner ability to set appropriate expectations about the role of the nurse. The novice to advanced beginner enters the workforce with a set of knowledge and skills that require continued growth, learning, and adaptation to the role (Billings & Halstead, 2020).

The shift to novice nurse is a critical time for the new graduate. It is important to consider the different settings that the learner comes into contact with and how those settings have the opportunity to enhance role socialization. The classroom, laboratory, and clinical setting are all crucial learning environments that can positively develop the professional characteristics of the learner. Faculty within the educational setting, including course instructors, clinical instructors, and advisors, all have an impact on enhancing role socialization. The clinical environment provides additional opportunity to socialize learners to the role as they interact with professionals practicing in the clinical role.

Classroom Learning Environment

The classroom setting is one learning environment that the learner is exposed to consistently. The classroom setting can be both a live classroom and include the online classroom through synchronous or asynchronous learning. The nurse educator has the opportunity to build socialization to the role into the curriculum. All nursing courses should integrate principles that address the norms, values, and beliefs of the profession. This can be done through creating lessons and activities that model the use of values and norms. Actively encouraging learners to participate in an activity together is a method that can be used to allow discussion about the role of nursing and exploration of norms and values.

One example of an activity to model role socialization can be role-playing an interaction between two nurses on a unit who are collaborating for the care of a complex patient who just received a terminal diagnosis. In this scenario, role-playing displays appropriate therapeutic communication and how clinical information is shared to develop a plan of care for a patient. The scenario socializes the learner to understand how the nurse behaves and practices in accordance with the standards of the role. Led by the course faculty, learners can then analyze the interaction to integrate their feelings and beliefs about the scenario. Role-play works well to explore emotions and understand more about human behavior (Billings & Halstead, 2020). It is crucial that any role-playing activity be well developed and specified to meet the intended outcome.

Online Learning Environment

One alternative to the traditional classroom setting can be the online environment. Although an online learning environment can be conducted in a much different manner, there is opportunity to use it as a form of role socialization. Online courses place a great deal of responsibility on the learner (Cannon & Boswell, 2016). Although materials are provided for learners, taking the time to obtain the materials and develop the knowledge base needed to apply the content is a skill that is immensely useful in the professional setting. Nurses are put in situations in which they must acquire new knowledge to handle situations, and seeking out those resources is a necessary skill. Online learners must take the information and apply it in a way that is meaningful and has relevance for them (Billings & Halstead, 2020). The use of technology and multiple platforms to assist in online learning are also helpful when considering the high use of technology in the practice setting. Nurses need to develop skills to adapt new technologies at a rapid pace.

Clinical Learning Environment

The clinical setting presents another opportunity to socialize the learner to the role and develop the critical thinking needed to make safe clinical judgments. This setting is perhaps one of the most formative, as learners can see the role on display through nurses they interact with and observe while in the clinical setting. Starting with the laboratory setting, nurse educators modeling appropriate behaviors can provide an introduction that sets learners up for success when moving into the clinical environment. Observing behaviors in the laboratory setting and having positive interactions with the educator set learners up for a role socialization experience that can be carried over to the clinical setting. Discovering affective skills can begin within the laboratory setting where learners can practice them (Billings & Halstead, 2020).

The educator in the clinical setting should serve as a liaison to build rapport between the school, students, and clinical staff. Creating a clinical environment with positive interaction allows learners to feel comfortable to safely practice and ask questions that enhance clinical judgment skills (Billings & Halstead, 2020). Having an educator who demonstrates the norms of the role and models expected behaviors is critical. The clinical environment allows learners to take the knowledge they are gaining in the classroom and apply it to real-world scenarios. The clinical instructor should facilitate those experiences and be a support system to allow learners to analyze and synthesize their unique experience.

Development of clinical judgment should grow throughout the experiences across different clinical settings. Clinical judgment ability is not developed overnight or even after one semester of school. The educator in the clinical setting takes on a role to help learners progress throughout their time in a program. Patient-centered care is a critical concept to model and assist the learner in developing. Taking details about a patient and applying them to past knowledge and the current patient situation is a skill that the educator can practice alongside the learner (Billings & Halstead, 2020). Time in the clinical setting, postconference, and clinical assignments should all be aligned to model the role the nurse plays in facilitating patient care.

Debriefing, or clinical postconference, is a critical element to clinical learning. Learners should have designated time when they can review their experiences to demonstrate critical thinking. Faculty should facilitate and listen to take the experiences and develop opportunities within the postconference to allow learners to start to expand on their clinical judgment. Postconference is a safe environment to analyze situations and encounters that can be tied directly back to the classroom. This also facilitates role socialization within learners as they review critical elements of the patient and how situations were handled from a professional standpoint. Clinical judgment can be explored more through asking questions such as, "Why were you concerned about that assessment finding?" or "What led you to make that decision?" Asking "what if" questions can also be a useful strategy to develop the critical thinking skills of the learner (Billings & Halstead, 2020). Discussing the emotions tied to patient care is also useful for delving into the values and norms of the professional role of nursing.

The clinical setting provides the opportunity to socialize to the reality of role expectations outside of the typical hands-on skill thinking that many learners focus on. Understanding more about the clinical setting can vary based on the type of model for clinical education that is used at any particular institution. The length of shifts that learners participate in and the timing can be one element to socializing the learner to the role. Understanding how a shift begins and ends and the responsibilities outside of direct patient care are all part of the role of being a nurse. Witnessing interactions between staff to coordinate patient care also provides another opportunity to understand the role. Nurses are part of an interprofessional team that is a critical element of socialization to the role. The clinical setting is just one piece of the puzzle to developing learners to become professionals.

The interprofessional model of patient care is tied to better patient outcomes (Billings & Halstead, 2020). Nurses are crucial members of the interprofessional team, and therefore it is part of the role that should be addressed in nursing education. Learning activities should be designed to allow the learner to gain the skills and knowledge of working in a team and to develop the attitudes and behaviors that go along with practicing collaboratively (Billings & Halstead, 2020). One example of facilitating role development of the nurse as part of the interprofessional team is to develop a simulation that intentionally is designed to include multiple members of the health care team. An interprofessional simulation allows the learners to practice in a safe environment and develop an understanding of what each member of the team does. Simulation also allows for further development of communication skills that are vital to the role of the nurse and the health care team as a whole.

Simulation, as noted in the earlier example, is another learning activity that provides the opportunity for role socialization. Although simulation is often part of clinical requirements, development of scenarios that demonstrate positive relationships among nurses and other health care professionals and that focus on more than just hands-on skills provides another growth opportunity. The learner can portray nurses in many different roles, all within the scope of practice (Billings & Halstead, 2020). Simulation allows the learner to take knowledge about socialization from the classroom and clinical setting to apply it in a safe environment. *Standardized patients* (SPs) can be used in simulation to provide human contact that can allow the learner to practice a higher level of interaction. Debriefing is a critical component to simulation and can also build on that opportunity to highlight the nuances of socialization and encourage learners to synthesize the situation to apply it to real-world practice. Asking questions to encourage deep thinking should be used in simulation just as it is in the clinical practice setting.

CNE®/CNE®n Key Point

Remember: Faculty have multiple avenues for demonstrating the role of professional nurse and building the reality of nursing through the many environments with which they interact. Working with learners on an individual basis and building a professional relationship that assists in the facilitation of experiences that help them reach their goals is an imperative part of the relationship that can develop role socialization.

TABLE **3.5**	Common Advisement Approaches	
Type of Advisement	**Goal**	**Methods/Tasks**
Prescriptive	Compliance and information sharing	Advisor provides information about: • General program curriculum • Selection and registration of courses
Developmental	Holistic personal development	Advisor shares responsibility and works with the learner to: • Select and schedule courses • Identify strengths and weaknesses • Respond to academic difficulties • Explore career options and life goals • Explore institutional and community resources

Data from He, Y., & Hutson, B. (2016). Appreciative assessment in academic advising. *Review of Higher Education, 39*(2), 213–240.

Learner Goal Setting

As learners progress through a program's curriculum, exposure to planned activities should include goal setting. Learners are often guided in the didactic and clinical settings to meet intentionally designed outcomes for success in a course. End-of-program learning outcomes and individual course outcomes are necessary to benchmark learners; however, these outcomes do not address the unique needs and characteristics of each individual learner.

As learners work with educators in various ways throughout the curriculum, educators have the opportunity to discuss which goals are meaningful and will benefit the learners professionally as they move forward. For example, learners can start working from the foundational level to set goals in areas where their knowledge is limited. Moving forward through each course, the goals can then change and be uniquely tailored for what is needed and the increasing complexity of the knowledge and skills. Educating early on how to set goals will provide a foundation that can be carried through a program.

The clinical setting provides an opportunity for the educator to often work more closely with learners and witness their judgment and skill level in practice. Clinical performance evaluations are critical to the growth of the learner. This type of evaluation should promote goal setting by the learner. The educator and learner should work together on appropriate goals and measuring regular progress toward those goals along with the outcomes of the clinical (Billings & Halstead, 2020). Setting goals within the clinical environment is an important skill to practice when preparing for the role of professional nurse.

Teaching and helping to facilitate goal setting are practices that can be carried into the professional world. Nurses have a responsibility to continually grow and learn as they progress in their career and perhaps change roles within the profession. A nurse can move from novice to expert in an area and then decide to change focus and have to start over as a novice in a new area. This provides an excellent opportunity to use the skills of goal setting to move toward that expert level in a new specialty area. Setting professional goals is an expectation of the role of nurse and should be integrated as faculty consider the ways that learners are socialized to the role of professional nurse.

Incivility

Incivility relates directly to role socialization of the learner. Incivility can take on various forms, including but not limited to:
• Bullying
• Disruptive conduct

- Lateral violence
- Horizontal violence

Learners are exposed to uncivil behavior, often starting while in school. Uncivil behavior can lead to poor learning environments (Cannon & Boswell, 2016). Learner to learner, faculty to learner, and even faculty to faculty are all types of incivility that learners may experience or witness. Uncivil behavior may also be experienced or witnessed in the clinical learning environment by staff. Uncivil behavior in the learning environment can lead to continued incivility when entering the professional environment.

Faculty face a major challenge to develop learners that are respectful and civil with peers, faculty, and the many professionals they come into contact with during their education. Cheating, lack of respect in the classroom or online environment, and making extreme demands are some of the more notable forms of incivility (Cannon & Boswell, 2016). Incivility does not begin in nursing school, but rather is often a behavior that has been developed throughout childhood and primary education. Behaviors are learned in many different ways throughout life and may be different for traditional learners versus learners returning to their education after having other work experience as an adult. The life experiences that learners bring with them can influence interpersonal interactions.

It is also important to consider the high-stress nature of nursing school. Experiencing high levels of stress and feeling underprepared for the challenges of nursing school can contribute to uncivil behaviors (Cannon & Boswell, 2016). The pressure and stakes of nursing school can lead to stress in ways that learners have not before had to experience or adapt to. Acclimating to the role of professional nurse is a transition that involves many emotions. Learners are often high achieving and may struggle with the many facets of learning that occur with the high-pressure element of caring for other individuals. On top of the demands of school, many learners have job obligations, financial pressures, and personal issues that can add to the stress. Uncivil behaviors driven as a result of stress can negatively affect the relationship between learners and faculty. Poor relationships between faculty and learners have the possibility to perpetuate uncivil behaviors and to create poor relationships that can hamper socialization to the role of professional.

Addressing incivility in nursing programs is imperative regardless of the level of student. Incivility exists in academia and in practice settings to which the learners are exposed. Uncivil behaviors are likely to spill over into professional practice. Socialization to the professional role includes education and strategies to prevent incivility. Empowerment to take part in and actively engage in methods to address and prevent incivility are important to instill in learners.

Programs should have policies that encourage the reporting of incivility and allow for that to occur without fear of repercussions. Such policies should be stressed as learners are admitted to programs, and education on incivility should occur regularly throughout the curriculum. Enforcement of any policies should hold learners accountable for their actions. Faculty should include language in the course syllabus that reflects expected behaviors and references policies (Cannon & Boswell, 2016). To create a culture without fear of reporting and one that takes seriously any acts of incivility, it must be embedded throughout the program.

Creating a welcoming learning environment where learners feel heard and respected is a start to modeling appropriate behaviors (Cannon & Boswell, 2016). As learners are taught about therapeutic communication and compassion, faculty must demonstrate those skills in order to model the behavior. Listening is an active skill that carries through all facets of life, and it is critical that faculty remember to listen in order to understand and respond appropriately to the needs and concerns of the learner. The classroom, laboratory, and clinical setting are all learning arenas where learners are acclimated to the professional role and where faculty should demonstrate high ethical standards and professional behavior.

Creating openness and a positive environment can look different online. Dialoguing through email, discussion boards, and text messages are a few of the ways that communication has changed. Learners may feel compelled to say things online that they otherwise would not say in person or at times do not understand appropriate communication and etiquette when communicating through typewritten ways. One tool to combat incivility in the virtual environment can be to teach learners what is appropriate and professional online (Cannon & Boswell, 2016). Showing examples and opening discussions via virtual methods to talk about what is appropriate and what is not can role-model professional behaviors.

Having open communication is another strategy to prevent incivility. Openly communicating expectations and the rationale behind decisions that are made allows for more transparency for the learner (Billings & Halstead, 2020). Communicating in a professional manner allows the learner to better understand expectations and why things are done a certain way. Therapeutic communication is vital to the role of the nurse, and educators should model this within their teaching to build on a positive environment for the learner.

The academic nurse educator is a role model for the learner. Learning environments extend beyond the confines of the classroom, clinical setting, and advisor–advisee relationship. Learners observe behaviors modeled by the educator, including interactions with other learners and other colleagues. It is an obligation for the educator to positively model the role that the learner is working toward. The support that educators provide should help learners as they encounter struggles or difficulties understanding the norms of the role. Faculty can also help instill values in learners that model the caring, compassionate nature of nursing. Educators should share the realities of the challenges of being a nurse while also sharing techniques on how to deal with situations that might be encountered. The actuality of being a nurse needs to be openly expressed to reduce reality shock and model for learners how to cope with the expectations. Educators foster the growth of learners in the role as they progress through the nursing program. Acting as a role model in the classroom and clinical settings helps with socializing learners to the role.

> **CNE®/CNE®n Key Point**
>
> *Remember:* The nurse educator is a role model for the learner. Learners observe behaviors modeled by the educator, including interactions with other learners and other colleagues, which can help prevent incivility.

Fostering Learner Development in Three Domains of Learning

The nurse educator has a responsibility to foster learner development while taking consideration for the three domains of learning. The cognitive, psychomotor, and affective domains of learning should all be used to develop activities for teaching and learning. Although learners may feel they learn better in certain ways, there is little evidence to support this (Billings & Halstead, 2020). It is important to incorporate activities and opportunities in each of the domains and to overlap them as necessary to meet learning outcomes. Table 2.1 in Chapter 2 provides examples of engaging student activities by learning domain. Nurses must be able to learn and receive knowledge in multiple ways and determine how to best analyze and use the information to deliver safe care.

Cognitive Domain

Bloom's revised taxonomy for the cognitive domain has six hierarchical levels in which learning occurs. The levels build from basic to higher levels of thinking and include:
- Remembering
- Understanding
- Applying
- Analyzing
- Evaluating
- Creating

The learner must first be able to recall knowledge (remembering) and understand a concept. Faculty should then allow the knowledge to be applied and analyzed to best achieve outcomes and move to a higher level. As learners progress and achieve higher outcomes, they can then evaluate and create new meanings where they can apply previous knowledge to situations.

The levels of the cognitive domain need to be considered when writing learning outcomes. Educators should use action verbs to describe the behavior that is wanted. Writing clear and concise outcomes guides the learner in what should be gained from the experience. Table 3.6 displays examples of learning outcomes at each level of the cognitive domain using a medical/surgical nursing topic.

Learning outcome 6 in Table 3.6 can further be analyzed to consider how the learner will design a plan of care. Faculty can use a concept map to have the learners apply their knowledge to create a plan that can be used to safely care for a patient experiencing an ST elevation myocardial infarction (STEMI). *Concept mapping* is a form of deep learning (Billings & Halstead, 2020). Faculty can provide demographic data, health history, current assessment, laboratory values, medications, and orders to allow formulation of a concept map. In this activity, basic knowledge of the data provided must be demonstrated along with taking that knowledge to apply to a specific patient scenario. This activity could be done in class to augment lecture or could be used in the clinical setting in postconference. Concept mapping can be adapted to multiple learning environments, including the online classroom. It is important to note that a concept map is most often used in the clinical setting, but can be adapted as noted in this example. Predicting what patients are available for learners during clinical can limit exposure to certain concepts. Therefore a predesigned concept mapping activity can provide learners with the opportunity to analyze data and draw from many learning experiences to mimic the real world.

Psychomotor Domain

The psychomotor domain primarily lends itself to the hands-on technical skills. This domain is largely used in the laboratory and clinical setting to help ensure competence for nursing practice. The psychomotor domain is critically important for patient safety and includes the following hierarchy of levels from more basic to more complex and challenging:

- Imitation
- Manipulation
- Precision
- Articulation
- Naturalization

TABLE 3.6 **Examples of Course Objectives With Cognitive Domain Level**

Course Objective (Student Learning Outcome)	Cognitive Domain Level
1. Define atherosclerosis and acute coronary artery disease.	Remembering
2. Explain the pathophysiology of atherosclerosis and acute coronary artery disease.	Understanding
3. Apply knowledge of the risk factors and signs/symptoms of acute coronary artery disease to the assessment of the high-acuity patient.	Applying
4. Compare the collaborative management of the patient with a non-ST elevation myocardial infarction (NSTEMI) versus the patient with an ST elevation myocardial infarction (STEMI).	Analyzing
5. Assess the effectiveness of nursing and interprofessional interventions for the patient experiencing a STEMI.	Evaluating
6. Design a plan of care for the patient experiencing a STEMI.	Creating

At the basic level, imitation and manipulation are used for the learner to develop hands-on skills. As skills are introduced at multiple levels, precision and articulation can develop. Learners may not internalize a skill until they have experience in practice and are able to easily adapt to a variety of situations (Billings & Halstead, 2020).

To reach the precision level, the learner must see a demonstration of the skill. Faculty can demonstrate skills in the laboratory setting, or the learner can be assigned a video to watch the skill. If assigning videos, it is important to note that they should be from a current, reputable source; the nurse educator should ensure the skill is appropriately demonstrated to achieve the learning outcome. The learner can also use course materials to prepare by reading about the skill and going through a list of steps, often accompanied by pictures. At the next level, the learner should then be able to manipulate the needed supplies for the skill. Handling the supplies allows practice and imitation to occur. As proficiency in demonstration of a skill develops, different scenarios can be provided for the learner to adapt the skill. In the case of an indwelling urinary catheter, a different type of catheter kit could be provided for the learner to alter the memorization of a particular brand of product and display how to use an unfamiliar kit. At the highest level, learners adapt their skill to the varied needs of particular patients, such as a patient who is unable to assume the appropriate position for urinary catheter insertion independently. Just like the cognitive domain, the skill level should progress throughout the program in a variety of contexts to ensure competence.

The laboratory setting is often used early in programs to socialize the learner to the supplies and skills that will be needed in clinical practice. Introduction of new skills should be done in the laboratory setting to allow the hands-on experience needed in order to perform the skill safely in the clinical setting. For example, advanced physical assessment skills should be practiced in the laboratory examination room before advanced practice learners assess actual patients in the clinical setting. It is not enough to perform a skill only one time. Programs should consider how skills are introduced and reintroduced over time, with the outcomes becoming more complex based on the psychomotor domain hierarchy and complexity of the patient.

The clinical setting and simulation using high-fidelity scenarios encourage further development in the psychomotor domain. The laboratory should prepare the learner to enter the clinical/simulation setting. Faculty should ensure repetition of skills in a safe, nonjudgmental environment to prepare the learner for clinical practice. Outcomes can reach a higher level of the psychomotor domain in the clinical setting. The learner will need to adapt skills to potentially meet the unique needs of the patient under the supervision of the nurse educator or preceptor.

Affective Domain

The affective domain incorporates the feelings, attitudes, and beliefs internalized by the learner. This domain has a strong emotional component and is closely tied to role identity as a nurse. The learner can acknowledge various feelings in this domain and move toward internalizing the values and feelings. It is important to note that clinical reasoning is related to the affective domain (Billings & Halstead, 2020). The affective domain includes the following hierarchy of levels:

- Receiving
- Responding
- Valuing
- Organizing
- Internalizing

The affective domain can be challenging for faculty to teach. Because this domain is closely tied to personal feelings and beliefs, it can create a challenge when considering assessment of outcomes. The levels of the affective domain are likely to grow and change throughout a program and as the learner enters practice and develops a unique identity. Learners can initially receive information about caring, altruism, and honesty, to name a few. Advancement to be able to discuss these concepts and eventually change behaviors can be achieved.

Values and beliefs are represented in the affective domain and are essential for learners in finding their professional identity. Providing learners with activities such as reflective journaling in which they can critically examine their own feelings and therefore develop values that can guide future practice is imperative. Although the cognitive and psychomotor domains may be regularly and more easily built into nursing curriculum, consideration of the affective domain is necessary to develop safe, caring nurses (Billings & Halstead, 2020). When developing activities for the cognitive and psychomotor domain, the educator should consider how an affective element can be added as the learner progresses through the curriculum.

> ### CNE®/CNE®n Key Point
>
> **Remember:** Although the cognitive and psychomotor domains may be regularly and more easily built into nursing curricula, consideration of the affective domain is necessary to develop safe, caring nurses (Billings & Halstead, 2020).

Assisting Learners to Engage in Self-Evaluation and Peer Evaluation

Evaluation is a critical element to learning and growth. Developing an identity as a professional nurse includes having the ability to critically evaluate oneself and one's peers. Self-evaluation and peer evaluation use the affective domain of learning to internalize the values of nursing and achieve continual improvement. Educators can model appropriate ways to engage in self-evaluation and peer evaluation by being approachable and available. Faculty serve as the role model for learners to mimic and eventually move toward being able to independently reflect and evaluate.

Before beginning the process of discussing reflection and evaluation, educators must teach about the rationale behind the purpose. Feedback and evaluation are needed to enhance success and allow for positive development in nursing. Understanding that feedback is not meant to be punitive is important to convey to learners. Using concepts from therapeutic communication is key to fostering feedback that is well received and able to be put into action. Reflecting on self can potentially enable the learner to develop new views (Billings & Halstead, 2020).

Reflection is a critical element toward the process of self-evaluation. Faculty should guide the learner in reflecting on experiences throughout the learning process. Guided reflection can help the learner move towards higher levels in the domains of learning to be able to create and extrapolate new ideas from past experiences and feelings. Reflection can be incorporated into class activities through group discussions or reflecting on role-play scenarios. Postconference or debriefing also provides the opportunity to openly reflect in a group setting that is guided by the educator. Group settings also allow the opportunity for the learner to begin engaging in peer evaluation.

Faculty can guide reflection and evaluation through the use of high-level questioning. Rather than simply asking a learner to describe a situation, the nurse educator should encourage the learner to further delve into the situation. Asking "how" and "what" questions can guide the learner to dive deeper into thinking about a situation (Billings & Halstead, 2020). Faculty can also take learner reflections and challenge the learner to move deeper. Journaling or online discussion boards can also offer the opportunity for faculty to pose questions that encourage a look from a different angle or to simply look deeper at a situation.

A positive, trusting environment and relationship are necessary to promote learners to feel open about sharing their thoughts and feelings. Reflection is not a matter of wrong versus right. Instead, it should be framed as the opportunity to continue to learn and grow, even in the midst of mistakes or actions. It may be helpful for educators to provide examples of how they use self-reflection. For example, academic nurse educators are evaluated by students, peers, and/or administration. Sharing how this feedback is used to perform the educator's self-evaluation is important to model.

As learners progress in their ability to reflect, educators can then put more responsibility on the learner to examine their own performance. One example could be that in addition to a faculty evaluation, learners could be required to write their own self-evaluation independently and review with faculty. Reviewing with faculty can allow additional opportunity for faculty to push learners outside of their "comfort zone" to reflect and develop further. This process can be used to support learners to internalize the values of nursing. Self-evaluation by the learner is tied directly to behavior changes and can be empowering (Billings & Halstead, 2020). Evaluating outcomes in the clinical setting, for example, through faculty and self-evaluation, while reviewing the feelings and values associated with that experience can progress learning in the affective domain.

As learners mature and grow in reflection and evaluation, adding peer evaluation can be a useful strategy. Professional nurses may be expected to evaluate peers in the future, so understanding how to provide constructive feedback and use appropriate communication to do so should begin while in school. Analyzing performance of others is necessary in a team environment. Feedback that is encouraging and points to concrete ways that improvements can be made represents a high level of learning in the affective domain and demonstrates maturity. One example of an activity to foster peer evaluation can be done through simulation. Recording a simulation can provide the opportunity for a learner to return to the video and conduct both self-evaluation and peer evaluation. It is important that faculty moderate and assist the learner through this process. A specified rubric should be used to demonstrate what outcomes are being evaluated. Feedback should be reviewed by faculty first so as to ensure professionalism, accuracy, and effective communication techniques.

As faculty coach learners in providing feedback for evaluation, they should model the following characteristics:

- Being honest
- Providing realistic feedback
- Being detail-oriented
- Being timely
- Providing concrete suggestions/demonstrations for improvement

Opportunities to actively practice these skills must be built in throughout a curriculum. Keep in mind the learning domains and increasing complexity as the learner matures. In coaching learners through the process of self-evaluation and peer evaluation, faculty must consider the needs of each individual. Diverse learners with unique needs may require more guidance in reflecting on and evaluating self and peers.

Encouraging Professional Development of Learners

Professional development is a hallmark of lifelong learning. Engagement in professional development should be fostered as a learner so that it can be carried into one's professional career. As has been discussed, the academic nurse educator serves as a role model for learners, and this includes modeling the values of lifelong learning and professional development.

One strategy to encourage professional development in learners is to discuss one's own journey. Educators should discuss what professional development looks like for them. Having realistic expectations set by the educator experience can encourage learners along their own journey in professional development. Sharing about professional development allows learners to see how professional development looks different among the many educators they will encounter. Learning about different ways to engage in development opportunities in addition to different nursing organizations can open new pathways for learners.

Engaging in professional development does not have to wait until a learner becomes a working professional. Having organizations on campus or nursing organizations that learners can join is important. Academic nurse educators should serve as sponsors for organizations and expand opportunities that are available on campus, such as the National Student Nurses' Association. Learners can also create their own organizations on many campuses and drive their own mission and vision. With educator support, such organizations can be a "stepping stone" for learners to engage in professional development. In addition to campus organizations, many states allow nursing students to join state nurses' associations in which they can engage with professional nurses. Learners should be encouraged to investigate professional organizations they are interested in to see if there is an option to join as a student. Engaging learners in organizations while they are still in school can highlight the benefits and provide opportunities for not just professional growth but also networking and scholarship opportunities.

The academic nurse educator often attends professional conferences. One option is to consider if learners are able to attend a conference with the educator. Attending a conference together can allow the learner to see the educator actively engaging in professional development and modeling appropriate behaviors. Networking is a skill that some learners need assistance with, and attending a conference together can allow the educator to model the behavior and facilitate networking for learners.

Professional development is part of the role of the professional nurse. Instilling the values around increasing knowledge and keeping up to date with the area of expertise that one chooses is another element of the role of the nurse. Advancing knowledge to keep current and safe is imperative for all nurses. It is important to remind the learner that reading and activities that access resources (often free) are useful for professional development. Reading journals, attending learning sessions at work, and using free continuing education available through nursing organizations are all professional development opportunities that are attainable for new nurses.

References

American Association of Colleges of Nursing (AACN). (2019). *Fact sheet: Enhancing diversity in the nursing workforce.* https://www.aacnnursing.org/Portals/42/News/Factsheets/Enhancing-Diversity-Factsheet.pdf.

American Association of Colleges of Nursing (AACN). (2021). *Latest data on diversity.* https://www.aacnnursing.org/Diversity-Inclusion/Latest-Data.

American Association of Colleges and Universities (AACU). (2008). *High impact educational practices.* https://www.aacu.org/node/4084.

American Nurses Association (ANA). (2015). *Code of ethics for nurses with interpretive statements.* https://www.nursingworld.org/coe-view-only.

Bastable, S. (2016). *Essentials of patient education.* Burlington, MA: Jones & Bartlett.

Benner, P. (1984). *From novice to expert: Excellence and power in clinical nursing practice.* Boston: Addison-Wesley.

Billings, D. M., & Halstead, J. A. (2020). *Teaching in nursing: A guide for faculty* (6th ed.). St. Louis: Elsevier.

Brower, A., & Inkelas, K. (2010). Living-learning programs: One high impact educational practice we now know a lot about. *Liberal Education, 96*(2), 36–43.

Cadet, M. J. (2021). Examining the learning characteristics of nursing students: A literature review. *Journal of Nursing Education, 60*(4), 209–215.

Cannon, S., & Boswell, C. (2016). *Evidence-based teaching in nursing: A foundation for educators* (2nd ed.). Burlington, MA: Jones & Bartlett Learning.

Chan, Z., Chan, H., Chow, H., Choy, Z., Ng, K., Wong, K., et al. (2019). Academic advising in undergraduate education: A systematic review. *Nurse Education Today, 75,* 58–74.

Chickering, A., & Gamson, Z. (1987). Seven principles for good practice in undergraduate education. *The Wingspread Journal, 9*(2), 1–5. https://files.eric.ed.gov/fulltext/ED282491.pdf.

Fleming, N. D., & Mills, C. (1992). Not another inventory, rather a catalyst for reflection. *To Improve the Academy, 11,* 137–155.

Frazer, C., Reilly, C. A., & Squellati, R. E. (2021). Instructional strategies: Teaching nursing in today's diverse and inclusive landscape. *Teaching and Learning in Nursing, 16*(3), 276–280.

Gardner, H. (1999). *Intelligence reframed: Multiple intelligences for the 21st century.* New York: Basic Books.

He, Y., & Hutson, B. (2016). Appreciative assessment in academic advising. *The Review of Higher Education, 39*(2), 213–240.

Keller, J. (2009). *ARCS model of motivational design.* https://www.learning-theories.com/kellers-arcs-model-of-motivational-design.html.

McLeod, S. A. (2017). *Kolb learning styles and experiential learning cycle.* https://www.simplypsychology.org/learning-kolb.html.

Metzger, M., Dowling, T., Guinn, J., & Wilson, D. (2020). Inclusivity in baccalaureate nursing education: A scoping study. *Journal of Professional Nursing, 36,* 5–14.

Murray, M., Sundlin, D., & Cope, V. (2019). New graduate nurses' understanding and attitudes about patient safety upon transition to practice. *Journal of Clinical Nursing, 28,* 2543–2552.

National Academic Advising Association (NACADA). (2017a). *NACADA academic advising core competencies model.* https://nacada.ksu.edu/Resources/Pillars/CoreCompetencies.aspx.

National Academic Advising Association (NACADA). (2017b). *NACADA core values of academic advising.* https://nacada.ksu.edu/Resources/Pillars/CoreValues.aspx.

National League for Nursing (NLN). (2016). *Achieving diversity and meaningful inclusion in nursing education: A living document from the National League for nursing.* http://www.nln.org/docs/default-source/about/vision-statement-achieving-diversity.pdf.

CHAPTER 3 Practice Questions

1. The nurse educator is preparing for academic advisement meetings and is planning to use the developmental advisement approach. What activity will the educator demonstrate using this approach?
   - **A.** Focus mostly on course and program information sharing during the advisement meeting.
   - **B.** Provide tutoring to the learner struggling with medication calculations.
   - **C.** Assume responsibility for learner course enrollment, progression, and graduation.
   - **D.** Collaborate with the learner on academic, personal, and professional goals during the meeting.

2. When deciding upon an academic advising approach, the nurse educator should consider which of the following behaviors?
   - **A.** Use a single advisement approach that best fits the educator's style.
   - **B.** Consider each learner's individual needs.
   - **C.** Use the developmental approach because it is most effective.
   - **D.** Use the prescriptive approach to help learners identify career goals.

3. The nurse educator is teaching a new concept and considering the use of classroom teaching strategies for a small group of visual (spatial) learners. Which learning activity should the nurse educator plan to use?
   - **A.** Diagrams and concept mapping
   - **B.** Small-group discussions
   - **C.** Slide presentations
   - **D.** Simulation

4. The nurse educator is teaching a course that is composed of learners from multiple generations. What approach should the nurse educator plan to use?
   - **A.** Use teaching strategies that focus primarily on the preferences of the generational majority.
   - **B.** Use mostly slide show presentations so that all learners have access to the information.
   - **C.** Use teaching-learning strategies that require technology and multitasking with group work.
   - **D.** Use a variety of interactive teaching-learning strategies, including use of technology, to appeal to multiple generations of learners.

5. To facilitate learning in students for whom English is an additional language (EAL), the academic nurse educator would avoid the use of which of the following teaching-learning strategies?
   - **A.** Allow students to record classroom sessions.
   - **B.** Use complex vocabulary to help increase their English capacity.
   - **C.** Place the students on teams with native English speakers.
   - **D.** Use role-playing exercises to practice communication with patients.

6. The nurse educator suspects that a student may have an undocumented learning disability after witnessing which behavior?
   - **A.** Making excessive spelling errors on written assignments like papers
   - **B.** Being late for both class and clinical practicum
   - **C.** Having high grades on examinations but poor clinical performance
   - **D.** Being disruptive in the classroom setting

7. The nurse educator is teaching a skills lab with mostly Millennial learners. When conducting the skills lab, the educator should consider which approach?
   A. Providing frequent feedback with clear goals and expectations
   B. Avoiding public acknowledgment of achievement
   C. Avoiding peer interaction and encouraging individual practice
   D. Remembering that they desire independence and informality

8. The novice nurse educator requires follow-up from the faculty mentor after making which of the following statements?
   A. "I should avoid using reflective journaling with adult students as it may bring up past traumas."
   B. "I will facilitate more group learning activities because adult students prefer collaborative learning."
   C. "I will develop learning contracts with the adult students so that they know exactly how their knowledge, skills, and attitudes will be evaluated."
   D. "I plan to incorporate more learning activities that encourage reflection and discussion of their past experiences."

9. The novice nurse educator knows that the most important principle for facilitating learning and engagement in learners is which of the following?
   A. To encourage competition among learners to create high achievers
   B. To maintain frequent contact with learners at regular intervals
   C. To initially set lower expectations to improve achievement and self-esteem
   D. To use a consistent method of teaching to promote classroom stability

10. To assess students for physical readiness to learn a new skill using the PEEK method, which factors would the educator include?
    A. Current knowledge base, presence of learning disabilities, and learning styles
    B. Coping mechanisms and level of orientation of the students
    C. Anxiety levels, motivation, and risk-taking behaviors
    D. Complexity of the skill and measure of students' abilities

11. After completing a learning style inventory, a student has been identified as being a convergent learner. Which activity would best help this student learn?
    A. By viewing instructional videos and demonstrations
    B. By reviewing slide presentations and diagrams
    C. By practicing technical tasks during simulation
    D. By listening to lectures and doing assigned textbook readings

12. The nurse educator is teaching a face-to-face course on campus. The educator should expect that learners from Generation X will primarily communicate using which of the following methods?
    A. Using social media because they prefer technology
    B. Face-to-face because they are social and friendly
    C. Through email using blunt and direct language
    D. Frequently with the educator using phone calls and voice mail

13. The novice nurse educator understands that the most significant barrier to academic advising is which of the following?
    A. Difficulty understanding the nursing program's policies and procedures
    B. Lack of time to complete academic advising
    C. Difficulty locating resources to improve learners' academic performance
    D. Communication and scheduling of academic advisement appointments with learners

14. During the first week of class a student notifies the instructor of a documented learning disability and that an accommodation is needed. How should the nurse educator respond to the student?
    A. Inform the student that all nursing students are held to the same standard; therefore accommodations are not usually permitted in nursing courses.
    B. Determine accommodations and inform other faculty of the disability to help monitor for medication and clinical judgment errors.
    C. Provide assignments mostly in the affective domain because the student will struggle with cognitive and psychomotor activities.
    D. Consult with the disability services office and provide the recommended accommodation.

15. The new nurse educator is designing learning activities to teach students about the renal system. Which of the following activities would be preferred by an individual with bodily/kinesthetic intelligence?
    A. Using simulation equipment to practice urinary catheter insertion
    B. Drawing pictures and creating designs of the renal system
    C. Collaborating in small groups to complete a renal case study
    D. Reading assignments and discussions

16. The nurse educator is designing learning activities for the classroom. There are several learners in the course for whom English is an additional language (EAL). Which statement by the educator about strategies to support EAL learners would require follow-up by the mentor?
    A. "I will highlight key words in the examination items, such as *most, least, best*."
    B. "I will try to use simple, common vocabulary on the examination questions."
    C. "I plan to allow extra time for completing assignments and examinations."
    D. "I will group together learners from similar cultural backgrounds so that they may speak their native language."

17. A mentor recognizes that a new nurse educator needs follow-up about accommodations for learners with documented learning disabilities after making which of the following statements?
    A. "Learners may need to take the exam in a separate, secure location to prevent cheating."
    B. "Learners who need a test reader may choose a friend to sit with them and read the exam questions."
    C. "Some learners with a disability may need someone else to take notes for them during class."
    D. "Additional time for test-taking may be permitted for learners with a documented learning disability."

18. A learner performs well in the clinical setting and on examinations but struggles with term papers and writing assignments. Which action should the nurse educator take to best assist this learner?
    A. Assign a short paper on the mechanics of writing and formatting.
    B. Refer the learner to the campus writing center for support.
    C. Provide weekly individual tutoring to strengthen writing skills.
    D. Refer the learner to the campus disability services office for assessment.

19. The new nurse educator is teaching a group of diverse learners. The nurse educator identifies which of the following learners as being most at risk for possible academic failure?
    A. The learner has a previous degree in psychology.
    B. The learner is considered a nontraditional adult learner.
    C. The learner has been identified as having an accommodative learning style.
    D. The learner is a first-generation college student.

20. A learner emailed a faculty advisor to make an initial appointment for help registering for classes. In the email the learner indicated being nervous about starting the nursing program after hearing that the examinations are very difficult. How should the faculty advisor proceed?
    A. Plan to incorporate both prescriptive and developmental advising during the first meeting.
    B. Plan to refer the learner to campus mental health services for additional assistance.
    C. Help the learner identify deadlines for academic scholarships to decrease financial stressors.
    D. Provide the learner with a list of appropriate courses in sequence, including the prerequisite courses.

21. The nurse educator is designing an interprofessional clinical simulation activity in which small groups of nursing students will manage a client scenario with social work students. The nurse educator understands that which of the following types of learners will function best in this environment?
    A. Learners from Generation X
    B. Learners with intrapersonal intelligence
    C. Learners from the Millennial generation
    D. Learners with visual/spatial intelligence

22. The nurse educator recognizes that individuals with the assimilative preference learn best through a combination of which of the following?
    A. Active experimentation and concrete experiences
    B. Active experimentation and abstract conceptualization
    C. Reflective observation and concrete experience
    D. Reflective observation and abstract conceptualization

23. To foster a sense of belonging in culturally diverse learners, which strategy would the nurse educator use?
    A. Avoid group work to decrease anxiety.
    B. Assign reflective journaling to high-risk learners.
    C. Meet with learners individually after class.
    D. Use inclusive language on exams and case studies.

24. The nurse educator is planning learning activities to teach a new concept to a group of learners. Using the PEEK method for readiness to learn, which of the following methods would the educator use to determine if the learners have the *knowledge* readiness to learn this new concept?
    A. Provide a short survey to learner to assess anxiety levels and motivation to learn.
    B. Use the ARCS model to assess if the learners are motivated to learn the new concept.
    C. Perform a cultural assessment to determine barriers to learning a new concept.
    D. Ask learners to complete a learning style inventory and a short quiz to determine concept knowledge.

25. The faculty has determined a need for increased student engagement and retention. Which statement by the nurse educator requires follow-up by the mentor?
    A. "Increase the number of high-stakes examinations throughout the semester."
    B. "Include service learning for students with good grades."
    C. "Change the admission criteria for the program."
    D. "Include more collaborative projects each semester."

26. Which statement by the novice nurse educator about the transition of learners to the professional role of nurse requires follow-up by the faculty mentor?
    A. "I should expect my learner to be experts upon graduation."
    B. "Learners enter the nursing profession at the novice to advanced beginner level."
    C. "Continued growth and adaptation in the role of nurse will take time."
    D. "Often the realities of practice are different from what learners encountered in school."

27. The nurse educator is planning an activity in the classroom to assist learners with socialization to the role. Which teaching/learning strategy would the nurse educator select?
    A. Case study
    B. Role-playing
    C. Lecture
    D. Debate

28. The novice nurse educator is teaching an online course. Which of the following statements about online learning is correct?
    A. "Teaching can be done the same online as it is in the classroom."
    B. "Learners will be able to manage online learning independently with little input from the nurse educator."
    C. "Online learning requires little work on the part of the educator and the learner."
    D. "The primary responsibility is placed on the learner in online education."

29. Which statement is true concerning socialization to the role of professional nurse?
    A. Learners will be socialized to the role of nursing once they learn the policies at their place of employment.
    B. Internalization of the norms, values, and beliefs is necessary to socialize to the role.
    C. Socialization to the role of nursing cannot be developed during an academic program.
    D. Formal education is all that is necessary to develop socialization to the role of nurse.

30. The novice nurse educator is exploring methods to best prepare students to enter the clinical setting. Which of the following statements by the nurse educator is accurate?
    A. "I should teach students all of the policies of the facility they will be going to."
    B. "Students do not need preparation to enter the clinical setting in our community."
    C. "I should model the behaviors that are expected of students in the clinical setting."
    D. "Students will learn what is appropriate and what is not once they start in the clinical setting."

31. The novice nurse educator is considering methods to integrate teaching about the values and norms of the profession. Which of the following statements requires follow-up by the faculty mentor?
    A. "Learning about values and norms in nursing can take place across the multiple learning environments that students interact with."
    B. "Nurse educators have a responsibility to role-model the values and norms of nursing."
    C. "The clinical setting is the only place for the student to develop the values and norms of nursing."
    D. "Simulation is just one area that students can have the opportunity to practice the norms of the role of the nurse."

32. The nurse educator finds that a nursing student is avoiding entering the room of any patients. The student is overheard stating the only reason for being in nursing school is to get a good job upon graduation. What is the appropriate response by the nurse educator to the student?
    A. Discuss the concerns with the student privately and stress the values of nursing.
    B. Tell the student that the student will be removed from the nursing program.
    C. Discuss the concerns with the student during clinical postconference.
    D. Report the student's comments to administration immediately.

33. The nurse educator is teaching a course about the professional role of the nurse. In reviewing the values of nursing, which of the following is *not* a value associated with the role of nursing?
    A. Caring
    B. Conceptualizing
    C. Diversity
    D. Integrity

34. The nurse educator is assessing learner characteristics of a group of online students. Which characteristic is needed for success in the online learning environment?
    A. Motivation
    B. Caring
    C. Inclusivity
    D. Organization

35. The nurse educator is developing a lesson on personal goal setting. Which of the following is true regarding goal setting for the learner?
    A. Outcomes for the course define the goals that the learner must achieve.
    B. Goals for the learner should be developed by the educator for each individual learner.
    C. There is no need to set goals while learning in any environment.
    D. Learners should set personal goals based on their own self-reflection and needs.

36. The novice nurse educator is learning about uncivil behaviors in students. Which of the following behaviors is an example of an uncivil behavior?
    A. Turning the camera off when online
    B. Regularly leaving class early without explanation
    C. Raising a hand to ask questions during class
    D. Requesting a change in due date for an assignment

37. The nurse educator witnesses an interaction between two learners who are openly discussing another learner in the cohort in a disparaging way while standing in front of a patient's open room. How should the nurse educator respond?
    A. Hold a conference with the two learners involved and the learner who the disparaging remarks were about so that all three can discuss their personal issues.
    B. Immediately take the two learners involved to a private setting to discuss the matter, and follow the incivility policy of the program.
    C. Notify the learner about whom others were making disparaging remarks what the remarks were about.
    D. Reprimand both learners immediately and send them home from the clinical learning environment.

38. Which of the following statements describes the rationale for including professional behavior expectations for learners in the course syllabus?
    A. Preventive actions can be an early intervention to avoid uncivil behavior.
    B. The educator should include a list of behaviors that are inappropriate.
    C. Learners inherently understand the expectations regarding professional behaviors.
    D. It is usually not necessary to include language regarding professional behaviors in the course syllabus.

39. The nurse educator is planning to use a case study during class. This teaching strategy represents which domain of learning?
    A. Diverging
    B. Psychomotor
    C. Cognitive
    D. Affective

40. The nurse educator plans a lesson with the following cognitive domain learning outcome, "Interpret data from the patient presenting with left-sided heart failure." Which hierarchy level does this outcome represent?
    A. Applying
    B. Remembering
    C. Evaluating
    D. Analyzing

41. The nurse educator is planning to teach sterile technique to a group of learners. Which teaching strategy would the nurse educator most likely select?
    A. High-fidelity simulation
    B. Lecture
    C. Reflective journal
    D. Skill demonstration

42. Which of the following learning outcomes represents the precision level hierarchy of the psychomotor domain of learning?
    A. Demonstrate safe technique in the insertion of an intravenous catheter in the assigned patient.
    B. Follow the list of steps to insert an intravenous catheter in the assigned patient.
    C. Analyze the steps to insert an intravenous catheter in the assigned patient.
    D. Describe the steps to insert an intravenous catheter in the assigned patient.

43. The nurse educator plans a learning activity about hospice care. The following outcome is planned, "Promote patient autonomy in the hospice setting." Which learning domain does this outcome represent?
    A. Cognitive
    B. Kinesthetic
    C. Psychomotor
    D. Affective

44. Which of the following learning outcomes represents the affective domain of learning?
    A. Demonstrate proper setup of an intravenous infusion piggyback.
    B. Discuss the values of the role of practical/vocational nursing.
    C. Apply the pathophysiologic process of heart failure to the care of the patient.
    D. Differentiate the risk factors for type 1 and type 2 diabetes.

45. The novice nurse educator is discussing providing feedback to learners. Which of the following statements regarding feedback requires follow-up by the mentor?
    A. "Feedback is meant to facilitate success of the learner."
    B. "Feedback should be timely and appropriate."
    C. "Feedback should provide concrete examples."
    D. "Feedback is meant to punish the learner."

46. Which of the following methods is appropriate to promote self-evaluation by learners?
    A. Allow learners to reflect on their clinical performance.
    B. Allow learners to grade their own course examination.
    C. Allow learners to grade their own unit quiz.
    D. Allow learners to evaluate peers in a simulation.

47. The nurse educator plans a learning activity to provide peer evaluation after an interprofessional simulation. Which of the following elements should the educator consider when planning the activity?
    A. Learners should be allowed to independently write out what they find to be important feedback.
    B. Learners should focus on what peers did wrong during the simulation.
    C. Learners should be provided with clear guidance and a rubric to use for evaluation.
    D. Learners should not be allowed to evaluate peers during the program.

48. The novice nurse educator needs further guidance after making which of the following statements regarding professional development in nursing?
    A. Learners do not need to engage in professional development; they are already in school.
    B. Learners should begin to engage in professional development as part of the socialization to the role.
    C. Learners should participate in service learning as a means to engage in professional development.
    D. Learners should engage in professional development alongside educators.

49. The nurse educator discusses membership in the state nurses' association. What is the purpose of sharing about professional organizations with the learner?
    A. Educators should share that professional organizations will teach the learner how to be a nurse.
    B. Educators should require that learners join the professional organization of their choice.
    C. Educators should model participation in professional organizations.
    D. Educators should discourage participation in professional organizations because learners do not have time.

50. The nurse educator is sharing with learners about a professional development activity regarding inclusivity and diversity in nursing education. This type of activity models which quality of the nurse?
    A. Caring
    B. Lifelong learning
    C. Dissemination of information
    D. Autonomy

Using Assessment and Evaluation Strategies

KAILEE BURDICK | SOMER NOURSE

LEARNING OUTCOMES

1. Discuss factors that influence the development and use of nursing program standards and policies regarding admission, progression, and graduation.

2. Identify formative and summative strategies to assess and evaluate learning in the cognitive, psychomotor, and affective domains.

3. Discuss methods for the development and use of evidence-based assessment tools to provide feedback to learners.

4. Describe the steps of the evaluation process for measuring student learning.

5. Analyze assessment data to measure learner outcomes and enhance the teaching-learning process.

6. Describe how to interpret relevant testing statistics to improve test development.

One of the most important roles of the nurse educator is assessment and evaluation of student learning. The National League for Nursing (NLN) *Academic Nurse Educator Scope of Practice* calls for nurse educators to implement a variety of strategies to assess and evaluate learning in classroom, online, laboratory, and clinical settings using evidence-based methods and practices (Christensen & Simmons, 2020). Nurse educators must evaluate learning in the cognitive, psychomotor, and affective domains while providing timely, constructive feedback to all learners.

Providing Input for and Enforcing the Development of Nursing Program Standards

Nursing programs must develop clear standards and policies for admission, progression, and graduation that are evidence-based to support learner outcomes. Creation of these policies should involve the entire faculty, and implementation should be consistent to ensure all student issues are handled fairly. National and state standards, in addition to local best practices, must be considered when developing program policies.

Admission Policies

The admission policies of nursing programs provide the criteria for which students may be accepted into a program of study. The policies must be clearly published and communicated to students before the application process. The admission criteria specifically detailed in the policy allow faculty to select candidates who are qualified and likely to be successful in the program of study. Depending on the type of nursing program, common admission policies typically include the following:

- Minimum grade point average (GPA) requirement from previous education
- Relevant prerequisite courses or degrees
- Graduation from an approved or accredited program (high school graduation for prelicensure programs; accredited undergraduate programs for application to graduate studies)
- Official school transcripts
- Standardized test scores (e.g., SAT or ACT for undergraduate education or GRE for graduate education)
- Minimum score on standardized entrance exam(s)
- Criminal background check
- Licensed practical nurse/licensed vocational nurse (LPN/LVN) or registered nurse (RN) licensure for degree completion or graduate programs
- Documentation of immunizations and health records
- Evidence of cardiopulmonary resuscitation (CPR) certification

Progression Policies

Progression policies are those used to standardize how learners may progress through a program. Academic nurse educators are obligated to follow these policies consistently to ensure that all learners are treated fairly and equally. Common progression policies may include the following:

- Maintaining a minimum GPA
- Achievement of minimum grade in nursing courses
- Achievement of minimum grade/score on standardized tests
- Number of times a learner may drop and repeat a nursing course
- Number of times a learner may fail a single nursing course
- Total number of times a learner may fail nursing courses
- Satisfactory performance of clinical skills

If learners are dismissed from a program for not meeting progression policy standards, there must also be a pathway for them to request reinstatement into the program. The readmission policy must be clearly stated so that learners know the expectations for reapplication to a program of study. Many readmission policies also include standards for learners transferring from other higher education institutions.

Graduation Policies

Graduation policies establish guidelines to ensure that learners have met all the criteria for completion of the program and are eligible to take licensure or certification examinations. Learners must meet all obligations to the educational institution and nursing program to achieve completion of the degree or certificate and graduate. Many prelicensure programs require learners to take a standardized exit examination as part of their graduation requirement. Other graduation policies include but are not limited to:

- Completion of credit requirements and all core courses
- Minimum GPA
- Achievement of program learning outcomes

Using a Variety of Strategies to Assess and Evaluate Learning

The terms *assessment* and *evaluation* are often used interchangeably, but there are key characteristics of each term that nurse educators must understand. *Assessment* refers to the gathering and interpreting of information to determine progress toward a desired outcome (Billings & Halstead, 2020). Educators can use the results of assessment to provide feedback to learners and make changes in the teaching-learning process to improve learner outcomes. *Evaluation* is the ongoing process of gathering information to make judgments based on predetermined criteria about the value of a nursing program, outcomes, or individual student learning.

Formative evaluation is the process of monitoring learner progress and providing meaningful feedback during a learning opportunity. Formative evaluation can help identify student learning needs and be used to improve learner performance. *Summative evaluation* is the process of making a judgment regarding a learner's performance at the end of an activity, course, or program. This type of evaluation necessitates quantifying learner achievement through assignment of a letter grade, score, pass/fail, or satisfactory/unsatisfactory rating. Therefore learners must be provided with formative assessments to allow them the opportunity to improve before summative evaluation is conducted.

> ### CNE®/CNE®n Key Point
>
> *Remember: Formative evaluation* is the process of monitoring learner progress and providing meaningful feedback during a learning opportunity. Formative evaluation can help identify student learning needs and be used to improve learner performance. *Summative evaluation* is the process of making a judgment regarding a learner's performance at the end of an activity, course, or program.

Measurement involves assigning numbers or scores to represent achievement or performance. To give a measurement meaning, the number must be referenced or compared with a predetermined standard (Oermann & Gaberson, 2021). *Grading* is an important component of both formative and summative evaluation and involves assigning a value to the completion of an assignment or course. Academic nurse educators must provide learners with grading criteria before completion of the learning activity, assignment, or course so that they are aware of the requirements for achievement. Grading criteria for activities and assignments may involve using grading rubrics. How learners will be assigned final grades for completion of a course should be clearly within the course syllabus. For some courses, grades are calculated using percentages; in other courses, grades are calculated based on a point system. Faculty should consider using a variety of strategies to evaluate the three domains of learning.

Learning Domains

Student learning outcomes provide the guidelines for educators to design instructional activities and evaluation methods in the cognitive, psychomotor, and affective learning domains. These outcomes describe the knowledge, skills, and values that learners should demonstrate upon evaluation. Learning outcomes can be written to evaluate learning at the program level, the course level, and the content level. Chapter 5 describes student learning outcome development in detail.

> ### CNE®/CNE®n Key Point
>
> *Remember:* Student learning outcomes provide the guidelines for educators to design instructional activities and evaluation methods in the cognitive, psychomotor, and affective learning domains.

The *cognitive learning domain* focuses on knowledge, understanding, and the higher-level thinking skills of clinical reasoning and critical thinking. The classic revised Bloom's taxonomy by Anderson and Krathwohl (2001) is commonly used to measure learning in the cognitive domain and includes these levels from low to higher order:

- Remembering (lowest cognitive level): Ability to recall specific information through memorization
- Understanding: Ability to explain information
- Applying: Use of information in a new situation
- Analyzing: Ability to break down information into parts and identify relationships between those parts

- Evaluating: Ability to make judgments based on criteria
- Creating (highest cognitive level): Ability to develop or combine pieces of information or elements to design a new product

Remembering and understanding are the least complex aspects of the cognitive domain and do not require critical thinking; therefore many student learning outcomes in nursing are written at the applying level or higher. Table 4.1 lists common verbs used to develop learning outcomes for each level of the cognitive taxonomy. Tests, written papers, and concept maps are effective methods for evaluation in the cognitive learning domain. Table 5.4 in Chapter 5 provides examples of additional evaluation methods to measure learning in the cognitive domain.

Because the *affective learning domain* features the development of attitudes and values within the practice of nursing, the levels of this domain progress from simple awareness of values to internalization and consistent practice of those values. The classic taxonomy by Krathwohl et al. (1964) is commonly used to measure learning in the affective domain and includes these levels from lowest to higher order and complexity (Oermann & Gaberson, 2021):

- Receiving: Awareness of and sensitivity to values and beliefs of others in a situation
- Responding: Reacting to a situation by choice
- Valuing: Accepting values and beliefs as a basis for behavior
- Organizing: Developing values or a set of values and beliefs
- Characterization by a value or value set: Internalizing values and beliefs

Reflective journaling, role-playing, and simulations can be used to evaluate learning in the affective learning domain. A list of action verbs that can be used to develop outcomes in the affective domain can be found in Table 4.2. Table 5.4 in Chapter 5 provides examples of additional evaluation methods to measure learning in the affective domain.

Learning in the *psychomotor learning domain* includes developing competency in performance of technical clinical skills and procedures. The simplest level of the psychomotor domain involves imitation of a skill. With practice, time, and increased knowledge, a learner can attain naturalization and carry out the skill with mastery and without having to think about it. Although Bloom developed a psychomotor taxonomy, the taxonomy by Dave (1970) is commonly used to measure learning in the psychomotor domain and includes these levels from low to higher order (Oermann & Gaberson, 2021):

TABLE 4.1 Action Verbs for the Cognitive Domain

Remembering	Understanding	Applying	Analyzing	Evaluating	Creating
Define	Explain	Apply	Analyze	Critique	Create
List	Describe	Use	Compare	Defend	Design
Select	Interpret	Relate	Contrast	Support	Develop
Recognize	Summarize	Demonstrate	Distinguish	Prioritize	Invent
Label	Discuss	Modify		Assess	Modify
Identify					

TABLE 4.2 Action Verbs for the Affective Domain

Receiving	Responding	Valuing	Organization	Characterization
Ask	Assist	Care for	Collaborate	Advocate
Acknowledge	Attempt	Contribute	Facilitate	Influence
Listen	Demonstrate	Support	Lead	Motivate
Attend to	Reply	Respect	Manage	Defend
	Respond	Foster	Recommend	Advance
	Offer	Encourage	Organize	Serve
		Value		

TABLE **4.3**	Action Verbs for the Psychomotor Domain			
Imitation	**Manipulation**	**Precision**	**Articulation**	**Naturalization**
Copy	Act	Demonstrate	Adapt	Develop
Repeat	Perform	Master	Carry out	Integrate
Mimic	Execute	Calibrate	Construct	Manage
Imitate	Build		Customize	Design
Reproduce			Modify	Invent

- Imitation: Ability to perform a skill after skill demonstration
- Manipulation: Ability to follow instructions rather than needing to observe a skill
- Precision: Ability to perform a skill accurately and independently
- Articulation: Ability to perform a skill efficiently within a reasonable time frame
- Naturalization: Ability to perform a skill with a high degree of proficiency

Return skill demonstration, role-playing, and simulation can be effective methods for evaluation in the psychomotor domain. Learners in a nursing program are not expected to function above the precision level. Efficiency and proficiency are developed after entry into nursing practice. Verbs for creating objectives in each level of the psychomotor domain can be found in Table 4.3. Table 5.4 in Chapter 5 provides examples of additional evaluation methods to measure learning in the psychomotor domain.

The levels of these taxonomies help provide a guiding framework for the development of instruction, assessment, and evaluation strategies. They also help ensure that assessment and evaluation methods and tools are appropriate for the intended learning outcomes.

CNE®/CNE®n Key Point

Remember: Tests, written papers, and concept maps are effective methods for evaluation in the *cognitive* learning domain. Reflective journaling, role-playing, and simulations can be used to evaluate learning in the *affective* learning domain. Learning in the *psychomotor* learning domain may be measured by return skill demonstration, role-playing, and simulation.

The Evaluation Process

Various philosophical approaches to evaluation may be selected by the nurse educator based on personal values and beliefs about the evaluation process. Academic nurse educators who use the *outcomes approach* typically rely on learning objectives and outcomes to evaluate courses, lessons, or programs (Billings & Halstead, 2020). Nurse educators who apply the *service approach* use a values-based, holistic perspective to identify strengths, weaknesses, and progress towards an outcome when evaluating learner performance. Evaluation from a *judgment approach* reflects a focus on assigning a numeric or letter grade or a pass/fail determination when evaluating learner performance. Those who use the *constructivist approach* focus heavily on the value of stakeholders who will be affected by program graduates, such as future employers and those who will be receiving nursing care. Most educators integrate multiple approaches to evaluation, although one particular philosophy may be more dominant.

Conducting an evaluation begins with first identifying the purpose of the evaluation and then systematically following a series of steps. Steps of the evaluation process include:

1. *Identify the purpose of the evaluation*: The purpose of an evaluation may be to identify learning needs, diagnose problems, make decisions regarding grades, judge the effectiveness of learning outcomes, or evaluate cost-effectiveness.
2. *Determine when to evaluate*: The academic nurse educator decides if formative or summative evaluation is needed and determines the frequency of the evaluation.
3. *Select an evaluator*: Educators need to decide whether to select an internal evaluator (someone directly involved in the learning, course, or program) or an external evaluator (someone not directly involved in what is being evaluated, such as a consultant or accrediting body).

4. *Select an evaluation design, framework, or model*: The model should be chosen based on the context of the evaluation and the needs of the stakeholders.
5. *Choose an evaluation instrument*: The reason for evaluation and its selected framework help guide the development of a measurement tool or instrument. Examples of tools include questionnaires, interviews, rating scales, checklists, attitude scales, and portfolios.
6. *Collect data*: The evaluator decides on how and when to use the instrument or tool for data collection.
7. *Interpret data*: The evaluator systematically organizes and analyzes the data.
8. *Report findings*: The evaluator decides how and when to communicate the findings to all appropriate persons.

Incorporating Current Research in Assessment and Evaluation Practices

Best current evidence is the foundation of professional nursing practice and education. For evidence-based practice to truly be effective, it must become standard routine in both teaching and clinical practice. Academic nurse educators have an obligation to incorporate current research and evidence-based educational methods into assessment and evaluation of student learning.

Academic nurse educators should use a variety of methods to evaluate learning outcomes. When deciding upon the best methods to evaluate learning outcomes, the nurse educator should consider the time it takes to create and implement the strategy, the purpose and setting, the cost, and the domain of learning. The learning outcomes must be measurable, and the evaluation methods must be reliable and valid to effectively measure outcome achievement.

Nurse educators need to be *information literate* and know how to adequately seek out knowledge using nursing and education-focused databases for evidence-based assessment and evaluation practices. The Cumulative Index to Nursing and Allied Health Literature (CINAHL), Education Resources Information Center (ERIC), PsychINFO, and Medline are commonly used databases for searching for education, health care literature, and systematic reviews. Systematic reviews, which synthesize knowledge on a particular topic using multiple studies, can also be found using the Cochrane Library database (www.thecochranelibrary.com) and the Campbell Collaboration (www.campbellcollaboration.org). Educators also have an obligation to conduct studies on assessment and evaluation practices and disseminate those findings to broaden the knowledge base in the science of nursing education.

Nurse educators should use current research to select assessment and evaluation tools that are valid and reliable. Although several types of validity can be established, the type that is most relevant for evaluation tools for nursing education is content-related evidence of measurement validity. *Content-related evidence of measurement validity* (formerly called *content validity*) refers to the degree to which an evaluation tool measures what it intends to measure.

Reliability indicates how accurate and consistent the results of measurement are and is related to those results and not to the individual instrument or tool. Reliability types vary depending on the characteristics of the cohort of learners being assessed and/or the measurement tool being used. In nursing, two types of reliability are most commonly needed: internal consistency and interrater reliability. *Internal consistency* refers to the degree to which consistent results are achieved from two halves of the same assessment, such as a unit examination. *Interrater reliability* is important when the same measurement tool is used by more than one rater evaluating the same group of learners (e.g., evaluation of learner clinical performance). High interrater reliability indicates that there is consistency and elimination of bias during assessments among different evaluators or raters. Interrater agreement of at least 90% is most desirable.

Academic nurse educators also need to be aware of how current research affects the selection of assessment and evaluation methods. For example, standardized testing of learners is an evidence-based method to determine their application of knowledge at various points in a nursing program, as discussed in the next section.

> **CNE®/CNE®n Key Point**
>
> *Remember: Interrater reliability* is important when the same measurement tool is used by more than one rater evaluating the same group of learners. High interrater reliability indicates that there is consistency and elimination of bias during assessments among different evaluators or raters.

Analyzing Resources for Learner Assessment and Evaluation

In addition to seeking out relevant nursing education literature, faculty must also consider analyzing other resources, such as guidelines from professional organizations, fair testing frameworks, and accreditation standards, when making decisions about assessment and evaluation practices (Billings & Halstead, 2020).

Standardized tests are often used in nursing programs to determine progression and readiness to take licensure or certification examinations. These tests can provide valuable information to learners and faculty about learner strengths and weaknesses. The National League for Nursing (NLN) developed guidelines to ensure that testing not only evaluates learner achievement and competency but also that tests are designed and implemented in a manner that provides the opportunity for all learners to demonstrate what they know. The Fair Testing Guidelines suggest that faculty have an ethical obligation to ensure that tests and the decisions based on the test results are valid and supported by evidence and that the tests are fair to learners from all backgrounds (NLN, 2020). Standardized tests should be selected based on evidence of reliability, content and predictive validity, and fairness and equity. Learners should be informed of the nature and content of the test, how the scores will be used, and procedures for test administration before taking the test. The NLN (2020) also recommends that to achieve a fair testing environment, a culturally and demographically diverse group of faculty, learners, and administrators should review the program's testing policy. Fair testing in nursing education should ensure that learners are given comparable opportunities to demonstrate competency and that testing results, especially if they are high-stakes, are used in an evidence-based manner to support learning, enhance teaching, and improve nursing programs (NLN, 2020).

> **CNE®/CNE®n Key Point**
>
> *Remember:* According to the NLN's Fair Testing Guidelines, educators have an obligation to ensure that tests and the decisions based on those tests are valid, supported by evidence, consistent across programs, and fair to test-takers from all backgrounds (NLN, 2020).

Creating, Using, and Implementing Assessment Tools and Strategies to Evaluate Outcomes

Faculty should plan to use a variety of evaluation methods and strategies to assess the knowledge, skills, and attitudes of nursing students. Faculty must consider all the domains of learning, the higher levels of the domain taxonomies, clinical reasoning, and learners' preparation for licensure and certification examinations when selecting evaluation methods (Billings & Halstead, 2020). The intended learning outcomes and setting of the instruction influence the type of evaluation methods needed. In addition to unit and final examinations, common methods to evaluate student learning include:

- Portfolios
- Papers and essays
- Journaling
- Concept maps
- Video and audio recordings
- Oral (verbal) questioning
- Patient simulation
- Service learning
- Classroom or online assessment techniques

Portfolios are used to determine admission, placement into a program, progression, or evidence of professional development. They allow learners to demonstrate competencies, progress, and accomplishments by providing an extensive collection of their work. When using portfolios as an evaluation method, the educator must first decide on the purpose of the portfolio. Portfolios can be used for both formative and summative evaluations and demonstrate learning in the cognitive and affective domains. Portfolios can be time consuming for the learner and for the educator, who must provide feedback and grading. However, they can be an effective method for identifying strengths and weaknesses during formative evaluation, which can provide opportunities for learners to make improvements. This method may also be used for summative evaluation at the end of the program to demonstrate achievement of graduate competencies.

Papers and essays can be used to evaluate learning in the higher levels of the cognitive and affective domains and can be used for formative and summative evaluation. Essays and papers can allow learners to demonstrate critical thinking, clinical reasoning, organization, writing skills, and creativity (Billings & Halstead, 2020). These assignments can be easy for the educator to create and administer but may be time-consuming to grade and evaluate using a grading rubric.

Journaling can be used to allow learners to self-assess and demonstrate critical thinking. Journals can help educators evaluate the high-level cognitive and affective domains. Journaling provides learners with the opportunity to reflect upon a topic or situation and articulate their knowledge, analysis, and feelings. As with other written assignments, journaling can be time-consuming for the learner to produce and the educator to grade using a grading rubric, but it allows for evaluation of deep self-reflection and clinical reasoning.

Concept maps are visual representations to express concepts and their relationships. They are used primarily to evaluate learning in the cognitive domain. Concepts maps can be created by hand or through the use of computer programs. Educators need to provide learners with guidance on how to develop concept maps for the method to be effective. The use of concept mapping can be particularly useful in the clinical setting; however, they can be used in the classroom or online to demonstrate how didactic and clinical concepts interrelate. Concept maps can be time-consuming for both learners and educators, but they are an effective method for formative evaluation to measure critical thinking development.

Video and audio recordings can be used to evaluate learning in cognitive, psychomotor, and affective domains. Recordings can be used for both formative and summative evaluation. Videos can be used to capture skills demonstrations and nonverbal behaviors for evaluation. As technology in education continues to improve, audio and video recordings continue to become easier to create and evaluate. Learners must be provided with the evaluation criteria before creating the recording and may need additional instruction on the use of technology for recording and uploading.

Oral questioning can be used to assess cognitive and affective domains. Use of Socratic questioning can allow for immediate feedback to learners and help determine mastery of content. It can be used in both classroom and clinical settings, is easy to use, and is useful for formative assessment. Allowing learners time to process and develop responses is an important part of using this technique.

Patient simulation is a method for evaluating all three domains of learning. It is effective for creating a safe learning environment in which learners can practice and refine a number of psychomotor, clinical reasoning, organizational, and communication skills. Patient simulation exposes learners to clinical scenarios that they may not have been able to experience in the clinical setting. Effective patient simulation requires extensive preparation by both the educator and learners. A standardized patient using a script or simulation equipment is typically used, and learners are scheduled for the experience in small groups. Coordination of scheduling, collaboration with other health care professionals, use of high-fidelity mannequins and other equipment, creation of patient scenarios, and time for debriefing must be considered by the faculty (Fig. 4.1).

Service-learning experiences are designed to help students achieve learning objectives in the cognitive and affective domains while helping to meet the needs of the community and develop

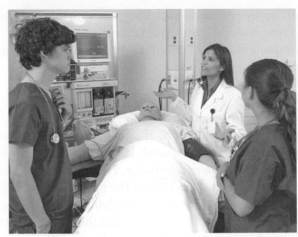

FIG. 4.1 Use of high-fidelity mannequins for clinical simulation. (From Black, B. P. [2020]. *Professional nursing* [9th ed.]. St. Louis: Elsevier.)

civic engagement. Service learning allows students to have hands-on, real-world experience and interact collaboratively with individuals and communities. Planning, organization, and evaluation of service-learning experiences require maintaining long-term relationships with community partners to facilitate meaningful student learning. Chapter 7 describes service learning in more detail.

Classroom or online assessment techniques can evaluate learning while it is in progress. These techniques enable learners to receive feedback while they are actively engaging with content and can promote learner success (Billings & Halstead, 2020). Classroom or online assessment techniques can also offer an active learning approach that promotes analysis of information at a higher cognitive level. These techniques also represent a method of formative assessment (Cannon & Boswell, 2016). Selected examples of these techniques include:

- *Muddiest point:* The learner identifies what information is not yet understood.
- *One-minute paper:* The learner has 60 seconds to write a response to a prompted question.
- *Background knowledge probe:* The nurse educator assesses learner knowledge before presenting information on a topic.
- *Pro/con grid:* The learner explores pros and cons of a particular situation; this technique can be used to connect clinical experiences with classroom content.

These techniques should take a short time and provide clarity for the nurse educator on which topics might need further development and review. Like other assessment and evaluation methods, classroom or online assessment techniques take advanced planning by the nurse educator.

Once the academic nurse educator develops measurable outcomes and selects the appropriate model and methods for evaluation, the process of developing and using evidence-based tools to evaluate outcomes begins. Learners should be provided with grading expectations before completing all tests, written papers, simulations, skills checkoffs, discussion boards, and other assignments. These expectations allow learners to know how they will be evaluated and how points and grades will be awarded. Developing and implementing rubrics, classroom tests, and clinical evaluations are the most common tools and strategies to effectively assess student achievement of learning outcomes.

Grading Rubrics

Grading rubrics are commonly used across different types of assignments and provide a clear system to evaluate learner performance (Billings & Halstead, 2020). Papers, concept maps, projects, and discussion boards are common assignments for which a rubric can be useful for both the learner and the academic nurse educator. The learner can use the rubric to identify what is expected in the assignment and understand how grading will occur. The nurse educator is guided by a rubric to consistently apply criteria to each assignment that is reviewed. The rubric must be concise and robust and communicate clear expectations.

The following four components make up a rubric and are usually outlined in a tabular format:

- Description of the assignment
- Scale
- Elements of the assignment
- Explanation of each level of performance

The description of the assignment should be succinct and identify how the assignment relates to the learning outcomes that are being measured. The grading scale provides clear terms for the learner and a specific way to delineate performance. For example, a scale could include exemplary, proficient, developing, and beginner criteria. The scale can also include numeric scores or ranges of scores. Elements of the assignment are then delineated, with each box representing an element of the assignment down the vertical column and the scale along the horizontal row. The descriptions within each box further explain the expectations of the assignment for each element and part of the scale. Table 4.4 provides a sample rubric for a written paper clinical assignment.

Testing

Tests in nursing education are most often used to evaluate learning in the cognitive domain and can be used to determine learners' admission, progression, and graduation. Careful consideration must be given to the planning, creation, and administration of examinations. The three most common types of examinations are *achievement tests, norm-referenced tests,* and *criterion-referenced tests.*

Achievement tests are a type of standardized test with very high reliability. These tests are usually created by a commercial vendor and measure clearly defined learning outcomes. Achievement tests are often used to assess learner performance throughout a program, identify learners at risk for failure of the licensure and certification examination, design remediation programs to improve performance, and determine progression (Oermann & Gaberson, 2021). Educators need to prepare learners for the test specifications before administration and must have a detailed plan for using the results.

Norm-referenced tests are constructed and interpreted to provide a ranking for all of the learners. One learner will receive the highest score and another learner the lowest; learners may be provided with information about how they ranked among their peers. These exams are useful for testing a broad range of learning while focusing on only a few test items per content area.

Criterion-referenced tests include specific test items that are designed to evaluate learning outcomes. Most faculty-created course examinations are considered criterion-referenced, although learners can achieve a variety of scores to "pass" and meet learning outcomes. These tests use a larger number of items per content area, including easy, moderate, and difficult items. Scoring is typically reported as a percentage or as points acquired. Criterion-referenced tests are used to evaluate specific knowledge, skills, and mastery of content using pre-established criteria.

> **CNE®/CNE®n Key Point**
>
> **Remember:** *Norm-referenced* tests measure learner performance in relation to other learners by ranking them. *Criterion-referenced* tests measure learner achievement of predetermined established learning outcomes. Most faculty-created course examinations are considered criterion-referenced, although learners can achieve a variety of scores to "pass" and meet learning outcomes.

Creating a Test Blueprint

Developing a test requires that considerable thought and planning be given to the type of test, design, administration, and use of the results. Tests may be given to determine admission into a program, to decide on appropriate academic placement, to evaluate learning progress, to

TABLE 4.4	Sample Rubric for Evidence-Based Practice Clinical Paper			
	Exemplary	**Average**	**Below Average**	**Poor**
Introduction— Describe patient's history and current status	Comprehensive description of patient's history, current medical status, and pathophysiology. Provides descriptive analysis of all pertinent data. **3 points**	Effective description of patient's history, current medical status, and pathophysiology. Provides some analysis of pertinent data. **2 points**	Limited description of patient's history, current medical status, and pathophysiology. Very limited in analysis of pertinent data. **1 point**	Poor description of patient's history, current medical status, and pathophysiology. No analysis of pertinent data. **0 points**
Evidence-based practice— Discuss current practice trends related to the current status of the patient	Comprehensively discusses three peer-reviewed, evidence-based practice articles. Articles relate directly to current patient condition. **3 points**	Effectively discusses three peer-reviewed, evidence-based practice articles. Articles relate directly to current patient condition. **2 points**	Provides a limited discussion of fewer than three peer-reviewed, evidence-based practice articles. Articles may relate directly to current patient condition. **1 point**	Does not discuss at least three peer-reviewed, evidence-based practice articles. Does not relate articles directly to current patient condition. **0 points**
Compare and contrast— Compare current care to the evidence discovered	Comprehensively compares and contrasts current patient care to three peer-reviewed, evidence-based practice articles, articulates opportunities for change. **3 points**	Effectively compares and contrasts current patient care to three peer-reviewed, evidence-based practice articles, provides developed opportunities for change. **2 points**	Provides a limited compare and contrast of current patient care to fewer than three peer-reviewed, evidence-based practice articles, provides minimal depth in discussing opportunities for change. **1 point**	Does not compare and contrast current patient care with peer-reviewed, evidence-based practice articles, does not discuss opportunities for change. **0 points**
APA format	Uses APA format with no mistakes. Includes title page, appropriate references in text, and formatted reference page. **3 points**	Uses APA format with minimal mistakes. Includes minimal mistakes within title page, references in text, and reference page. **2 points**	Uses APA format with several mistakes. Includes several mistakes within title page, references in text, and reference page. **1 point**	Uses APA format with numerous mistakes. Includes numerous mistakes within title page, references in text, and reference page and missing some elements. **0 points**

determine summative mastery of content, or to determine achievement of program outcomes. Once the academic nurse educator decides on the type of test to administer, the next step in the planning stage is to develop a *test blueprint,* also called a *test plan,* which ensures content-related evidence of measurement validity of the test. Classroom or online examinations are designed to evaluate learning in the cognitive domain.

A basic test blueprint displays the distribution of test items for each learning outcome and content area. A more complex test blueprint, particularly for prelicensure learners who will take the NCLEX®, may also include the level of the cognitive taxonomy, type of question, NCLEX® integrated process, and NCLEX® client needs category. Many programs have a testing policy for faculty that specifies the percentage of test items that should be written at the applying or higher level of the cognitive domain taxonomy. The number of items to include on the examination is dependent on the number of outcomes to be evaluated, the types of items being used, and the length of time learners will need to complete the examination. Table 4.5 illustrates part of a basic test blueprint for a unit exam on assessment of the respiratory system.

Test Item Development

After the blueprint is constructed, the academic nurse educator needs to decide on which types of test items to use. Educators may choose or revise items from a test bank or may develop their own test items based on selected content learning outcomes, also referred to as *course objectives*. Examples of test items (also called *test questions*) include:

- Multiple choice
- Multiple response (Select all that apply or Select *N*)
- True/false
- Hot spot
- Fill in the blank
- Matching
- Short answer
- Essay
- Priority/ordered response
- Exhibit questions

Multiple-choice test items are the most commonly used questions on nursing program exams, licensure exams, and certification exams and are the focus of this discussion. When constructed properly and written clearly, the multiple-choice question can measure critical thinking, elements of clinical judgment, and the higher levels of the cognitive domain (Billings & Halstead, 2020). A multiple-choice test item consists of three parts: the stem, the answer, and the distractors. The *test item stem* presents a question, problem, or clinical situation that relates to the learning outcome being assessed. This information is followed by a question or an incomplete statement with a list of possible answer options. The *test item distractors* are the incorrect options and should attract test-takers who are not knowledgeable or who cannot critically think to determine the correct response. Each choice (also called *option*) for a test item should be distinct and different from the other choices.

TABLE 4.5	Sample Partial Blueprint for a Unit Examination on the Respiratory System		
Learning Outcomes	**Concept/Topic**	**Level of Cognitive Domain**	**Question Number**
Assess client's thorax and lungs	Chest landmarks	Applying	1
	Normal breath sounds	Understanding	3
	Adventitious breath sounds	Analyzing	4
Assess client's subjective data for respiratory system	Common symptoms	Applying	2
Analyze subjective and objective data to formulate plan of care	Risk factors	Applying	7
	Pneumothorax	Evaluating	5
	Pneumonia	Analyzing	6

Nurse educators should construct the multiple-choice test item so that the correct answer and distractors are approximately the same length, using grammar consistent with each option, and labeled in alphabetical or numeric order. Multiple-choice questions written at the remembering and understanding levels of cognition do not adequately assess a learner's ability to think critically and make clinical decisions. The following is an example of a multiple-choice test item written at the remembering level of the cognitive learning domain. This test item measures the ability of learners to memorize content, but does not ensure that the learner understands the process of summative evaluation.

Example of Multiple-Choice Test Item Written at the Remembering Cognitive Level

Which of the following statements describes the process of summative evaluation?
A. Monitoring learner progress and providing meaningful feedback during a learning opportunity
B. Gathering and interpreting information to determine progress towards a desired outcome
C. Assigning numbers to represent achievement or performance of learners on an evaluation tool
D. Making a judgment regarding a learner's performance at the end of an activity, course, or program.
Answer: D

Test items to measure critical thinking should be written at the applying or analyzing cognitive level. Critical thinking items require learners to examine their previous nursing knowledge, approach the situation from more than one viewpoint, and then apply that knowledge to make a decision (McDonald, 2018). The following is an example of a multiple-choice test item written at the applying level of the cognitive learning domain.

Example of Multiple-Choice Test Item Written at the Applying Cognitive Level

Which of the following methods is the most appropriate for the nurse educator to use for summative evaluation of learners?
A. Online quiz on reading assignment
B. Concept map on pain management
C. Final course examination
D. *Jeopardy* activity during class
Answer: C

CNE®/CNE®n Key Point

Remember: The nurse educator should develop multiple-choice test items at the applying or higher cognitive level to evaluate critical thinking to make appropriate decisions.

Test Administration

Tests may be administered using paper and pencil or taken electronically. All tests should include clear instructions to inform learners of the number of items, point values, and the amount of time permitted to take the exam. Academic nurse educators should provide ample time for learners to complete the entire test. Nurse educators have an obligation to maintain an appropriate physical testing environment with adequate physical space, lighting, temperature, and minimal distractions. Facilitating a quiet testing environment free from distractions can help ease learners' anxiety during the testing process. Educators also have an obligation to maintain a secure test and testing environment. Faculty should remind learners of the academic honesty policy before testing. To prevent cheating, learners should not be allowed to exit the testing room before submitting the exam and should not be allowed to access phones or other electronic devices during an exam. Faculty need at least two proctors in the classroom during testing and require all learners to place all personal items, including bags, phones, watches, and hats, at the front of the classroom.

For online testing, learners should be required to use a lockdown browser that prevents them from looking up answers on the Internet during an examination. Remote proctoring may also be a consideration for those taking exams in an online environment. Educators may permit learners to raise their hands and ask questions during an exam but should take care to not provide hints or clues to the correct answer when doing so.

Nurse educators may elect to use collaborative testing methods when administering exams. *Collaborative testing* allows small groups or pairs of students to work together on a test as a learning experience. Although there are several ways to test collaboratively, a commonly used method is described here. First, learners take the examination individually and submit their answers electronically or on paper. Then groups or pairs meet to discuss test items and retake the same examination. These exams may be graded by taking the sum or mean scores from both tests. Another option is to award points to the tests of those individuals who got an "A" or "B" on the collaborative test. The collaborative testing environment mimics many of the collaborative working environments for nurses in the clinical setting. Collaborative testing fosters teamwork and communication and may reduce test anxiety in learners. However, it requires more class or online time to complete, which must be considered during planning.

There is limited evidence supporting best practices for the recommended length of tests, the mode of testing (paper or computerized), or the frequency of exams. Educators must consider their program's testing policy, the length of the class time, the program level of the learners, and the characteristics of the cohort when deciding on length, frequency, and types of tests to administer each academic term.

Evaluation of Learner Clinical Performance

Assessment of clinical performance is important to develop each learner's growth within the practice of nursing. Assessing clinical performance involves all domains of learning. Feedback to the learner in the clinical setting should occur regularly throughout the experience as part of formative evaluation. Summative evaluation is documented using a formal clinical evaluation tool (CET) at the end of the clinical learning experience, such as the example in Table 4.6. The tools used for evaluation of learners' clinical performance should be made available and discussed with learners at the beginning of the experience. Learners must be aware of what they are being evaluated on and how. The nurse educator can set expectations for levels of performance and assist learners in understanding how they will achieve clinical learning outcomes. A rating scale like the one shown in Table 4.6 can be used to determine the learner's level of performance, or the CET criteria can be scored as "Met" or "Not Met."

The CET should include specific and measurable learner behaviors or competencies. The knowledge and skills that are expected of learners should be clearly defined within the CET (Billings & Halstead, 2020). The nurse educator should also strive to create and implement a tool that is as objective as possible to evaluate learners. The learner can be evaluated using observation, oral communication, written communication, self-evaluation, and simulation (Billings & Halstead, 2020). However, the educator's observation of learner performance is the best method for assessing clinical competence of learners at all levels of education.

CNE®/CNE®n Key Point

Remember: Evaluating clinical performance involves assessing the learner in the cognitive, psychomotor, and affective domains. The educator's observation of learner performance is the best method for assessing clinical competence of learners at all levels of education.

TABLE 4.6	Sample Clinical Evaluation Tool

Final Obstetric Nursing Clinical Evaluation

Clinical faculty will fill in a numeric score on all clinical learning outcomes. Learner must obtain a 75% grade or more on the final clinical evaluation to pass the course.

Scoring:

4—Exceeds expectations

3—Meets expectations

2—Below expectations

1—Does not meet expectations

Learning Outcome	Final Evaluation	
	Learner	**Faculty**
	Score self 1–4 in each box.	Score learner 1–4 in each box.
Use the nursing process to create and implement a plan of care for the obstetric patient.		
Integrate knowledge of pathophysiology into the care of the obstetric patient.		
Demonstrate an assessment of the obstetric patient.		
Verbally communicate effectively with the interprofessional team about data relating to the obstetric patient.		
Demonstrate appropriate and thorough documentation of the obstetric patient in the electronic health record.		
Demonstrate caring, family-centered care to the obstetric patient.		
Demonstrate safe, timely care of the obstetric patient appropriate to the period.		
Engage in active self-evaluation and demonstrate responsibility for one's own learning.		
Communicate effectively with peers and faculty to analyze clinical data and situations related to the obstetric patient.		

Learner Comments

In the space provided address scores given to self earlier and provide examples of performance:

Identify three areas for improvement:

Identify three strengths:

Faculty Comments

In the space provided address the scores given to the learner earlier and provide examples of performance:

Identify areas for improvement:

Identify strengths:

Final comments:

Learner signature: _____

Date: _____

Faculty signature: _____

Date: _____

Clinical Observation

Evaluating the learner in the clinical environment includes many different formats. The first way to evaluate a learner is through direct observation. The nurse educator should make an effort to spend time with each learner in the clinical setting to observe performance. Observation should include the following interactions:

- Learner and faculty
- Learner and patient
- Learner and patient visitors/support system
- Learner and staff
- Learner and peers

Observing the learner requires the nurse educator to develop an organized system to keep notes. Because there are often many different learners within a group and the educator may have multiple groups at one time, a tracking system to keep notes about each learner is imperative. Any tracking of data about learners must be kept secure and confidential. Keeping detailed notes can be useful to provide specific examples to the learner when evaluating performance (Billings & Halstead, 2020). The nurse educator must be intentional about observing each learner in the clinical setting and devoting adequate time to evaluate practices and behaviors that are expected to meet clinical competencies.

Written Clinical Assignments and Oral Communication

Evaluation of the learner in the clinical setting should also include any written assignments. Learners are usually assigned a variety of written assignments such as care plans, concept maps, patient assessments, and/or written papers. Written work can provide evidence of critical thinking and clinical reasoning and can allow learners to articulate their own understanding of patient or community care. Written assignments should be graded using a rubric and included in the formative evaluation process.

Learners may also complete reflective assignments, which can be useful in evaluating the affective domain. For example, *journaling* can be an effective clinical assignment that allows for intentional reflection and demonstrates evidence of learning in the affective domain.

Learners can also be evaluated on the effectiveness of their oral communication. Professional communication is an essential skill for the learner to develop for nursing practice. The nurse educator can evaluate the learner on communication skills through clinical conferences, formal discussions, and assigned case presentations (Billings & Halstead, 2020). Providing learners the opportunity to articulate clinical information through multiple formats also allows the educator to analyze their critical thinking.

Interprofessional Collaboration and Simulation

Learners should be provided the opportunity to actively engage and collaborate with other health professionals while in the clinical setting. For example, learners can present interprofessional clinical cases that focus on ensuring the safety and quality of patient care. Simulation is another example in which learners from various health professions can work together to achieve shared learning outcomes and practice collaborative communication and patient care.

Simulation is an effective and controlled method for evaluating learner clinical performance, critical thinking, and clinical judgment. Simulation experiences can be low-fidelity to high-fidelity and can involve standardized patients. Clinical scenarios in the simulation lab are designed to meet expected learning outcomes and should be appropriate for the level of the learner. Expectations for each scenario should be clearly communicated in advance such that learners can be adequately prepared for each experience. Learners should also be aware that simulation is a safe space where they can practice patient care without fear of making errors as part of formative evaluation.

In some programs, simulation is also used as part of summative evaluation through successful completion of an *objective structured clinical examination (OSCE)*, a type of clinical performance examination. Learners must pass this evaluation to pass a clinical course or other learning experience.

Learner self-evaluation should also be included as part of comprehensive clinical performance evaluation. Promoting self-reflection on clinical learning is an important skill for learners in all types of nursing programs, as discussed in Chapter 3. Using a tool to allow learners to self-evaluate can allow a deep level of reflection on their own strengths and weaknesses (Billings & Halstead, 2020). Learners may not always be open and honest for fear of negative effects on their course grade. Nurse educators need to assure learners that their fear is not valid.

Preceptorship Experiences

Using a preceptor model for clinical learning involves assigning each learner to a predetermined and well-qualified clinical preceptor. In this model the faculty is usually not onsite on a daily or weekly basis. The nurse educator, preceptor, and learner all work together to facilitate the learning experience.

The nurse educator needs to consider that regular contact with the preceptor is necessary to successfully evaluate the learner. Using methods of contact such as telephone, email, online sessions, and onsite visits are all ways to connect and dialogue about ongoing progress toward specified objectives (Cannon & Boswell, 2016). Preceptors need coaching on providing feedback on learner progress and should be mentored by nurse educators as they work with learners. Although the preceptor should provide regular verbal and written feedback to the nurse educator, the nurse educator is responsible for conducting the learner's summative clinical performance evaluation. At the end of the preceptor experience, learners should be given the opportunity to evaluate their preceptors, the clinical site, and the overall preceptor experience.

> **CNE®/CNE®n Key Point**
>
> *Remember:* Although the preceptor should provide regular verbal and written feedback to the nurse educator, the nurse educator is responsible for conducting the learner's summative clinical performance evaluation.

Course Evaluation Calculation

After reviewing the syllabus, program objectives, and program curriculum, the nurse educator can begin the process of developing a systematic course evaluation. Assigning course grades is a critical component of learner progression in a nursing program. Faculty must provide learners with a detailed plan for how course grades will be assigned and rubrics for how individual assignments and examinations will be graded. Additional information about assignment due dates, policies for late assignments, and make-up tests should also be available to learners in the course syllabus. Grading scales may vary slightly from institution to institution, but a typical course grading scale can be found here:

- A = 90% to 100%
- B = 80% to 89%
- C = 75% minimum passing percentage
- C– = 70% to 74%
- D = 60% to 69%
- F = 59% and below

Final course grade calculation should be displayed in the syllabus and show percentages or points for each component used to determine the final grade. Table 4.7 shows an example of course grade calculation. Final course grades are provided as evidence of achievement of course outcomes.

Analyzing Assessment and Evaluation Data

Analysis of assessment and evaluation data is a necessary part of teaching and learning. The academic nurse educator must ensure the instrument being used to measure student learning outcomes is both valid and reliable. Verifying that what is being taught aligns with the defined outcomes is

TABLE **4.7**   Course Grade Calculation
Course grades will be calculated using the following points. This course is worth a total of 400 possible points.

Four 50-point unit exams (50% of total grade):	200 points
Final exam (25% of total grade):	100 points
Geriatric care plan (15% of total grade):	60 points
Dementia reflection paper (10% of total grade):	40 points
	————
	400 points total

a critical element of teaching. Construction of assessment tools that are valid and reliable is a skill that can require a great deal of time for the educator. This section focuses on analyzing tests in nursing education. Statistical analysis occurs after a test has been administered; testing statistics are available from software or web-based platforms. Nurse educators need to know how to interpret these data to make appropriate decisions about test items for continuous quality improvement.

Validity

Validity ensures that inferences from test scores are appropriate, meaningful, and useful (Billings & Halstead, 2020). As defined earlier, the nurse educator needs to establish content-related evidence of measurement validity to determine whether a test is measuring what was intended to be measured. A test blueprint, discussed earlier, is one of the best ways to establish an exam's validity. Another method the nurse educator can consider to assist with determining content-related validity is to request peer reviews by content experts in the area being tested.

Validity can be affected by many different factors. During the development and implementation of a test, the nurse educator should consider its quality and design. Lack of clear directions, poor sampling of content represented, and inadequately written test items can all negatively affect validity (Billings & Halstead, 2020). The nurse educator should analyze the multiple factors associated with validity on an ongoing basis to maintain high standards and rigor.

CNE®/CNE®n Key Point

Remember: A test blueprint is one of the best ways to establish an exam's content-related validity. Another method is to request peer reviews by content experts in the area being tested.

Reliability

Reliability refers to whether the test produces scores that are consistent and dependable (Billings & Halstead, 2020). Reliability is about the scores on the exam from a specified sample and therefore differs from validity. The ability to replicate the results on the same sample can indicate reliability (McDonald, 2018).

To assess the reliability of test scores from a single administration, the *Kuder-Richardson formula (KR-20)*, a measure of internal consistency, can be calculated. KR-20 values range from 0 to 1.00, with 0 meaning there is no reliability and 1.00 meaning the test is perfect, an unachievable expectation. A high KR-20 value establishes good test reliability; conversely, a low value demonstrates poor reliability. A standardized test usually has a KR-20 of 0.90 or higher. An *ideal* KR-20 for a course test would be greater than 0.80, but very few faculty-developed tests achieve this level. Some sources suggest that any value above 0.70 is considered acceptable (Billings & Halstead, 2020). Many nursing programs agree that any KR-20 value above 0.50 is acceptable. Software data or a testing office can supply these data. Several factors can affect the reliability of a test and therefore the KR-20. See Table 4.8 for factors that can negatively affect the KR-20 value and strategies that may improve that value.

TABLE 4.8	Factors Affecting Test Reliability and Strategies for Improvement
Factors Affecting Test Reliability	**Strategies for Improvement**
Inadequate test length (fewer than 40 test items)	Add more items to the test
Inadequate sample size (fewer than 20–25 test-takers)	Increase the number of test-takers if possible by combining sections or another method
Too many easy questions *or* too many hard questions	Increase or decrease the difficulty level based on content
Poorly written questions	Enhance the discrimination level

Measures of Central Tendency

Measures of central tendency—the mean, median, and mode—can be calculated for each test. The *mean* is the average score for the test. It is a simple statistic to calculate based on this formula: Mean = Sum of all scores ÷ Number of scores. Knowing the mean score of a test can provide the nurse educator with knowledge about the overall score of the test. However, the mean can be skewed by outliers of very high or very low scores.

The *median* divides all of the scores for a test in the middle to determine the midpoint. This means that 50% of scores on the test are above the median and 50% of scores on the test are below the median. The median can be more useful when the test scores are skewed by outliers. Looking at both the mean and the median can help the nurse educator better understand how scores on the test are distributed.

The *mode* is the most frequently occurring test score. The mode is simple to determine because it involves reviewing all of a test's scores to identify the most frequently occurring score(s).

Test Item Analysis

In addition to reviewing the overall scores on a test, the KR-20 value, and measures of central tendency, the nurse educator should review each individual test item on an examination for distribution of learner responses, difficulty level, and item discrimination. This *item analysis* allows the educator to analyze each test item to determine if revisions are needed when the item is used in the future.

The educator should first review each test item for how many learners selected each potential option. Consider these multiple-choice test items and which options a class of 48 learners selected. The correct answers are indicated with an asterisk (*).

Example of Learners' Responses for Multiple-Choice Test Items				
	A	**B**	**C**	**D**
1.	0	8	28*	12
2.	20*	7	10	11

In Item #1, the majority of test takers selected the correct answer; others selected two of the distractors—B and D. However, no learner selected A. For this test item, the nurse educator would consider revising Choice A if this item is used again on future tests. In Item #2, a significant number of learners chose each option. The test item distractors were attractive to many learners who may not have been as knowledgeable or able to critically think when compared with learners who selected the correct option (A).

Test Item Difficulty

The first statistic for the nurse educator to review for each item is its *difficulty level,* which may be presented as a percentage of learners who got the item correct. To calculate the percentage of learners who got an item correct, divide the number of learners who selected the correct response by the total number of test takers. For example, in Item #1, 28 learners selected the correct response and 48 learners took the test. The calculation is 28/48 for a percentage of learners who got Item #1 correct as 58%. The difficulty level for Item #2 is calculated as 20/48, or 42%.

Some software or web-based programs report test item difficulty as a *p level,* which represents the percentage of learners who got the item correct expressed as a decimal. The range for the p level is 0.00 (no test scorers selected the correct response) to 1.00 (all test scorers selected the correct response). For example, a p level of 0.58 means that 58% of learners taking the test got that item correct. Experts vary about which p value range is acceptable, but these ranges are commonly used by many nursing programs:

- 0.90 and above: Test item may be too easy
- 0.50–0.89: Test item difficulty is acceptable
- 0.49 and below: Test item may be too difficult

An item that is too easy or too difficult should be determined by the nurse educator based on the test content and expectations. It is generally accepted that a p level of 0.50 and above is a satisfactory test item. An item that is considered too easy or too difficult should be evaluated for revision by the nurse educator.

> **CNE®/CNE®n Key Point**
>
> *Remember:* It is generally accepted that a p level of 0.50 and above is a satisfactory test item.

Test Item Discrimination

After reviewing test item difficulty, the nurse educator needs to interpret the ability of each item to discriminate between those learners who are knowledgeable and can critically think and those who cannot. Item discrimination can be measured using several statistics, but a *point biserial* (PBS) correlation coefficient is most frequently used for multiple-choice objective tests. A PBS can measure how a learner performed on a particular test item compared with the learner's overall test score (Billings & Halstead, 2020). Learners who score high on the exam and got a specific test item correct are compared with learners who score low on the exam and got the same test item correct. Like other testing statistics, it is essential for the nurse educator to be able to interpret item discrimination data provided by either testing software or a testing center rather than using complex formulas to perform the calculation.

Analysis of the PBS should be done for the correct answer and each incorrect response, with a focus on test items that are more difficult. The PBS for the correct response to a test item is generally accepted as the overall PBS for the item. PBS values range from −1.00 to 1.00. To discriminate, the correct answer should be overwhelmingly positive. A positive PBS shows that the learners who scored high on the test were able to answer that test item correctly more than the learners who scored low on the test. Conversely, a very low or negative PBS demonstrates that the learners who scored low on the test answered the test item correctly more than the learners who scored high on the test. The following is a guide to interpreting PBS values:

- 0.30 and above: Excellent test item
- 0.20 to 0.29: Good test item
- 0.09 to 0.19: Reasonable test item
- <0.09 and negative values: Poor test item

> **CNE®/CNE®n Key Point**
>
> *Remember:* Test item discrimination for objective-style tests is best determined using the PBS coefficient. The PBS for the correct response to a test item should be 0.09 or higher, with the preferred PBS at 0.20 or greater.

A PBS that is closer to 0.00 demonstrates that the same number of learners in the high-scoring group versus the low-scoring group answered the question correctly (Oermann & Gaberson, 2021).

Therefore the item does not discriminate because it did not show a difference in learners. The other possibility to consider is a negative PBS. A negative PBS for the correct item should warrant special review by the nurse educator. This finding indicates that learners who scored high on the test answered the item incorrectly. High test scorers answering an item incorrectly could be related to the quality of the test item and options, which requires further analysis of the test item, including analyzing the distractors. A PBS below 0.09 should be carefully reviewed by the nurse educator because this item shows poor discrimination. It is appropriate to consider nullifying a difficult item with a low PBS. *Nullification* means that the nurse educator accepts all choices for the item because it is difficult and has poor discrimination.

It is important to note that there are limitations to the PBS. The ability to discriminate a test item appropriately relates to the item difficulty. For test items that either a very high or a very low number of learners answered correctly, the PBS can be skewed to a lower value (Oermann & Gaberson, 2021). A very challenging test item in which no learners are able to answer correctly could also create a PBS that is 0.00 and therefore is not able to discriminate. After considering the PBS for the correct choice, the next step in analysis is to review the PBS for each distractor.

CNE®/CNE®n Key Point

Remember: The nurse educator should consider nullifying an item with a PBS below 0.09.

The PBS values for distractors in a multiple-choice test item should be negative or extremely low. A negative value demonstrates that low-scoring learners chose one of the distractors on the test item. Ideally the distractors on a test item should attract the low-scoring learners. The nurse educator should analyze each distractor individually. If there is a distractor that no learners choose, the PBS will be 0.00. This means that the distractor did not function as intended because the learner already knew the choice was incorrect. This situation can increase the chances that a low-scoring learner can achieve the correct answer by guessing (Billings & Halstead, 2020).

Consider this example to interpret the PBS values for options for a multiple-choice test item. The correct response is indicated with an asterisk (*).

Example of Multiple-Choice Item With Difficulty and Point Biserial Values

	Choice p Level	PBS Value
A.	0.27	−0.10
B.	*0.35	0.29
C.	0.14	0.02
D.	0.24	−0.08

In this example, the PBS for the entire test item is 0.29 because it is the PBS for the correct response. This value indicates that the high-scoring learners selected the correct response. The PBS values for the distractors are either very low or negative, indicating that low-scoring learners selected the wrong choices, which is the desired outcome. This item appears to discriminate well between high scorers and low scorers. The nurse educator would not change any option if the test item were used as part of future tests.

In the next test item example, the PBS values are different.

Example of Multiple-Choice Item With Difficulty and Point Biserial Values

	Choice p Level	PBS Value
A.	0.27	−0.10
B.	*0.35	−0.29
C.	0.14	0.02
D.	0.24	0.28

The PBS for this test item is −0.29, which is the PBS for the correct response. This value indicates that the low-scoring learners selected the correct response, an undesirable finding showing that the test item poorly discriminates between high- and low-scoring learners. As a result, for this test administration, the nurse educator would nullify the test item. High scorers selected Choice D, an incorrect response. The other distractors have negative PBS values, which indicate that low scorers selected these choices. The nurse educator would need to change Choices B and D if this item were used again as part of future testing because their PBS values were the opposite of what was desired.

Using Assessment and Evaluation Data to Enhance the Teaching-Learning Process

Assessment and evaluation data should be used by the nurse educator to enhance the teaching-learning process. Course assessment and evaluation data reflect whether learners met the learning outcomes. Data may be shared with other nurse educators and learners. Sharing with educators can be very useful, particularly if multiple sections of a course are being taught by different nurse educators.

Special consideration should be given to sharing assessment and evaluation data with learners. The nurse educator should reflect on what is necessary and pertinent for the learner to know. For example, for a course exam, learners often only need to know their overall score. Feedback should be specific to the type of assessment used and what is necessary for the learner to interpret and understand.

Learners should be given adequate feedback as part of their evaluation and the opportunity to ask questions. This feedback can be conducted in a group format or individually with learners. Determining the most effective method is based on the course components that were evaluated and the method that most effectively addresses learners.

The nurse educator should consider how well assessment and evaluation data measured what was intended and if revisions should be made. Improving assessment and evaluation tools can be completed over time with intentional feedback and continuous review. Enhancing the teaching-learning process is not a one-time event and should be done as part of continuous quality improvement to refine reliable and valid methods of assessing and evaluating student learning.

Some programs may choose to use a standardized testing product to supplement the course evaluations used in each course. It is important that these exams not replace the expert teaching, assessment, and evaluation conducted by nurse educators. If a program chooses to use a standardized testing product, remediation is a critical element for the learner. The nurse educator should facilitate the use of such products as part of the evaluation plan to continue to make improvements (Billings & Halstead, 2020).

Advising Learners Regarding Assessment and Evaluation Criteria

It is the responsibility of the nurse educator to ensure that learners know the details regarding how they will be assessed and evaluated. Grades are very important to learners because they allow progression within a program. Depending on the types of assessments, there may be several ways to inform learners about expectations.

As an overall nursing program, the nursing student handbook provides the retention and progression policies as a critical first step to informing learners about the criteria for assessment and evaluation. In addition to these policies, student handbooks should include information about testing, including what technology is needed and how tests are developed and graded. The handbook should also include the grading scale and information about grade rounding (or not). Ensuring consistency in grading throughout a program is critical for the learner to clearly understand and respect program expectations.

At a course level, the syllabus is an important tool that the nurse educator should use for communicating specific assessment and evaluation criteria. The syllabus should clearly outline what is essential to pass a particular course (Billings & Halstead, 2020). Inclusion of grading scales and assessment and evaluation method weighting is imperative. Tables and charts that are easy to read and reference are useful to the learner. The nurse educator should make the syllabus readily available and review the syllabus with learners to ensure understanding on the first day of the course.

The nurse educator is responsible to provide all assignment expectations in a clear format. These expectations include rubrics, evaluation tools, and test blueprints. Information about how assessment will occur for all evaluation methods should be provided well in advance to the learners. All documents and tools should be easily accessible to learners using the institution's learning management system. Evaluation criteria should be assessed regularly by the nurse educator and learners for effectiveness and clarity. This allows the nurse educator to make edits as necessary to ensure that expectations are reasonable and clear for learners. Setting clear and up-front expectations can help decrease learner anxiety, questions, and disputes over assessment and evaluation criteria.

> ### CNE®/CNE®n Key Point
>
> *Remember:* The syllabus should clearly outline what is essential to pass a particular course (Billings & Halstead, 2020). Inclusion of grading scales and assessment and evaluation method weighting is imperative.

Providing Feedback to Learners

Providing feedback to learners regarding assessment and evaluation allows the opportunity for learners to improve and set clear, realistic goals moving forward. Formative evaluation can be used to provide feedback that encourages growth while learning continues. Feedback given to learners should be specific, timely, and practical for the learner to understand the modifications needed immediately and how to make changes for the future.

Learner feedback can be provided through the use of formal evaluation tools and/or in an informal manner, providing verbal feedback in a classroom or faculty office. Regardless of the format, the nurse educator should regularly implement constructive ways to provide feedback during a course. Using the evaluation and assessment techniques previously discussed allows the nurse educator the opportunity to formatively provide feedback while learners are still engaged. Feedback should include both learner strengths and weaknesses. Being specific when providing feedback is necessary to help learners achieve success and make improvements moving forward.

Timeliness is important in providing feedback. In a classroom setting where in-class activities or verbal interaction is occurring, feedback can be immediate. The learner can quickly take the response and note it to make improvements. Written work assignments often require more time to grade. Depending on the length of what is assigned, 1 to 2 weeks can be a standard turn-around time to provide learner feedback (grades). The nurse educator explains when learners should expect feedback and when grading might take longer than usual.

The nurse educator should be aware that providing meaningful constructive feedback to learners is a skill that takes intentional practice to improve. Developing trusting relationships with learners can facilitate the process of providing feedback. Constructive feedback not only enhances learners' growth but also allows nurse educators the opportunity to track their own progress and growth.

References

Anderson, L. W., & Krathwohl, D. R. (2001). *A taxonomy for learning, teaching, and assessing: A revision of Bloom's taxonomy of educational objectives.* Boston: Allyn & Bacon.

Billings, D. M., & Halstead, J. A. (2020). *Teaching in nursing: A guide for faculty* (6th ed.). St. Louis: Elsevier.

Cannon, S., & Boswell, C. (2016). *Evidence-based teaching in nursing: A foundation for educators* (2nd ed.). Burlington, MA: Jones & Bartlett Learning.

Christensen, L. S., & Simmons, L. E. (2020). *The scope of practice for academic nurse educators and academic clinical nurse educators.* Washington, DC: National League for Nursing.

Dave, R. H. (1970). Psychomotor levels. In R. J. Armstrong (Ed.), *Developing and writing behavioral objectives* (pp. 20–21). Tucson: Educational Innovators Press.

Krathwohl, D. R., Bloom, B. S., & Masia, B. B. (1964). *Taxonomy of educational objectives: Handbook II: Affective domain.* New York: David McKay.

McDonald, M. (2018). *The nurse educator's guide to assessing learning outcomes.* Burlington, MA: Jones & Bartlett Learning.

National League for Nursing. (2020). *NLN fair testing guidelines for nursing education.* www.nln.org/fairtestingguidelines.

Oermann, M., & Gaberson, K. (2021). *Evaluation and testing in nursing education* (6th ed.). New York: Springer Publishing.

CHAPTER 4 Practice Questions

1. When conducting an evaluation, the nurse educator recognizes that the first step in the evaluation process is which of the following?
   A. Selecting an internal or external evaluator
   B. Choosing an evaluation framework or model
   C. Selecting an evaluation instrument
   D. Identifying the purpose of the evaluation

2. The nurse educator is observing learners in the clinical lab practicing a new skill. As the learners practice performing the skill, the educator observes and provides feedback. The educator is conducting which type of evaluation?
   A. Norm-referenced evaluation
   B. Formative evaluation
   C. Summative evaluation
   D. High-stakes evaluation

3. A group of three faculty members are team-teaching a nursing course. Which of the following is necessary for maintaining fairness and eliminating bias in the grading of assignments?
   A. Interrater reliability
   B. Instrument validity
   C. Formative evaluation
   D. Learner evaluations

4. The new nurse educator wants to design an activity to assess learning in the cognitive, affective, and psychomotor domains. Which of the following would be the best method for concurrently assessing learning in all three domains?
   A. Reflective journaling
   B. Essay
   C. Patient simulation
   D. Concept mapping

5. A new nurse educator needs follow-up from the mentor after making which of the following statements?
   A. "I will use summative evaluation to determine achievement of course objectives."
   B. "I will use classroom assessment techniques for formative assessments of learning."
   C. "I can use formative assessments to adapt my teaching to better accommodate student learning."
   D. "I will use formative assessments to determine final course grades for my students."

6. The nurse educator is designing a reflection paper assignment to evaluate learning. Which of the following does the nurse educator know to be true regarding reflection papers?
   A. Reflection papers can be used to effectively evaluate learning in the psychomotor domain.
   B. Reflection papers can be used to evaluate high-level cognitive and affective domains of learning.
   C. Reflection papers can foster collaboration and interaction among learner groups.
   D. Reflection papers do not allow for assessment of critical thinking skills needed for nursing practice.

7. The nurse educator is developing muddiest points as a classroom activity to assess what is still unclear to learners after content is presented. This activity represents which type of evaluation?
   A. Summative evaluation
   B. Norm-referenced evaluation
   C. Formative evaluation
   D. Criterion-referenced evaluation

8. Which of the following would be the most important consideration for a nurse educator when deciding which assessment tools to use in a course?
   A. The assessment tools measure the course learning outcomes.
   B. The assessment tools measure the program learning outcomes.
   C. The assessment tools measure what the nurse educator thinks is important.
   D. The assessment tools measure specified outcomes from the accrediting body.

9. The nurse educator is designing a grading rubric for a concept map assignment. Which of the following is a critical component that must be included in a rubric?
   A. Measurement of affective behaviors
   B. Evidence of observation
   C. Multiple-choice items
   D. Explanation of each level of performance

10. The nurse educator is discussing facilitating a clinical group with another faculty member. The nurse educator states, "I do not know how to keep track of all of the observational data I gather." What would be the best response by the faculty member?
    A. "You should not keep any notes; address any concerns with learners immediately."
    B. "You do not need to keep track of observational data for clinical performance."
    C. "Keep detailed notes in a secure location regarding each learner."
    D. "You should always have your phone available to keep notes on each learner."

11. A nurse educator has asked colleagues to collaborate on creating a grading rubric for a shared assessment. What is the most important reason that the nurse educators should work together to create the rubric?
    A. To avoid using the same rubric
    B. To establish interrater reliability
    C. To ensure that faculty members can create their own rubric
    D. To ensure the statistics are appropriate

12. Graduate nursing faculty are considering methods to conduct summative evaluation on nurse practitioner students for their clinical experience in a course. Which of the following assessment methods is the best choice?
    A. Portfolio showing learning in each course
    B. Final clinical evaluation tool
    C. Self-evaluation tool
    D. Grading rubric

13. The novice nurse educator is developing clinical learning outcomes for a course. Which of the following outcomes is appropriate for the clinical learning environment?
    A. Demonstrate skill in using patient care technologies.
    B. Develop advanced knowledge and skills in caring for patients across the lifespan.
    C. Demonstrate safe, holistic care of the patient with chronic heart failure.
    D. Independently administer medications to a group of older patients.

14. The nurse educator is evaluating a learner in the clinical setting through observation. The learner disregards aseptic technique while working with a patient. What is the appropriate action by the nurse educator?
    A. Document this instance to review with the learner in the final clinical evaluation tool.
    B. Wait to address the issue in postconference with the clinical group.
    C. Immediately give the learner feedback in front of the patient.
    D. Ensure privacy for the learner to provide feedback.

15. The nurse educator is mentoring a novice educator regarding clinical evaluation. Which statement by the novice educator requires follow-up from the mentor?
    A. "I should keep secure notes to help me adequately evaluate learners."
    B. "Learners should be receiving regular feedback as they progress through their clinical experience."
    C. "The clinical setting only evaluates learners in the psychomotor domain."
    D. "I should discuss clinical objectives with the learners to foster understanding."

16. The nurse educator is analyzing a unit exam. The KR-20 for the exam is 0.81. How should the nurse educator interpret the KR-20 value?
    A. This exam is reliable.
    B. This exam requires major revision.
    C. This exam requires revision for a few items.
    D. This exam is valid.

17. The nurse educator is concerned about the reliability of an exam. Which of the following characteristics could cause poor reliability?
    A. 40 questions on the exam
    B. 15 learners taking the exam
    C. 60 minutes to take the exam
    D. 77% average score on the exam

18. The nurse educator is analyzing exam statistics. The KR-20 for the exam is 0.49. How should the nurse educator interpret this KR-20?
    A. Good exam reliability
    B. Adequate exam validity
    C. Poor exam reliability
    D. Poor exam discrimination

19. The nurse educator is sharing with the novice nurse educator how to create an exam blueprint. The novice nurse educator asks, "Why is it necessary to create an exam blueprint when I know what I want to ask on the exam?" What is the appropriate response?
    A. "It is nice to have an exam blueprint in case administration needs it."
    B. "An exam blueprint can tell if reliability is met."
    C. "An exam blueprint can provide item discrimination."
    D. "An exam blueprint can help ensure content-related validity."

20. The nurse educator is monitoring continuous assessment of exam validity over several semesters and notes that learners seem to score poorly on alternate format items. What factor should the nurse educator consider to increase validity?
    A. Provide clearer directions.
    B. Remove alternate format items.
    C. Rewrite alternate format items.
    D. Poor scores on items do not affect validity.

21. The novice nurse educator is learning about analysis of exams. Which statement by the educator is incorrect regarding exam analysis?
    A. "I should make necessary adjustments to individual items based on analysis."
    B. "I should use the data gathered to improve the exam."
    C. "I should ensure that all learners pass the exam."
    D. "I should conduct an analysis on each individual exam item."

22. The nurse educator reviews the following statistics for a multiple-choice test item:

Test Item Choice	p Level	Point Biserial
A	0.18	−0.09
B	0.11	0.15
C (CORRECT RESPONSE)	0.62	0.23
D	0.09	−0.30

What choice should the nurse educator change before using this test item again?
    A. Choice A
    B. Choice B
    C. Choice C
    D. Choice D

23. The nurse educator reviews the following statistics for a multiple-choice test item:

Test Item Choice	p Level	Point Biserial
A (CORRECT RESPONSE)	0.56	0.41
B	0.20	0.01
C	0.12	−0.24
D	0.12	−0.37

Based on the item analysis, which statement by the nurse educator is correct?
    A. This item requires no revision.
    B. The distractors for this item should be revised.
    C. This item should be nullified.
    D. The correct response for this item should be revised.

24. During an exam analysis, the nurse educator notes that a test item has a p level of 0.35. How should this p level be interpreted?
    A. The item needs to be nullified.
    B. 65% of learners answered the item correctly.
    C. 35% of learners answered the item correctly.
    D. This is an acceptable p value.

25. The nurse educator notes that the mean score on an exam is 90%. How should the nurse educator interpret this finding?
    A. This is an appropriate finding.
    B. This indicates the exam was too difficult.
    C. This indicates the exam was too easy.
    D. The exam should be nullified.

26. The nurse reviews the following statistics regarding a multiple-choice test item:

Test Item Choice	p Level	Point Biserial
A	0.00	0.00
B (CORRECT RESPONSE)	1.00	0.00
C	0.00	0.00
D	0.00	0.00

What action should the nurse educator take based on the statistics for this test item before using it again?
A. Revise the distractors.
B. Take no action, as learners scored well.
C. Revise the correct response.
D. Nullify this item.

27. The novice nurse educator is discussing the KR-20 of an exam. Which statement by the novice nurse educator requires intervention?
A. "Test reliability is good if it is above 0.70."
B. "The KR-20 will help me predict exam validity."
C. "A KR-20 can range from 0.00 to 1.00."
D. "A KR-20 can help me understand exam consistency."

28. The nurse educator reviews the following statistics for a multiple-choice test item:

Test Item Choice	p Level	Point Biserial
A	0.13	−0.40
B (CORRECT RESPONSE)	0.57	0.34
C	0.14	−0.31
D	0.16	−0.27

Which of the following statements is true regarding these test item statistics?
A. 57% of learners got this test item incorrect.
B. This test item shows a high level of validity.
C. Low-scoring learners chose Choice B.
D. This is a highly discriminating test item.

29. The nurse educator reviews the following statistics for a multiple-choice test item:

Test Item Choice	p Value	Point Biserial
A	0.06	−0.14
B	0.20	0.19
C (CORRECT RESPONSE)	0.64	0.31
D	0.10	−0.27

Which choice should the nurse educator revise based on these statistics?
A. Choice A
B. Choice B
C. Choice C
D. Choice D

30. A nurse educator who relies on learning outcomes and objectives to evaluate courses, lessons, or programs uses which of the following philosophical approaches to evaluation?
A. Service approach
B. Constructivist approach
C. Judgment approach
D. Outcomes approach

31. The nurse educator is designing evaluation methods for the course student learning outcome "Distinguish between personal and professional values and legal/ethical responsibilities in practice." Which of these evaluation strategies would be most appropriate to use?
A. Checklist
B. Test question
C. Paper
D. Questionnaire

32. The new nurse educator is designing an activity to evaluate mastery of the learning outcomes. Which of the following activities would be most appropriate to use?
A. Criterion-referenced test
B. Reflection journal
C. Formative assessment
D. Norm-referenced test

33. The nurse educator uses the following test item to evaluate which level of the cognitive domain:

A client is reporting a cough for 2 weeks and discomfort in the chest when taking a deep breath. Which action will the nurse take first?
A. *Notify the physician immediately.*
B. *Encourage the client to cough and deep-breathe once every hour.*
C. *Perform a respiratory assessment on the client.*
D. *Provide pain medicine to alleviate discomfort.*

A. Remembering
B. Understanding
C. Applying
D. Analyzing

34. The nurse educator wants to assess student learning after teaching a didactic lesson on nursing theorists. What type of assessment should the educator perform at this time?
A. Summative assessment
B. Formative assessment
C. Criterion-referenced assessment
D. Norm-referenced assessment

35. The nurse educator is designing learning activities for student learning outcomes. Which of the following student learning outcomes is written at the understanding level of the cognitive domain?
A. Describe the signs and symptoms of Bell palsy.
B. Formulate a plan of care for the pregnant client.
C. Summarize how to conduct a health history.
D. Identify screening tests for colorectal cancer.

36. The nurse educator is using the test blueprint to create a unit examination. What is the purpose of using a test blueprint?
    A. It confirms interrater reliability of the test.
    B. It helps assess the students' readiness to learn.
    C. It provides evidence of item discrimination.
    D. It helps establish content-related validity.

37. A new nurse educator needs additional mentoring after making which of the following statements?
    A. "I have created a reflective journal activity to evaluate the affective domain."
    B. "I plan to evaluate critical thinking using test questions in the high-level cognitive domain."
    C. "I have developed a checklist for evaluating skills in the psychomotor domain."
    D. "I will have learners develop a concept map so that I can evaluate the psychomotor domain."

38. The instructor wants to assess the learning objective, "The learner will be able to demonstrate the technique of inserting a urinary catheter." Which is the best method for assessment of this objective?
    A. Give a short quiz on sterile catheter insertion.
    B. Place learners in small groups for discussion.
    C. Ask learners to perform insertion on a simulation mannequin.
    D. Have learners write a short essay on catheter insertion.

39. The course coordinator wants to ensure that all instructors are grading the learners' scholarly papers fairly and equally. Which of the following evaluation methods would be most appropriate to use?
    A. Grading rubric
    B. Likert scale
    C. Test blueprint
    D. Peer evaluation

40. The nurse educator designs a summative clinical evaluation tool. Which of the following assessments would be appropriate for this tool?
    A. Performance of clinical skills at midterm
    B. Achievement of learning outcomes at the end of the semester
    C. Learners' perceptions of the clinical site
    D. Learning after providing a lesson on sterile technique

41. The new nurse educator is creating assignments to assess the objective, "The learner will identify factors that can affect or alter mobility." Which assignment would be best in assessing this objective?
    A. Have learners demonstrate the proper use of canes and walkers.
    B. Have learners create a care plan for a client with a hip replacement.
    C. Provide a quiz that includes factors that can alter mobility.
    D. Have learners perform active range of motion on a partner.

42. The nurse educator is writing test questions to evaluate that the medication administration objective was met. Which type of test question would be best for assessing at the application level of the cognitive domain?
    A. Calculate the proper dose of acetaminophen for a pediatric patient.
    B. Match the name of the pediatric medication with the correct classification.
    C. Identify the side effects of common pediatric antibiotics.
    D. List the common administration sites for pediatric intramuscular injections.

43. The novice educator and mentor are creating a test to assess student learning. Which of the following statements made by the novice educator requires further guidance from the mentor?
    A. "I will use the test blueprint to make sure I am testing the appropriate content objectives."
    B. "I will make sure the distractor options are reasonable and viable."
    C. "I will use action verbs that are consistent with the cognitive process being measured."
    D. "I will develop a test blueprint after writing the test questions and provide it to the students."

44. Nursing faculty want to ensure that learners have achieved the program learning outcomes. What would be the best method for summative evaluation of learning outcomes at the end of a program?
    A. Require learners to take a comprehensive final exam to evaluate learning in the cognitive domain.
    B. Have learners maintain a comprehensive portfolio of assignments throughout the program.
    C. Require achievement of a benchmark score on a high-stakes examination before graduation.
    D. Require learners to submit a self-reflection paper of their achievement of program outcomes.

45. What is the primary characteristic of admission policies for a nursing program?
    A. Policies are necessary to prevent learners from filing grade grievances.
    B. Policies are only modified based on changes in health care delivery.
    C. Policies must be ethically sound and based on current evidence.
    D. Policies help provide feedback to learners about their progress in the program.

46. The nurse educator has an obligation to incorporate current research and evidence-based education methods. What is the primary purpose of incorporating current evidence into the nursing student's education?
    A. To ensure that students receive an education that prepares them to be competent in practice
    B. To demonstrate nurse educator scholarship for promotion and tcnurc
    C. To help develop student competencies in the clinical setting to meet accreditation standards
    D. To help demonstrate expertise in all methods of assessment and evaluation

47. The nurse educator is designing evaluation strategies for a new course in a graduate program. To evaluate student learning, the most significant factor influencing the development of evaluation strategies would be which of the following?
    A. Most recent pass rates on the certification exam
    B. Current trends in the health care system
    C. Student learning outcomes
    D. Students' learning styles

48. Classroom assessment techniques can effectively be used for which of the following?
    A. For summative assessment of course learning outcomes
    B. To determine final course grades
    C. As an alternative to a comprehensive final examination
    D. As a formative assessment of student learning

49. A nurse educator who tends to use the judgment philosophical perspective when evaluating learners in the clinical laboratory setting would do which of the following?
    A. Evaluate the learners on the achievement of course objectives.
    B. Use a holistic approach to identify the strengths and weaknesses of learners.
    C. Focus on evaluation of learners using a pass/fail approach.
    D. Use peer evaluations for learner performance.

50. The nurse educator is reviewing a multiple-choice test item with the following statistics:

Test Item Choice	p Level	Point Biserial
A	0.00	0.00
B	0.00	0.00
C	0.49	0.15
D (CORRECT RESPONSE)	0.51	0.20

Which of the following statements is true regarding this test item?
    A. This is an acceptable test item.
    B. The learners were able to guess the correct answer.
    C. This item requires revision of all of the choices.
    D. This item is highly discriminating.

51. The nurse educator is reviewing a multiple-choice test item with the following statistics:

Test Item Choice	p Level	Point Biserial
A	0.11	−0.36
B	0.12	−0.07
C (CORRECT RESPONSE)	0.59	−0.14
D	0.18	0.20

Which of the following statements is true regarding this test item?
    A. Learners who scored lower on the exam got this test item correct.
    B. Learners were able to guess the correct answer to this test item.
    C. This is a highly discriminating test item.
    D. This test item demonstrates a high level of validity.

52. The nurse educator is reviewing a multiple-choice test item with the following statistics:

Test Item Choice	p Level	Point Biserial
A (CORRECT RESPONSE)	0.37	−0.36
B	0.00	0.00
C	0.40	0.14
D	0.23	−0.21

Which of the following actions should the nurse educator take based on these statistics?
    A. This test item is appropriate and does not require any action.
    B. Accept Choices A and C.
    C. Nullify this test item.
    D. Change the correct response to C.

53. The novice nurse educator states, "I can discard all of my learner assessment and evaluation data at the end of each course." What is the best response by the mentor?
    A. "You are correct, there is no need to keep data, as it is not necessary."
    B. "You should keep data to turn in to the university at the end of each semester."
    C. "You should wait 1 year to throw out all data regarding assessment and evaluation."
    D. "You should keep data to compare over time to enhance the teaching and learning process."

54. A novice nurse educator is unsure whether a new exam is valid and should be used. Which of the following options should the nurse educator consider in helping to evaluate validity?
    A. Consult with the academic affairs unit on campus.
    B. Consult with a clinical expert in the area being tested.
    C. Consult with faculty outside of nursing.
    D. Consult with learners after the exam is administered.

55. A nursing program is investigating the use of standardized testing as an addition to the curriculum. Which of the following factors is most important to consider when analyzing standardized testing products?
   A. A standardized testing product should be chosen based on cost to learners.
   B. Programs can choose a standardized testing company based on their own personal preferences.
   C. Standardized tests can replace the testing created and administered by nurse educators, which will save time on preparing exams.
   D. Testing, administration, and evaluation information must be available for learners.

56. The novice nurse educator tells the mentor that assessment grading rubrics for papers are not provided to learners until they have feedback. How should the mentor respond to this situation?
   A. "It is important to provide clear evaluation data early so that learners know how to achieve the objectives."
   B. "Learners do not need access to rubrics. You are correct to keep them confidential."
   C. "You should provide the rubric to learners 1 week in advance of the paper due date."
   D. "Provide the evaluation data to the learners who ask because they are the ones who care about their grade."

Participating in Curricular Design and Evaluation of Program Outcomes

SUSAN ANDERSEN

LEARNING OUTCOMES

1. Describe components of the curriculum development and revision process.
2. Discuss the role of the academic nurse educator in curricular design and revision.
3. Explain the program assessment process, including the systematic plan for program evaluation.
4. Identify relevant sources of evidence for informing curriculum and program assessment.

The academic nurse educator is responsible for participating in curriculum design that reflects current health care trends, focuses on societal needs, reflects current issues in nursing, and prepares graduates to function effectively as generalist or advanced practice nurses in today's complex and dynamic health care environment. Curriculum design must be grounded in evidence and incorporate current educational principles and theories of adult learning. The educator is also responsible for continuous, data-driven evaluation of the curriculum to ensure quality and achievement of learning outcomes. This evaluation process drives curricular revision when indicated.

Demonstrating Knowledge of Curriculum Development

One of the most important responsibilities of the academic nurse educator is curriculum development and revision. Educators need to be skilled at designing an effective curriculum that guides learners toward achievement of desired end-of-program learning outcomes (EOPLOs) and reflects current nursing practice trends such that graduates are adequately prepared for generalist or advanced practice. The nursing curriculum should be faculty-driven and begins with a review of the mission/vision of the educational institution and nursing program. Faculty then outline their beliefs and values about nursing and nursing education into a program, department, or college of nursing philosophy, as discussed later in this chapter. The *philosophy* should flow from the mission/vision and direct the development or revision of the curriculum (DeBoor, 2023). The nursing faculty may decide to also create a *conceptual* or *organizing framework* to identify core themes or concepts that are emphasized in the curriculum. Nursing programs often build their curriculum in alignment with Quality and Safety Education for Nursing (QSEN) competencies, including patient-centered care, evidence-based practice, and safety. These competencies can then be aligned with the EOPLOs for new graduates.

After developing these foundational components, the academic nurse educator develops a curricular road map that guides learners through the program toward achievement of the EOPLOs. Desired competencies that reflect the knowledge, skills, and attitudes learners need to develop to attain EOPLOs are leveled throughout the program. Learning activities, clinical activities, and evaluation strategies are selected that are appropriate for the level of the learner, engage the learner, and adequately measure achievement of learning. The nurse educator must demonstrate knowledge in all areas of curriculum design and evaluation to build a relevant, leveled, and effective curriculum.

Identifying Program Outcomes

Program outcomes (POs) include curricular outcomes that are achieved by learners by the end of the program (EOPLOs) and additional outcomes that indicate program effectiveness and are measured after graduation. All state and accreditation standards for nursing education programs require that programs measure both types of POs on the systematic plan for evaluation (SPE). This quality improvement process is described later in this chapter.

Identifying *EOPLOs* for the learners to achieve by graduation is one of the first steps in the curricular design process. EOPLOs are broad competency statements that reflect the philosophy and conceptual/organizing framework for the program and define learning expectations for graduates (Billings & Halstead, 2020; DeBoor, 2023). EOPLOs are most often referred to as *program learning outcomes* (PLOs). Depending on the type of program, a nursing program usually has between 6 and 10 PLOs. The essential knowledge, skills, and attitudes expected for contemporary practice may change over time based on new practices and trends, but PLOs are generally broad enough to remain current (Billings & Halstead, 2020; Iwasiw et al., 2020). Examples of typical PLOs for varying levels of nursing programs are shown in Table 5.1.

Academic nurse educators should examine a variety of sources when developing PLOs. National standards relevant to the type of program are often reviewed and used as a basis for developing PLOs. For example, baccalaureate and graduate nursing programs typically use the American Association of Colleges of Nursing (AACN) *Essentials: Core Competencies for Professional Nursing Education* (2021) and incorporate the broad competency areas delineated in this document into the PLOs. The National League for Nursing (NLN) developed *Outcomes and Competencies for Graduates of Practical/Vocational, Associate, Baccalaureate, Master's Practice Doctorate, and Research Doctorate in Nursing* (2012), which defines nursing outcomes, competencies, skills, and behaviors for programs at each of these levels.

TABLE 5.1	Program Learning Outcome Examples Related to Patient Safety and Quality From Varying Levels of Nursing Education
Type of Program	**Program Learning Outcome**
Practical/Vocational Nursing	Demonstrate safety and effectiveness in performance of nursing skills. Jersey College
Associate Degree in Nursing	Apply clinical competence in the provision of patient-centered care. Denver College of Nursing
Baccalaureate of Science in Nursing	Provide safe, high-quality nursing care using principles of leadership, quality improvement, and patient safety to improve patient outcomes. New York University Rory Meyers College of Nursing
Master of Science Degree in Nursing	Guide the planning, development, and evaluation of exemplary patient-centered care that values the dignity of all humans and reflects advanced, comprehensive knowledge, insight, and commitment to culturally competent care of unique individuals in a global society. Elms College School of Nursing
Doctor of Nursing Practice	Design, implement, and evaluate evidence-based quality improvement methods to promote safe, ethical, and equitable patient care. Bay Path University

CNE®/CNE®n Key Point

Remember: Program learning outcomes (PLOs) are broad competency statements that reflect the philosophy and conceptual/organizing framework for a nursing program and define learning expectations for graduates.

Review of accreditation requirements is also important when developing curricular outcomes to ensure the ability to meet all required standards. For example, the Accreditation Commission for Education in Nursing (ACEN, 2020) requires that the curriculum and its PLOs incorporate national standards, guidelines, and competencies. The ACEN also requires that the curriculum and PLOs be developed and regularly reviewed by faculty and:

- Incorporate cultural, ethnic, and socially diverse concepts
- Reflect regional, national, and global perspectives
- Be grounded in educational theory
- Include interprofessional collaboration

Academic nurse educators should review the relevant scope of practice for the state in which the program is approved when designing PLOs. Each state board of nursing outlines guidelines and expectations for nursing programs and graduates. Some states have a core curriculum for certain types of programs and/or a required list of PLOs. For example, Kansas has developed and mandated PLOs for both the state's practical nursing and associate degree nursing programs. These outcomes were developed by the Kansas State Board of Regents (KBOR) with participation by program advisory committee members from Kansas colleges and employers of new graduates to create preferred sets of outcomes for new graduates. Accreditation guidelines and national standards were integrated into these outcomes.

Nurse educators should meet with external stakeholders such as clinical partners, community organizations, faculty, and student alumni to gain perspective on current practice expectations and community needs. This information helps educators develop PLOs that are relevant and future focused. Societal trends should be examined to lend guidance for developing relevant PLOs. For example, the COVID-19 pandemic greatly increased the need for telehealth and e-health resources for providing care. It is expected that this method for providing care will continue to be implemented beyond the pandemic, as many have found this an effective and efficient method for providing care. It is important to identify PLOs that include requiring new graduate competence in implementing a variety of technologies to provide care in the current complex health care environment.

To be effective, PLOs need to be evidence-based, informed by key stakeholders, meet state and accreditation standards, reflect current societal and health care trends, and maintain congruence with both the institution and program for which they are developed. Once developed, faculty must then create a *plan of study* (often called a *degree plan*) with observable, measurable course outcomes that describe the actual knowledge, skills, and attitudes the learners should demonstrate as they progress toward achievement of PLOs. The plan of study outlines the sequence of courses, with credit allocations for each course, that must be completed before graduation from the program.

Additional POs that measure program effectiveness include first-time pass rates on either the NCLEX® (for prelicensure graduates) or certification exams (for advanced practice graduates), employment rates, and program completion rates. These outcomes are discussed later in this chapter as part of program assessment and evaluation.

Developing Competency Statements

Competency statements are the actual knowledge, skills, and attitudes that learners need to demonstrate achievement of the PLOs. These competencies are stated as course, clinical, and content student learning outcomes and are typically listed on each course syllabus. Learners must meet these competencies to pass the course (Iwasiw et al., 2020).

Developing course outcomes requires careful planning and input from all faculty across the program. Each nursing course must provide the best context for achieving the desired outcomes. For example, if a course does not include care of intrapartum patients, it would not be appropriate to require an outcome for assessment and care of a laboring patient. Outcomes for each course are leveled as they build across the curriculum toward final achievement of the PLOs. In leveling these outcomes, the academic nurse educator needs to consider the level of the learner, the level of behavior appropriate for that learner, and the context in which the learner will demonstrate the competency (Billings & Halstead, 2020). The learner needs to have multiple opportunities to develop the competency at increasing levels of complexity throughout the program to become proficient at the desired end-of-program level.

The academic nurse educator selects the desired behavior or competency suitable for each level of learner in the program (Iwasiw et al., 2020). For example, the nurse educator would not create a competency for first-semester learners that require them to evaluate a plan of care for a patient in the critical care unit because *evaluate* is a high-level taxonomic verb and the patient requires complex care. Instead, it may be more appropriate to ask the first-semester learner to describe basic nursing care to meet the needs of the healthy older adult. *Describe* is a remembering/understanding taxonomic verb and is more appropriate for this level of learner. Providing care for older adults is a common experience for first-semester learners and a relevant context for this type of patient. Table 5.2 displays an example of course outcome leveling, demonstrates increasing levels of Bloom's revised cognitive taxonomy, and shows how each course outcome aligns with a PLO.

After creating outcomes for all courses, the nurse educator teaching each course identifies the content topics and develops content learning outcomes, often referred to as *course objectives*. Course objectives delineate the competencies for learners to demonstrate related to specific course content. Learning activities are then carefully selected that allow learners the opportunity to achieve these objectives.

Writing Course Objectives

Once course outcomes have been delineated, course objectives need to be developed. These objectives are placed in the syllabus or topical outline to communicate to learners the expectations they will need to achieve in the course for each content topic. The objectives operationalize the curriculum and direct all learning activities (Billings & Halstead, 2020). Fig. 5.1 shows the relationship between course objectives, course outcomes, and PLOs within a curriculum.

TABLE 5.2   **Example of Leveling and Alignment of Course Outcomes With Program Learning Outcome for Associate Degree in Nursing Program**

Program Learning Outcome	Semester 1	Semester 2	Semester 3	Semester 4
Prioritize safe, quality, evidence-based nursing care for patients across the lifespan in a variety of health care settings.	Identify the role of the nurse in adhering to safety and quality standards when providing patient care.	Explain the most common national safety and quality standards that guide the delivery of safe, quality, evidence-based nursing care.	Apply knowledge of safety and quality standards to provide evidence-based care for infants, children, and adolescents in acute and community care settings.	Develop a nursing plan of care for a group of patients to ensure safe, quality evidence-based care.
Action Verb	Identify	Explain	Apply	Develop
Level of Bloom's Revised Cognitive Taxonomy	Remembering	Understanding	Applying	Creating

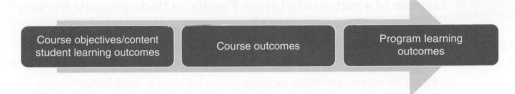

FIG. 5.1 Competency statements: Relationship between course objectives, course learning outcomes, and program learning outcomes.

Course objectives are much more specific than course outcomes. In some institutions, course objectives are referred to as *content student learning outcomes (SLOs), unit objectives, modular objectives,* or *class objectives. Course objectives* should provide the opportunity for achievement of course outcomes and show alignment with one or more of those outcomes. Table 5.3 shows a portion of a faculty plan for teaching the gas exchange exemplar of chronic obstructive pulmonary disease (COPD) in a classroom. This document can be used as a lesson plan for the nurse educator and a study guide for learners; it also specifies how the objectives align with the course outcomes.

One method for developing course objectives is to use the *SMART* acronym. This acronym represents objectives that are Specific, Measurable, Achievable, Relevant, and Timely (University of Buffalo, n.d.). The desired outcome is specific to the desired knowledge, skill, or attitude to be achieved. The outcome is easily measurable. For example, a poor clinical outcome might state: *Students will learn about safety as part of older adult care.* A more appropriate and measurable clinical outcome could state: *Students will apply principles of safety while caring for older adult patients.* Outcomes should be achievable and specify learner competencies. Objectives should be relevant for the desired learning. Finally, SMART objectives are timely and achievable by the end of the course.

Like course outcomes, objectives need to be leveled throughout the program. Course objectives also need to be specified for each context or learning environment—theory (classroom or online), skills laboratory, simulation experience, or clinical experience in a health care agency. Learners need multiple opportunities to develop and advance their knowledge of a particular concept or content topic and should be provided opportunities for applying the content in lab or clinical learning experiences. For didactic course content, use of the revised Bloom's cognitive taxonomy can aid the academic nurse educator in selecting verbs for the objective that are appropriate for the level of learner. All course objectives must be learner-centered and focus on what the learner will achieve in the course rather than what the instructor will do. After course objectives have been developed, the nurse educator can then proceed to determining appropriate learning activities to aid students in their achievement.

Selecting Appropriate Learning Activities

Once course outcomes and objectives have been developed, it is then important for the academic nurse educator to select and/or develop learning activities that are appropriate for helping learners meet the content or clinical objectives. This is an opportunity for the educator to use creativity to develop activities that inspire learning and actively engage the learner in achieving the objectives (Iwasiw et al., 2020). Learners need to participate in activities that help them advance their thinking and determine the link between theory and clinical practice (Billings & Halstead, 2020).

The educator needs to ensure the selected *learning activities* promote achievement of desired course objectives. Learners should be informed through the lesson plan why the learning activity was selected and how it aligns with course objectives (see Table 5.3). Additionally, if a learning activity is evaluated or graded, learners should be provided a grading rubric or other grading system.

Many factors should be considered when selecting learning activities most appropriate for the desired course objective. Case studies, simulation scenarios, in-class or online discussions,

TABLE 5.3	**Example of a Portion of a Lesson Plan for an Undergraduate Nursing Program**[a]			
Exemplar/ Topic	Course Objectives/Content Student Learning Outcome	Related Course Outcomes	Learning Activities/Assessment	Evaluation Methods
Gas exchange: COPD	1. Recall the introduction to gas exchange, including anatomy and physiology. 2. Explain the pathophysiology of COPD as it affects gas exchange, including risk factors. 3. Outline the role of the nurse in caring for patients with COPD having diagnostic testing to measure gas exchange. 4. Apply knowledge of pathophysiology to document assessment findings for the patient with COPD to determine the status of gas exchange. 5. Use nursing judgment to plan safe, evidence-based care to promote gas exchange in the patient with COPD. 6. Apply knowledge of pharmacology to delineate nursing implications for administering drug therapy used to promote gas exchange in the patient with COPD. 7. Plan collaborative care with the health care team to coordinate and improve gas exchange in the patient with COPD. 8. Apply knowledge of pathophysiology to reduce potentially life-threatening complications of COPD that affect gas exchange and perfusion. 9. Plan health teaching for the patient and family to manage transitions in care, including smoking cessation if applicable, to promote gas exchange. 10. Explain the professional role of the nurse in assisting patients and families with end-of-life and palliative care for patients with COPD.	1, 2, 5	Before class: • Complete gas exchange worksheet and bring to class #1). (NOTE: May use as an admit ticket.) • Review respiratory system with focus on ventilation and diffusion of gases. • Read COPD section in textbook. • Review chapter on end of life in textbook. During class: • Have learners pair up and draw a graphic to demonstrate what happens with the pathophysiology of COPD. Be prepared to explain this graphic in class. (#2) • Use audience response questions. (#3) • Assign an unfolding case study in small groups. (#4–#6, #8, #9) • Create drug cards for assigned selected prototype bronchodilators. (#6) • Take NCLEX® Practice Test Items. (#6–#7) • Assign 3Rs (Recognize, Respond, and Rescue) activity on cor pulmonale in small groups. (#8) After class: • Participate in the online discussion forum about ethics and end-of-life care. (#10)	• Worksheet worth a possible 1 point • Unit exam questions on Exam #1 • Discussion forum due before next class; 3 points possible (see rubric)

[a]Courtesy Donna Ignatavicius.
COPD, Chronic obstructive pulmonary disease.

concept maps, skills demonstrations, pair activities, and group work are just some of the many options available to nurse educators. Additionally, there are many virtual and online activities that allow students to apply learning in a simulated environment. Questions to consider include: What is the mode or setting for instruction: online, class, clinical, or laboratory? Does the activity match the program's educational philosophy? What type of activity is most appropriate for teaching the identified content? For example, journaling in the clinical learning environment is a very effective method for aiding learners in developing and recognizing professional attitudes and beliefs for nursing. What learning activity is most appropriate for each level of student? What technology and/or software is required, and are there any barriers or extreme expenses for learners related to the activity? What type of equipment might be needed, and is it easily available?

Learning activities should be varied to maintain interest and appeal to a wide range of diverse learners. It is widely known in higher education that active strategies promote increased learning and long-term retention of material for retrieval when needed. Learning activities should be selected that provide an environment for active engagement of the student in applying the information learned. See Chapter 2 for further information on facilitating learning and learning activities.

Selecting Appropriate Clinical Experiences

Once competencies are developed for clinical courses, the nurse educator must select experiences that provide the opportunity for learners to meet these outcomes. In clinical practice, students apply the theory they have learned so that they may engage in developing the essential knowledge, skills, and attitudes needed for generalist or advanced practice. Clinical experiences should be leveled across the curriculum, increasing in complexity over time. For example, early in a prelicensure program learners may care for one patient and by the end of the program may coordinate care for multiple patients. Learners in the first nursing semester provide care for patients with common and predictable health care conditions, whereas learners near the end of the program care for patients who are experiencing multisystem and complex health care conditions. In advanced practice nursing programs such as those preparing nurse practitioners, students begin learning primary diagnoses for less complex patients and then progress to managing patients who have multiple health problems, often complicated by challenging social and psychological issues.

Clinical nurse educators need to prepare for the wide range of diverse learners in most nursing programs. Learners differ in cultural backgrounds, age-groups, racial/ethnic groups, gender identity, health care experience, prior degrees, technologic backgrounds, and preferred learning styles. It is important for the nurse educator to balance these varying learner attributes and preferences while maintaining experiences that ensure *inclusivity* and align with the curriculum (Billings & Halstead, 2020). (See Chapter 3 for further discussion.)

Clinical experiences for learners need to be provided in the setting with the most appropriate type of patient that supports achievement of course outcomes. For example, if the course outcome is to use clinical judgment to care for multiple complex-care patients, an outpatient clinic setting would not likely help learners meet this outcome. Learners need the opportunity to care for a wide range of diverse populations to gain experience in effectively working with patients of all types of backgrounds.

Objectives for *interprofessional collaboration* require that learners be provided the opportunity to observe, discuss, and participate in this activity during their clinical experience. It is widely expected that nurses be effective in collaborating and communicating with the interprofessional team to provide optimal patient care.

Clinical learning activities are determined by the clinical objectives for the day or as a focused learning activity (FLA) in which a specific skill is selected for learners to perform for a particular day (Billings & Halstead, 2020; Ignatavicius, 2019). A clinical objective for the clinical experience could be to develop five patient priority needs based on data from a head-to-toe assessment, review of diagnostic tests, and review of health history. An FLA could be to complete Morse Fall Risk Scales for five different patients to determine risk and develop plans for patient safety. Clinical objectives and FLAs should directly align with a course outcome or objective and provide students the opportunity to apply what they have learned in class to the clinical area.

Selecting Appropriate Evaluation Strategies

Evaluation of student learning involves gathering data from a variety of strategies to make a judgment about the learner's achievements. To be effective and comprehensive, the evaluation process includes the need to (Billings & Halstead, 2020; Oermann & Gaberson, 2021):
- Identify the purpose of the learning objectives to be assessed
- Match the evaluation strategy to the learning outcome (e.g., skill performance cannot be demonstrated with multiple-choice exams)

- Consider the setting in which the learning and evaluation will occur (e.g., a chaotic clinical breakroom may not be the best environment for a drug calculation quiz that requires concentration and focus)
- Determine the best procedure for the evaluation (e.g., for an online test, consider how test integrity will be maintained)
- Be valid, reliable, and overall effective (e.g., consider how test item performance will be evaluated to determine effectiveness)
- Meet learner needs and provide ongoing feedback on progress
- Use multiple evaluation strategies for each course outcome and course objective, and consider limitations of assessment; keep in mind the limitations of assessment when interpreting the results (e.g., one exam does not fully describe a learner's achievement of a particular course outcome)

Educators should also consider the advantages and disadvantages of using each evaluation strategy. For example, is the strategy time-consuming to implement or too costly? When selecting appropriate evaluation strategies, educators also need to consider which domain of learning is being measured: cognitive, psychomotor, or affective. All domains of learning should be evaluated over the course of the program. Table 5.4 lists examples of evaluation strategies appropriate for each domain.

Evaluation of learning should replicate what the learner will be expected to perform in the real world (Billings & Halstead, 2020). The educator determines whether evaluation should be formative, which occurs throughout the course, or summative, which is an overall evaluation of how the learner performed upon completion of the course or program. Selecting the appropriate evaluation strategy for each course outcome is key in performing accurate measurement of both learner competence and program effectiveness. See Chapter 4 for a more in-depth discussion of student evaluation strategies.

Participating Actively in Curricular Design and Considerations

In addition to teaching responsibilities, all academic nurse educators are responsible for the development and assessment of the nursing curriculum. The curriculum requires continuous review to ensure relevance, currency, and alignment with the mission and philosophy of the institution and academic division. Academic nurse educators must examine their beliefs about teaching/learning and nursing and design a curriculum that is consistent and reflective of this philosophy. The curriculum needs to be evidence-based and reflect educational theory, current nursing standards, and research. Trends in nursing and health care must be considered and

TABLE **5.4** Examples of Evaluation Methods for Each Learning Domain	
Learning Domain	**Examples of Evaluation Methods**
Cognitive: Knowledge/Thinking	Scholarly paper Concept map Quiz Unit examination Discussion board Oral presentation Case study
Psychomotor: Technical "Hands-on" Skills	Direct observation of skill performance in lab, simulation, or clinical agency
Affective: Attitudes/Feelings	Reflective journaling Reflection paper Ethical debate Discussion board

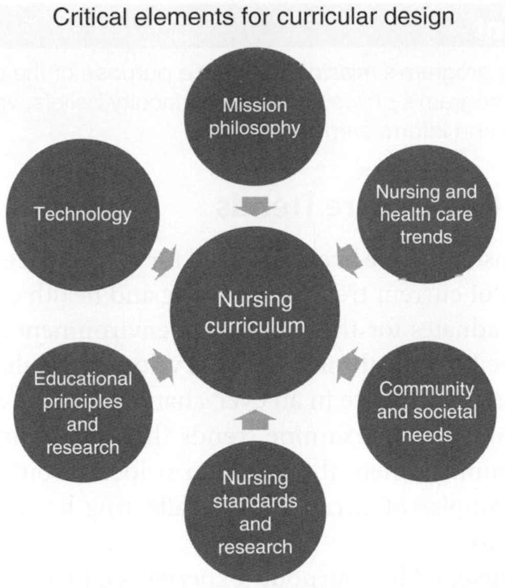

Critical elements for curricular design

FIG. 5.2   Critical elements of an effective nursing curriculum.

addressed. Current societal needs and the status of health in the community must be examined and addressed with the curriculum. Learners need to be able to engage in relevant health care technology for current nursing practice. Fig. 5.2 shows critical elements needed for an effective curricular design.

Philosophy and Mission: Institutional vs. Program

When participating in curricular design, the nurse educator is responsible for regular review of the mission and philosophy statements for the nursing program. Developing or revising the mission and philosophy for a nursing program is a comprehensive process that requires input from the entire faculty. During the review process for the nursing program, the faculty must also review the mission and philosophy statements for the institution and academic division or college to ensure congruence with those of the nursing program or department.

The institutional *mission* statement is a broad statement that describes the purpose for the entire college or university. This statement describes the beliefs and purpose of the institution in preparing graduates. The institutional mission often focuses on education, service, scholarship, and/or research. A nursing program may also be part of an academic division, school, or college that may have an additional mission statement. The nursing program mission statement describes the purpose of the program in preparing nursing graduates to provide care for and improve the health of the community.

The *philosophy* statement for an institution emerges from the mission statement and reflects the beliefs, values, and attitudes of the institution, academic division, or nursing program. It provides the rationale for an organization's existence. Some schools may use value statements to describe their institutional philosophy. The institutional definitions for education, service, scholarship, and/or research are further defined within the philosophy.

As mentioned earlier in this chapter, the nursing program *philosophy statement* is reflective of the faculty's beliefs, values, and attitudes about nursing and serves as a guide to the development of the curriculum. It is not only based on beliefs about nursing but also incorporates faculty beliefs regarding educational theory, nursing theory, evidence-based practices, and standards. These philosophical beliefs and values should be evident throughout the curriculum and reflected in the mission statement, organizing framework, PLOs, and course outcomes. Typical components included in a nursing education *philosophy statement* include faculty's beliefs about professional nursing, adult learning, and the role of the nursing graduate for each program type (Ignatavicius, 2019).

CNE®/CNE®n Key Point

Remember: The nursing program's *mission* states the purpose of the program in preparing nursing graduates. The program's *philosophy* reflects faculty beliefs, values, and attitudes about nursing that guide and inform curriculum.

Current Nursing and Health Care Trends

Once the mission and philosophy have been reviewed for congruence, the academic nurse educator participates in a review of current trends in nursing and health care to develop a curriculum that effectively prepares graduates for the health care environment in which they will practice. Nurse educators need to be forward thinking and develop curriculum that is future focused to anticipate challenges graduates may face in an ever-changing health care environment.

Academic nurse educators should examine trends that are occurring in nursing and health care not only in the community where the program is located but in their state, country, and across the globe. Some examples of current trends affecting health care and nursing practice include but are not limited to:

- Shortage of nurses worsened by "burnout" experienced by new nurses
- Limited growth of nursing school graduates; not keeping pace with societal need for new nurses (programs are often limited by the number of clinical sites they can provide and number of qualified faculty)
- Physician shortages creating high demand for advanced practice nurses
- Outcomes-focused nursing care, quality measures, and patient safety goals
- Collaborative nursing care with the interprofessional team
- Incivility experienced by nurses from patients and colleagues
- Rapid pace of changing patient care technology
- Increased focus on community-based nursing and health care
- Increased focus on health equity, diversity, and inclusivity

Nurse educators also need to examine health care practice trends in their community, nationally, and globally to ensure currency and relevancy of the curriculum for the learners. Current health care practice trends that need to be addressed in the curriculum may include (Billings & Halstead, 2020):

- Health care reform, including access to care, health equity, and inclusivity
- Health care policy, both at the state and national levels
- Global disaster events such as the COVID-19 pandemic of 2020–2022
- Globalization and increased interactions among the world's populations
- Economic issues facing hospitals and health care providers; increasing costs of health care
- Explosion of telehealth and other health care technology
- Health care worker safety
- Ever-changing health care challenges such as emergence of new microbes, resistance of antibiotics, and shortages of needed supplies or medication

Community and Societal Needs

When designing a curriculum, the academic nurse educator must consider the needs of the community and society where graduates will be practicing to adequately prepare them to address those needs. For the curriculum to be relevant and current, the nurse educator needs to incorporate the current needs of the community and society into the curriculum. Examples of community health needs that should be addressed may include:

- Current trends in the health of diverse community residents
- Crime rates and violence
- Prevalence of chronic conditions and types of conditions
- Prevalence of mental health conditions and access to care within the community; risk for suicide

- Health care available within the community and equity and access to care
- Substance use and abuse
- Malnutrition and food insecurity

In addition to local community health-related needs, the educator needs to consider the broader perspective of the societal context in which the graduate will practice. *Healthy People 2030* defines the *social determinants of health (SDOH)* as conditions in the environments where people live that affect health, well-being, and quality of life. *Healthy People 2030* describes examples of SDOH, which include (https://health.gov/healthypeople/objectives-and-data/social-determinants-health):

- Safe housing, transportation, and neighborhoods
- Racism, discrimination, and violence
- Education, job opportunities, and income
- Access to nutritious foods and physical activity opportunities
- Polluted air and water
- Language and literacy skills

CNE®/CNE®n Key Point

Remember: When designing a curriculum, the academic nurse educator must consider the needs of the community and society where graduates will be practicing to adequately prepare them to address those needs. For the curriculum to be relevant and current, the nurse educator needs to incorporate the current needs of the community and society into the curriculum.

Nursing Standards, Theory, and Research

When designing a curriculum, it is important the academic nurse educator incorporate current and relevant nursing standards, theory, and research to design a curriculum that will prepare graduates for successful entry into generalist or advanced practice, as applicable. *Nursing standards* that should be reviewed include but are not limited to (Iwasiw et al., 2020):

- NCLEX® or national certification exam test plan
- Legal and ethical standards
- State approval and accreditation organization standards
- Quality improvement measures
- Evidence-based practice standards for care including national guidelines
- Scope of practice statements for the state or province where the program is located
- White papers and other official statements from national nursing organizations and accrediting bodies
- Reports on nursing from groups such as foundations, governmental agencies, or commissions that make recommendations about nursing practice or nursing education (such as the *Future of Nursing* reports)
- Competencies for *interprofessional collaboration (IPC) and education (IPE)*, including the Interprofessional Education Collaborative (IPEC) Core Competencies

The curriculum needs to be grounded in nursing theory, and an evidence-based *curricular theory* may need to be selected on which to base the curriculum. A traditional approach to organizing curriculum is to use a particular *nursing theory* on which to build the curriculum (Billings & Halstead, 2020). However, nursing theory as a basis for nursing curriculum is not required by most nursing regulatory or accrediting agencies (Ignatavicius, 2019). Examples of nursing theories that may be utilized as theoretical frameworks include *Watson's Theory of Caring* and *Benner's Novice to Expert*. Some programs may use an eclectic framework and a combination of multiple theories on which to base curriculum (Billings & Halstead, 2020). For example, faculty may determine that a combination of both the *Theory of Caring* and *Novice to Expert* provides key principles that would provide a relevant foundation on which to build a prelicensure nursing curriculum.

To develop a curriculum that is contemporary and evidence based, the curriculum must be grounded in *nursing research*. Research of both nursing educational principles and current nursing practice needs to be reviewed. Research of nursing practice and standards ensures the curriculum will adequately prepare the graduate for practice and should include a review of topics such as:

- Concepts related to patient safety
- Coordinated care/transitions of care
- Evidence-based practice
- Leadership skills required for practice
- Nursing care trends
- National standards for care
- Core measures and bundles
- Clinical practice guidelines

Research on nursing educational principles and best practices is also crucial to promote development of a curriculum that is based on best practices in contemporary nursing education. For example, the nurse educator needs to examine nursing educational research when designing a curriculum to determine the best type of curricular model to use to structure the program. Faculty may decide to select a traditional model in which content is blocked around focal areas or a model that may be concept-based. A concept-based model is an evidence-based approach to nursing curriculum that focuses on carefully identified key concepts and exemplars (examples of the desired concept). This method is shown to focus learning by helping students apply patterns of learning and thinking across concepts, thereby preventing nursing content overload (Ignatavicius, 2019).

Educational Principles, Theory, and Research

The nurse educator should incorporate educational principles, theory, and research for adult learning and higher education into any new curricular design. Review of current trends in these areas ensures that the curriculum is based on contemporary and evidence-based teaching methods and is relevant for the adult learner in higher education. Selected educational theories for use in curricular design often seen in contemporary nursing education are briefly summarized in Table 5.5. Chapter 2 describes these theories in more detail.

The educator must research educational literature for best practices in *andragogy* (the education of adults) when developing nursing curriculum. Additionally, educators need to research best practices in teaching and learning to design a curriculum that aligns with these principles. The educator should select the educational principles that best align with the desired curriculum and learning to be achieved. Examples of current practices in andragogy often incorporated into nursing curricula are briefly summarized in Table 5.6.

Use of Technology

One of the more critical and challenging aspects in curricular design is the integration of relevant health care and educational technologies that support student learning and prepare learners to be able to be ready for the technology they will experience upon entry into practice. Nurse educators should research technologies both for nursing practice and to support the design and implementation of the curriculum. When designing the curriculum, the nurse educator must consider where technology can be best integrated to support desired course learning outcomes and ultimately assist learners in achieving PLOs. Technology selection and integration for support of the curriculum takes advanced planning and requires:

- Examination of curriculum for appropriate integration
- Consultation with technology representatives
- Budget development and securing of funding
- Planning for physical space for implementation of technology and storing of equipment
- Faculty and staff positions to implement
- Training for faculty and staff
- Maintenance and upkeep of technologies

TABLE 5.5	Examples of Educational Theories to Support Curriculum Design
Educational Theory	**Defining Characteristics**
Constructivism	Knowledge is created by the learner with the faculty as a guide, builds on prior learning, and requires active engagement by the learner in the learning. An example of a constructivist curriculum is leveling a curriculum so that it would increase in complexity over the length of the program.
Narrative pedagogy	The focus is on the experiences created for students and to help students interpret learning. This theory uses dialogue to help learners process and gain knowledge from experiences. An example of a curriculum that encourages narrative pedagogy would include providing a time for reflection for learners during clinical education to assist them to process the experience of providing patient care.
Adult learning theory	Adult learners are self-motivated, prefer to apply new knowledge to solve real-life problems, and must view the learning as personally relevant. An example of a curriculum grounded in adult learning theory would be providing a curriculum that allows learners to engage in clinical practice to apply their didactic learning to a real-life patient care scenario.
Experiential learning theory	Providing experiences that demand reflection and review about the experience, use abstract thinking to reach conclusions, lead to a decision to act, and allow for engagement in active experimentation or being able to try what was learned. An example of experiential learning theory would be providing simulation experiences for students to practice making clinical judgments.

TABLE 5.6	Examples of Learning Practices in Andragogy for Nursing Education Curriculum Design
Learning Practice Strategy	**Defining Characteristics**
Active learning	The student participates or engages in the learning as opposed to being passive, where the teacher imparts information to be learned.
Concept-based teaching/learning	Concepts are identified for learners to focus on in the clinical environment. The focus is not only on direct patient care but also on critical thinking about the concept being studied. For example, each learner may be asked to assess a patient related to a key concept such as oxygenation. Learners are engaged in a comprehensive examination of the pathophysiology, pharmacology, treatment, and response to patient care through discussion and analysis rather than focusing simply on the nursing skills to be implemented for patients (Billings & Halstead, 2020).
Flipped/scrambled classroom	Learners complete a significant amount of preclass preparation and spend class time in engagement in application of learning material rather than lecture. An adaptation of the flipped classroom is the scrambled classroom, in which small segments of lecture are interspersed with active application activities.
Problem-based learning/team-based learning	Learners work as a team to solve a problem through group interaction and discussion to develop communication and collaboration skills while in class.

Health care technology needs to be selected to aid in preparing learners for the technologic environment in which they will practice. For example, prelicensure students need the opportunity to engage in use of an electronic health record (EHR). Oftentimes clinical sites are unable to grant access to learners to utilize and become familiar with this vital tool. Programs can be prepared for this barrier by purchasing a simulated EHR. The simulated EHR can provide learners unlimited opportunities for researching patient data and developing documentation that can be reviewed by the instructor for feedback. Additionally, learners need to be prepared for patient care technologies, including telehealth and e-health resources. Learners need to be prepared not only to utilize these resources but also to be able to educate patients in the use of these resources.

Simulated clinical care experiences are essential for most nursing education programs due to lack of available clinical experiences and limitations for learners in the actual patient care environment. Simulation replicates practice situations and is an evidence-based alternative to actual clinical experiences (Billings & Halstead, 2020). *Simulation* provides an opportunity for active, experiential learning that helps the student transfer classroom and skills knowledge to a realistic patient care setting in a controlled and safe environment (Billings & Halstead, 2020). The simulation learning environment provides students the opportunity for applying knowledge, solving problems, and developing clinical judgment. Simulation can provide students invaluable learning opportunities for caring for computerized mannequins, manipulating and practicing with equipment such as IV smart pumps, and utilizing computerized documentation. Learners can also practice communication, assessment, and collaboration skills and receive real-time feedback for performance improvement, especially when caring for standardized patients. *Standardized patients* follow a script and allow learners to practice in an authentic relationship. Simulations can be varying levels of fidelity or realism. Levels of fidelity and examples of types of technology are described in Table 5.7.

Creating a simulation environment can be highly complex and expensive. Faculty and staff require significant development on operating, maintaining, and troubleshooting all types of simulation equipment and technology. This environment requires high levels of technologic abilities for educators who may not have a background in this area (Billings & Halstead, 2020).

As previously stated, the cost is steep for this technology, and the technology can become quickly outdated. For example, the recent renovation and update for a community college Simulation Center in Kansas City, KS exceeded $500,000. The life of the computerized mannequin and recording equipment is roughly 4 to 5 years and requires continual upkeep and plans for replacement. The educator must review a wide range of equipment for the simulation environment and search for sources of funding. In addition to high-fidelity mannequins, cameras, microphones, video recording equipment, patient care equipment, and equipment for a simulated clinical setting are also required. The equipment requires a large amount of physical space, not only to conduct simulation but also for storage. Smaller hospital equipment such as IV smart pumps and tubing is also needed and requires additional updates and maintenance. Partnerships with area clinical facilities can aid in providing space or funding so that both agencies can utilize the equipment and simulation center staff. Grant funding can sometimes be obtained.

TABLE **5.7** Levels of Simulation Fidelity and Examples of Technology	
Level of Fidelity	**Examples of Technology**
Low fidelity	Case studies, role-play, task trainers for skill practice (e.g., IV arm), static mannequins; provides learners the opportunity to practice psychomotor/technical skills.
Mid fidelity	Mannequins that have heartbeat and lung sounds but do not have chest rise/fall; provides learners the opportunity to perform psychomotor/technical skills and make decisions as needed.
High fidelity	Human patient simulators, virtual reality, standardized patients; provides learners the opportunity to be fully immersed in realistic clinical care situations.

The academic nurse educator must also research what type of educational technology best supports the design of the curriculum. The educator needs to examine to what extent the technology will be used, the capabilities of the organizational technologic environment, the available funding or space, and what faculty development is needed to implement (DeBoor, 2023). A *Learning Management System* (LMS) needs to be selected and integrated. The LMS provides organization for the course and the learning and provides a standardized and consistent look across courses, which aids students' familiarity with the program learning environment (Iwasiw et al., 2020).

> **CNE®/CNE®n Key Point**
>
> *Remember:* Simulation provides an opportunity for active, experiential learning that helps the student transfer classroom and skills knowledge to a realistic patient care setting in a controlled and safe environment (Billings & Halstead, 2020).

The COVID-19 pandemic created an explosion of technology as educators were suddenly forced to quickly determine methods for delivering nursing education in a distance learning and simulated patient care environment. *Distance learning* is defined as a learner receiving education in a different location than faculty. It may be held synchronously with classmates and faculty or asynchronously where work is assigned; learners often progress at their own pace while meeting assigned deadlines for work. The technology for distance learning requires advanced planning. Faculty need training to be prepared to coordinate the course in this format; faculty and learners need technologic support. Distance learning can include video conferencing, audioconferencing, recorded lectures, asynchronous discussion boards, and podcasts.

Flipped or scrambled classrooms require educational technology to engage students in active learning activities inside and outside of class. Various educational technologies that can be used for learning are widespread and ever changing. Three examples being used currently include Kahoot, Poll Anywhere, and Socrative Questioning. These learning technologies are examples that can aid educators in providing interactive sessions with live learner response on mobile devices during class, where the educator can frequently evaluate the level of learning while engaging learners. When effectively implemented, technology can have a very positive impact on promoting student learning.

Leading the Development of Curriculum Design

Leading the development of curriculum design begins with identification of the leadership structure needed. A single faculty or nurse administrator may be identified as the leader. An outside consultant expert in nursing education may be secured to provide leadership to the process. Or a small group of nurse educators may be identified to lead the process. Nursing faculty are charged with development and/or revision of nursing curriculum, which should be part of their role description in organizational job descriptions (Ignatavicius, 2019). The leader needs to examine potential barriers to and facilitators of curriculum development or revision (Billings & Halstead, 2020). The leader must determine how the work will be completed: by the faculty as a whole or by small subgroups. A model for change might be selected to serve as a framework for implementing the desired changes. See Chapter 6 for further information on functioning as a change agent and leader.

The leader should begin by (Billings & Halstead, 2020; Ignatavicius, 2019):

- Gaining support of both the institution and program administrator for the change
- Establishing norms for the change
- Identifying benefits and risk for change
- Determining what must change and what must stay the same
- Identifying resources needed

Potential barriers leaders may face in leading curriculum revision or design include but are not limited to:

- Faculty who feel they do not have time to develop curriculum
- Inexperienced faculty
- Faculty who do not have a background in curriculum design
- Faculty who are insecure with changing curriculum
- Lack of trust for the new curriculum and/or leader
- Faculty resistance to change
- Unfamiliarity with new content or curricular model
- Faculty not completing assigned work by due dates

It is important for the leader to anticipate these barriers in preparation for the design and be prepared with potential solutions, such as:

- Refer faculty to job descriptions and remind them of their importance in the development of the curriculum.
- Develop a timeline for submission of work and set up agreed-upon goals for completion.
- Establish check-in points to determine that the work is being completed and the timeline is followed.
- Pair inexperienced faculty or those without curricular backgrounds with those experienced in curriculum design when making assignments so that they can be mentored.
- Provide evidence to faculty that demonstrates the need for change and professional development for faculty on curriculum design and revision.
- If possible, provide release time so that faculty can fully engage in the design of curriculum without being overwhelmed by teaching responsibilities.
- Involve key faculty in all curricular decisions.

Leading the Development of Course Design

The development of course design follows a process that begins with course learning outcomes and ends with the development of lesson plans. The process should be methodical and allow time for writing, modifying, critiquing, and revising before finalizing (Iwasiw et al., 2020). In leading the course design process, identifying a leader or small group of experienced nurse educators can be helpful in coordinating the work of course design.

The leaders should ensure that the *course design* (Iwasiw et al., 2020):

- Adheres to curriculum philosophy and educational approach
- Facilitates achievement of learning outcomes
- Is effective within the context of the program
- Fits within the parameters of both the course and the program

Leading course design requires a predesign phase in which faculty must consider the following (Billings & Halstead, 2020):

- Educational background and level of learner
- Course alignment with curricular PLOs and competencies
- Review of evidence on nursing care standards, nursing education research, state regulations and accreditation requirements, as well as review of the NCLEX® or national certification requirements for what is to be included
- Determination of the number of hours and content for the course
- How the course supports or builds upon learning from other courses; what the relationship will be between courses

The design of courses for a nursing curriculum is usually done in the order the curriculum is implemented (Iwasiw et al., 2020). For example, it is best to begin with the early courses in the program and end with the final course because faculty can develop courses in sequence and build on prior learning. The design process requires extensive communication between all faculty members so that courses are not developed in a "silo" manner, but rather fit together as parts of a whole. The group can provide ongoing review to determine (Iwasiw et al., 2020):

- Are the curricular courses what was intended?
- Does the curriculum align with all courses?
- Are the courses properly leveled; do they build upon prior knowledge and prepare the learner for the next level?
- Is it possible for students to achieve the established learning outcomes?
- Does the curriculum have reasonable workload expectations for faculty and learners?

The process of designing a course begins with the syllabus, including developing course outcomes and aligning these outcomes with PLOs and a brief course description. Course content and concepts are selected, and a course calendar is designed for implementation. Lesson plans are then drafted and learning activities selected. Lesson plans must be aligned with course outcomes. Lesson plans describe the purpose of the lesson, outcomes for the lesson, learning activities and assignments (aligned with course outcomes), and evaluation strategies (Billings & Halstead, 2020). Learning activities need to be selected to appeal to a variety of student learning styles. The final step is selection of evaluative methods for the course to determine effectiveness of teaching and learner achievement of course objectives (see Table 5.3). Some nursing faculty share their lesson plans with learners to communicate expectations for learning and evaluation.

When leading course design, the academic nurse educator needs to anticipate faculty, learner, time, and resource constraints that may be faced (Billings & Halstead, 2020). Faculty must be identified to develop the course. It is important to select faculty members who have course design experience and expertise in the course content or specialty. Novice faculty or those inexperienced with course design should be mentored through this process. Learner constraints must be considered, such as: How many learners will be in the course? What prerequisite knowledge do learners have? What strategies will engage varying types of learners? Time constraints need to be considered so that outcomes for course development are achievable in the desired time frame. Resource constraints also need to be considered. What physical, fiscal, and technologic resources are needed to implement the desired course design? And finally, time must be allowed for the lengthy approval process for the course. Most often, new courses must be approved by some or all the following:

- Curriculum committee for the nursing program
- Nursing faculty committee for the program
- Academic division for the program
- Institution
- State boards of nursing and/or other higher education regulatory body
- Nursing accrediting agencies

This approval process can take up to a year. Educators need to be prepared well in advance of implementation. Additionally, each step of the approval process may require editing of course information, and the approval process may need to start over. It is most important that the course design has been extensively evaluated and reviewed by faculty before initiation of the approval process so that the design that is presented is robust and does not require major edits throughout the approval process.

Revising the Curriculum and Considerations

The academic nurse educator must recognize that the curriculum requires ongoing review and development on a regular basis. This review requires faculty to extend their knowledge beyond experiences and preferences. Faculty need to continually consider and adapt the curriculum to address the future of nursing practice, technologic trends, external stakeholder feedback, learner feedback, changes in health care, societal considerations, and new educational research (Billings & Halstead, 2020).

The curricular revision process requires input and discussion with the full faculty about the need for the change and requires the support of the institutional and program administration (Ignatavicius, 2019). The revision may be led by a curriculum committee or task group or, if the faculty is small, it may be coordinated by the entire faculty. Not all faculty have formal preparation in curriculum development and evaluation. The minimum required degree for faculty teaching in a practical or vocational nursing curriculum in many states is a bachelor's degree, which does not provide preparation in curriculum development or evaluation. Faculty who are master's-prepared or higher may also not have a background in curriculum development/revision and evaluation. The faculty may need to be provided resources to aid in revision of curriculum.

CNE®/CNE®n Key Point

Remember: The curricular revision process requires input and discussion with the full faculty about the need for the change and requires the support of the institutional and program administration (Ignatavicius, 2019).

One of the first steps in revising the curriculum is selection of the leader and champion for the revision. This leader might be an external consultant who is experienced in nursing education. The external consultant is responsible for guiding the faculty through the revision process and providing information on national trends in nursing, nursing education, and curriculum development (Ignatavicius, 2019). Or the leader might be an appointed faculty member. Co-leaders might be appointed or volunteer to share the responsibility for leading the change (Billings & Halstead, 2020). The leader then needs to determine who should be assigned the various tasks of revision. The leader may need to determine a change model or theory for the revision process to successfully enlist all faculty in the shared vision of change. Change theories are described in detail in Chapter 6 of this book.

The leader should anticipate possible barriers to the change process, such as faculty who feel they do not have time to complete the revision; faculty who are inexperienced with curricular design; or limitation of available resources needed for the design, such as release time for faculty or access to needed evidence for development of materials. The leader needs to develop strategies for mitigating these barriers by setting agreed-upon goals with the design team, being transparent throughout the revision process, creating an environment of respect for safe sharing of ideas, providing for needed resources, and creating and maintaining feasible timelines for completion of revision work (Billings & Halstead, 2020).

The leader may need to be prepared that emerging redesign might result in changes in how the program is implemented and may be met with resistance. The redesign or revision may require (Iwasiw et al., 2020):

- Changes in teaching assignments
- Faculty development
- Increased clinical experiences
- Increased or decreased number of courses
- Reduction of faculty if no longer needed
- Increased number of faculty
- Increased/decreased faculty hours

Curricular revisions begin with approval by the nursing department or program, health sciences division, and/or college (within large universities). After approval at these levels, the revision is reviewed by the school, college, or university curriculum body. Substantial curricular changes may then require approval by state educational governing or regulatory agencies, boards of nursing, and/or nursing accrediting bodies. The nurse educator needs to seek relevant approvals for changes to any of the following formal curricular components, including:

- EOPLOs
- Overall program credits, including required prerequisites
- Course descriptions
- Course outcomes
- Course credits/hours
- Clinical requirements

The leader must consider that approvals of curricular changes are a lengthy process that can exceed a year to complete before any implementation of revised curriculum.

The leader reviews all requirements for each approval agency and presents curriculum for approval that fully meets all requirements. The desired outcome is that the curriculum be approved without recommendations for change. If the curriculum is changed at any point in these approval processes, the entire approval process may need to restart, likely for all involved agencies. It is the leader's responsibility to be aware of all timelines and deadlines for approval agencies so that the curriculum is ready to implement at the desired implementation date.

Additionally, it is important to consider the implementation process for the new curriculum. In collaboration with faculty and nursing administration, the leader determines a teach-out timeline for the "old" curriculum and a timeline for implementation of the new curriculum. Many factors need to be considered during this time: adequate faculty for teaching both curriculum during overlap time, adequate clinical and lab resources during the overlap period, adequate classroom space, and a plan for continuing to provide "old" curriculum courses for learners who may need to repeat failed coursework.

The need for a curriculum revision is often triggered by program data that are collected and analyzed as part of the SPE. For example, if a program establishes an expected outcome for licensure or certification examination to be an 80% first-time pass rate and the actual outcomes have been below 80% for the past 2 years, the faculty may want to review the curriculum for possible revision. In other words, program data inform program decisions by faculty and nursing administration.

Program Learning Outcomes/Program Outcomes

As stated earlier, PLOs are broad statements that delineate the new graduate competencies that learners need to achieve by the end of the program and often remain current over a long period. More specific knowledge, skills, and attitudes that learners need to develop to achieve those outcomes change more frequently (Billings & Halstead, 2020). PLOs are somewhat similar among nursing programs because they are based on national standards for nursing and education, accreditation criteria, and state regulations. However, some PLOs may remain somewhat unique in that they reflect the philosophy of the program and the institution (Iwasiw et al., 2020). For example, nursing programs in faith-based institutions include PLOs that incorporate the unique values of the college or university.

Other POs are delineated to determine the effectiveness of the nursing program. For example, most nursing accreditation criteria require reporting POs related to licensure or certification pass rates, new graduate employment, program completion rate, and graduate satisfaction with the program. Data from all types of PLOs and POs are considered when determining whether a curriculum revision is needed.

PLOs and POs need ongoing measurement using both internal and external measures to determine the effectiveness of curriculum and are summarized on the program's SPE and described later in this chapter. Examples of external measures include first-time NCLEX® or certification exam pass rates, scores on standardized tests, and employer surveys. Internal measures include assessment of learner work, graduation rates, attrition rates, learner satisfaction, learner self-perception of readiness, employment rates, and pursuit of higher degrees (Oermann & Gaberson, 2021).

National guidelines for nursing education should be considered when evaluating currency of PLOs and curriculum revision. For example, BSN and graduate PLOs are guided by the AACN's *Essentials: Core Competencies for Professional Nursing Education* (2021), which is updated regularly. Upon each update of this document, each essential needs to be reviewed for incorporation into the PLOs.

Learner Needs

When revising a curriculum, student learner needs must be considered throughout its development. The curriculum should be revised in a manner that reflects relevant nursing practice and current evidence-based practice in education. Learner perceptions about the curriculum are informative and need to be considered. Students learning about the curriculum revision may experience anxiety related to what this change may mean for them or how this revision may affect them. Learners should be informed and supported throughout the curricular revision process.

Ongoing input from learners should be sought to determine whether the curriculum is meeting their needs. Learners need an ongoing survey of their perceptions about the program and whether they feel that the program is adequately preparing them for entry into generalist or advanced nursing practice. Faculty should seek input from learners by having learner representatives attend committee meetings and provide feedback on their experiences with the curriculum.

Multiple measures throughout the program can help identify learner needs. For example, a comprehensive exam at the program's midpoint might be implemented to inform faculty of learner performance. Review of a variety of assignments at set points throughout the program can demonstrate learner achievement of desired objectives. A portfolio of learner work can be reviewed at the end of the program to determine achievement of objectives. Additionally, a journal assignment in which learners self-report achievement of objectives at the end of the program can be helpful.

CNE®/CNE®n Key Point

Remember: Ongoing input from learners should be sought to determine whether the curriculum is meeting their needs. Learners need an ongoing survey of their perceptions about the program and whether they feel that the program is adequately preparing them for entry into generalist or advanced nursing practice.

Faculty need to maintain transparency throughout the revision process with learners. It is usually helpful for faculty to engage learner representatives or leaders in the curricular revision process (Iwasiw et al., 2020). Learners in the current curriculum need to be informed about what the change in curriculum means for them. They should be reassured those expectations described at their admission to the program will not change and they will remain in the curriculum as expected. If there are any modifications to the curriculum, these must be clearly communicated to learners with as much advance notice as possible. Learners need to be reassured that they will have every opportunity to complete their current curriculum, including offering the option for repeating courses if needed.

Once the curriculum is revised, faculty need to provide reassurance to learners in the existing curriculum to promote confidence in a curriculum that is under revision. Faculty should avoid referring to the curriculum as "old" versus "new" when talking with learners so that the curriculum under revision is not deemed to be negative or inadequate. Nurse educators can demonstrate confidence in both the teach-out curriculum and the newly revised curriculum so that learners can feel confident as well.

Communication regarding the revised curriculum must be shared with the public and potential applicants to the program through advising appointments, websites, and program information documents. Keeping public information current during the curriculum revision process is essential. Chapter 7 discusses the process for notifying learners about program changes.

Societal and Health Care Trends

Societal and health care trends are constantly changing, particularly in technology. A nursing curriculum needs to be constantly informed by these trends. Ongoing monitoring of these trends needs to be done to inform any necessary revisions of the curriculum so that it remains continually current and relevant. Billings and Halstead (2020) describe six dominant trends for nursing educators to monitor to ensure currency of curriculum. These areas include:

- Health care reform
- Global violence and natural disasters
- Changing population demographics

- Continuing growth of technology
- Globalization and global health
- Environmental challenges

Faculty must conduct research on external factors that have the potential to influence curriculum in the community, region, country, and world. In addition to the factors listed earlier, it is recommended that faculty be regularly informed on professional *standards and trends in health care*, nursing practice, and nursing education (Iwasiw et al., 2020).

Changes in technology are often the greatest challenge to address in the curriculum because of the rapid pace of change in this area. Academic nurse educators need to revise and update the curriculum so that it keeps pace with current nursing practice. The curriculum must provide learners the opportunity to practice use of technology for communication with the health care team, retrieval of health care information, and use of technology to inform clinical decision making (Billings & Halstead, 2020).

Many external factors need to be considered for a curriculum revision. Ongoing data collection must be implemented so that the curriculum is responsive to current societal and health care trends. Faculty must work to determine which trends are most significant and obtain data on these trends through literature and Internet surveys, document and website reviews, key stakeholder interviews or advisory committee meetings, surveys, and consultations with subject matter experts (Iwasiw et al., 2020). A faculty session should be held in which these data are reviewed and discussed to determine how they influence and inform curriculum revision.

Stakeholder Feedback

Ongoing evaluation of both internal and external stakeholder feedback is crucial in informing and evaluating the curriculum for potential revision. *Internal stakeholders* include program faculty, program administration, staff, and learners. Examples of *external stakeholders* include clinical preceptors, advisory committee members, community members, consultants, area health care administrators, state and accreditation representatives, and area nursing leaders. It is important for nurse educators to spend time in consultation with both internal and external groups to determine effectiveness of the curriculum and to drive any needed revisions.

Internal stakeholders provide data on the effectiveness of the curriculum and identify potential areas of concern for revision. Program faculty report on learner achievement of course outcomes to help evaluate curriculum effectiveness. Program administration report areas of concern identified through review of program documents or report of learner concerns regarding curriculum. Staff provide valuable feedback to faculty to inform curriculum decisions based on interactions with learners in the program.

External stakeholders inform faculty on the current state of nursing in the area, the region, and the nation. Area health care leaders, practicing nurses, and clinical partners should be surveyed to determine the current state of nursing practice at area clinical locations. Community members and clinical partners surveyed through the program's advisory committee aid in informing the program regarding nursing practice in the area. Graduate and employer surveys also provide data that drive decisions about curricular revisions (Ignatavicius, 2019). Expert consultants in nursing education provide review of the status of a curriculum and recommendations for curricular improvement based on best practices in nursing education, national trends, accreditation standards, and regulatory requirements. State boards of nursing provide regulations about how prelicensure nursing curricula should be developed (Ignatavicius, 2019). External regulatory leaders (such as educational specialists at state boards of nursing) and accreditors provide information on changes in state regulations or accreditation guidelines that inform curricular changes.

Academic nurse educators need to inform external stakeholders about curriculum revision. Nurse preceptors need to be informed of any revised objectives for learners or changes in expectations for clinical education. Faculty should provide orientation for any curricular changes through presentations or written materials to clinical sites and clinical preceptors. Faculty must enter discussion with the clinical partner to determine whether the revised curricular outcomes are achievable in the clinical site or if modifications need to be made (Iwasiw et al., 2020). It is important to consult with state regulatory representatives to determine compliance of curriculum with state scope of practice. Regulatory bodies need to be consulted and informed of any curricular changes so that the program remains in constant compliance with all regulations and guidelines. Accrediting bodies must also be informed of curricular changes being implemented and may need to approve any changes.

Implementing Curricular Revisions Using Appropriate Change Theories and Strategies

Implementation of the curriculum is the responsibility of all faculty in the program under the guide of a designated nurse leader or committee (DeBoor, 2023). A revised curriculum is a significant change for the culture of the nursing program faculty. Curriculum revision and implementation can lead to shifts in dynamics within the culture of the nursing program, which can result in faculty power struggles, incivility, and uncertainty and lack of faculty buy-in to the proposed revised curriculum (Iwasiw et al., 2020). The designated nurse leader or program administrator needs to be prepared for these feelings of uncertainty and potential distress. A *model of change* should be selected to aid with implementation of this curriculum while appropriately engaging the support of the entire nursing faculty team. Faculty need leadership and assistance with transitioning from a previous way of implementing the "old" curriculum to a new understanding of how to implement the new curriculum. This process of supporting change and specific change theories are discussed further in Chapter 6.

For the successful implementation of a revised curriculum, all faculty must be fully informed and supportive of all key elements of the new curriculum for it to be successfully operationalized. Full-time faculty should be aware of all curricular components and how they fit together. Part-time faculty should be aware of how the relationship of the course they teach fits with the curriculum and PLOs (DeBoor, 2023). Program faculty need to be aware of how their program corresponds with others at the organization. For example, undergraduate program faculty need to be aware of how the curriculum prepares learners for potential advancement to graduate programs. It is critical for faculty to understand how the curriculum works together within the framework of the program and institution so that faculty are less likely to make any unnecessary changes to the curriculum (DeBoor, 2023).

Faculty need orientation to their assigned course and the course relationship to the curriculum by the nurse leader or course leader. The leader also must conduct periodic assessment of the course and delivery of course content to ensure faculty are meeting desired course objectives (DeBoor, 2023). Additionally, any newly hired faculty who may have not been present for the revision process should be oriented and mentored to the curricular revisions.

CNE®/CNE®n Key Point

Remember: For the successful implementation and operation of a revised curriculum, all faculty must be fully informed and supportive of all key elements of the new curriculum. Full-time faculty should be aware of all curricular components and how they fit together. Part-time faculty should be aware of how the relationship of the course they teach fits with the curriculum and PLOs (DeBoor, 2023).

Collaborating With Community and Clinical Partners

Providing clinical experiential learning is one of the most effective active learning components of a nursing curriculum in which learners are engaged in applying and translating their theoretical learning into practice (Ignatavicius, 2019). This opportunity to practice in the clinical environment not only promotes skill development but also promotes development of professional role identity as a nurse generalist or advanced practice nurse (Billings & Halstead, 2020; Ignatavicius, 2019). Additionally, students learn about today's practice environment and have the opportunity to observe and engage in interprofessional collaboration. Learners use clinical health care technology to become familiar with these tools to be prepared for practice. This opportunity for clinical practice engages learners in developing their clinical judgment and clinical reasoning skills.

Depending on the type of nursing program, clinical experiences can be provided in a variety of settings, including:

- Skills laboratory/examination suite
- Simulation center
- Acute care
- Long-term acute care (LTAC)
- Long-term care (LTC)
- Ambulatory care
- Public health clinic
- School
- Correctional facility
- Day care setting/preschool
- Homeless shelter

Typically, clinical experiences begin in a skills laboratory, examination room, and/or simulation setting and proceed to live patient care environments once learners have had the opportunity to develop the essential skills needed for practice. Clinical practice settings, faculty, and preceptors may be scarce, unavailable, and/or difficult to secure. Because of the complexity of providing a comprehensive clinical experience throughout the curriculum with often scarce resources, the nurse educator must be very innovative to develop clinical experiences that meet the learner's objectives.

The academic nurse educator has the responsibility for selecting clinical sites or experiences for the students that create a learning environment that promotes achievement of desired clinical and course objectives. When selecting a site, the educator must consider whether the site has the regulatory or accreditation status that is appropriate for clinical learning. Staffing, patient population, and physical resources must be evaluated. Questions to consider are: Does the site have adequate numbers of patients that provide learning experiences that aid achievement of objectives? Is the site appropriate for the level of the learner? For example, it would not be appropriate to send first-level prelicensure students to an intensive care unit to provide direct patient care.

In addition to providing opportunities for learning, the environment should be welcoming, supportive, and respectful of learners (Billings & Halstead, 2020). Extensive orientation to the clinical site needs to be provided to prepare learners to provide care in a confident manner.

> ### CNE®/CNE®n Key Point
>
> *Remember:* The academic nurse educator has the responsibility for selecting clinical sites or experiences for the students to create a learning environment that promotes achievement of desired clinical and course objectives.

To build an effective clinical learning environment, a nurse educator must create a collaborative partnership and positive relationship with the clinical agency and staff. It is important that the educator has a clear understanding of the clinical environment, roles and responsibilities of various clinical agency staff, and the routine/schedule of the unit (Billings & Halstead, 2020). The educator must work to establish a relationship with the agency and staff by clearly communicating student outcomes for learning, expectations for learners, expectations for staff working with learners, and the schedule for the learners. The educator should obtain ongoing feedback from agency leaders and staff as to the progress of the learners and the overall experience for the facility. The educator must become familiar with the agency mission and values and incorporate these into the learning activities. This action demonstrates the educator's commitment to and support of the goals of the clinical agency and further enhances the relationship with the clinical partner (Billings & Halstead, 2020).

Creation of learner clinical experiences is often the most complex piece of curriculum implementation. Clinical units or agencies must limit the number of learners they can accommodate, making it necessary for programs to find and manage large numbers of sites to accommodate all learners. Clinical partnerships require legal agreements, and attaining and updating these agreements can take months. Providing skills laboratory and simulation experiences is extremely costly, requiring both fiscal and physical resources and large numbers of faculty. The academic nurse educator must create innovative solutions to providing this critical learning opportunity for students. Some examples of innovative solutions include:

- Creative scheduling for clinical experiences, skills labs, and simulation labs to include evenings and weekends to use these facilities to their maximum potential
- Partnerships with clinical or educational partners to provide needed resources (i.e., a joint simulation laboratory developed, staffed, and funded by a partnership between a hospital and a school that can be used by both)
- Partnership with an agency to provide lab space for skills practice or vice versa
- Library or community setting to provide a space for clinical postconference for a clinical setting that does not have conference space
- A *dedicated educational unit (DEU)* developed as a partnership between a program and a clinical agency
- Partnership with a community agency to provide opportunities for service learning
- Partnership with an international group to provide health services abroad

Designing Program Assessment Plans That Promote Continuous Quality Improvement

Nursing program quality improvement is driven by a well-documented, comprehensive assessment plan for data collection, analysis, and implementation and is commonly referred to as the *SPE*. The SPE is designed to measure both the processes of the program and the abilities of the graduates upon completion of the program (Iwasiw et al., 2020). The assessment plan is critical not only for program quality improvement but also to ensure adherence to accreditation standards. The SPE provides a roadmap to guide faculty in managing continual evaluation of program effectiveness and implementation of program improvement.

Program data are provided not only for decisions that result in program change but also may provide a rationale for not changing current practices and processes (Oermann, 2017). Although the SPE may be grounded in accreditation or regulatory standards, it needs to also be useful for improving the program; its value needs to be demonstrated to faculty to encourage active participation in this evaluation process. The process of data collection and documentation can be coordinated by a program director or a committee such as a program assessment committee, but all faculty need to be informed of the data and participate in the analysis and action plan based on the data review. Discussions of the data, analysis, and plan of action need to be documented in the faculty meeting minutes. The SPE is not a tool that a program develops shortly before an accreditation visit, but is a dynamic, living document that continuously informs faculty and guides the direction of the program (Iwasiw et al., 2020).

Although the faculty make the decision about what to include in an SPE, accreditation bodies and state boards of nursing usually specify the minimum outcomes that should be part of an ongoing assessment. For example, in Standard IV on Program Effectiveness, the Commission on Collegiate Nursing Education (CCNE) requires ongoing assessment of:

- Program completion rates
- Licensure/certification exam first-time pass rates
- Employment rates
- Aggregate faculty outcomes
- Program outcomes (curricular outcomes)

In addition to accreditation standards, state regulators typically set requirements for measurement of specified POs (employment rate, first-time NCLEX® pass rates, program completion rates) and curricular outcomes (PLOs). These outcomes are required to be reported by graduating cohort and program option. The expected levels of achievement (ELAs), also called *expected outcomes*, for faculty credentialing may be established by accreditors or state regulators, whereas ELAs for scholarship, tenure, and promotion are set by the institution. Credentials and progress toward scholarship, tenure, and promotion need to be measured, documented, and analyzed to demonstrate faculty achievement or to identify potential barriers to completion of desired outcomes, such as a teaching workload that is too heavy to allow time for completion of scholarship activities.

Each assessment focus included on the SPE may contain the following components (Ignatavicius, 2019):

- Description of assessment focus being measured
- ELA or expected outcome
- How the outcome is measured, including frequency of assessment
- Person(s) responsible for the data collection
- Actual data or outcome obtained (results)
- Analysis of data
- Action plan for improvement, if needed
- Follow-up on action plan

In most cases, the faculty may determine which data are used to measure the outcomes on the SPE, including the PLOs. PLOs are often assessed by direct and indirect measures of performance. Direct measures include specific assessments performed by learners, such as scores on end-of-program standardized exams or evaluation tools for clinical performance in a capstone/preceptor course. Indirect measures are opinions, such as learner perceptions using a course survey to determine whether students believe they have met the desired objectives for learning. Another indirect measure is feedback from external stakeholders, such as surveys of advisory committee members or employers on graduate performance in the clinical setting. Direct measures are more informative and data driven; however, it is also important to consider learner and external stakeholder perceptions when making program decisions. When selecting assessment methods and ELAs or expected outcomes, it is essential to make them reasonable and, when possible, based on historical trends. One or two methods of collecting data for each measure is usually sufficient (Oermann, 2017). The person or committee responsible for collecting and documenting the data is set by the program. The analysis, action plan, and follow-up are the responsibility of all faculty. Additionally, a schedule or calendar for review and analysis of the data is set by the faculty so that all outcomes are scheduled for regular assessment. Table 5.8 displays an example of part of an SPE for assessing a PLO.

In addition to assessing curricular and program outcomes as part of the SPE, nursing faculty must evaluate the effectiveness of the processes and resources for the program, including (Ignatavicius, 2019; Oermann, 2017):

- Performance on course SLOs
- Support course performance (prerequisites, general education courses) in providing preparation for successful completion of the nursing curriculum
- Teaching methods and strategies
- Clinical experiences
- Program policies for admission, retention, and program completion
- Partnerships with external agencies
- Fiscal, physical, and human resources for the program
- Alumni and employer satisfaction

CNE®/CNE®n Key Point

Remember: Nursing program quality improvement is driven by a well-documented, comprehensive assessment plan for data collection, analysis, and implementation and is commonly referred to as the SPE. The SPE is designed to measure both the processes of the program and the abilities of the graduates upon completion of the program (Iwasiw et al., 2020).

TABLE **5.8**	Sample of a Portion of a Systematic Plan for Evaluation

Systemic Plan of Evaluation: Assessment of Program Learning Outcomes (PLOs)					
PLO	**Assessment Method**	**Frequency of Data Collection and Assessment**	**Expected Outcome**	**Data Results**	**Analysis and Action Plan**
PLO 1: Graduates will collaborate effectively with members of the interprofessional health care team.	Direct measure of learners' scores on the standardized exit exam	Every January and June for each graduating cohort; data will be reviewed every August and April	75% of final-semester learners will score 70% or higher on the interprofessional collaboration indicator on the standardized exit exam.	**2021** **4/2021:** 80% of learners achieved 70% score or greater **2020** **4/2020:** 79% scored 70% or greater **8/2020:** 77% scored 70% or greater **2019** **4/2019:** 82% scored 70% or greater **8/2019:** 82% scored 70% or greater	**2021** **4/2021:** Analysis: Expected outcome consistently met ×3 years. Action plan: Continue to monitor; incorporate interprofessional simulation for senior students into curriculum. **2020** **4/2020:** Analysis/plan of action: Expected outcome consistently met ×3 years; continue to monitor. **8/2020:** Analysis/plan of action: Expected outcome consistently met ×3 years; continue to monitor. **2019** **4/2019** Analysis/plan of action: Expected outcome consistently met ×3 years; continue to monitor. **8/2019** Analysis/plan of action: Expected outcome consistently met ×3 years; continue to monitor.

Implementing the Program Assessment Plan

Implementation of the *program assessment plan* is the responsibility of nursing administration and nursing faculty. The program assessment plan may be coordinated in a variety of ways. Some large programs or departments have a designated evaluation position or an Office of Evaluation that prescribes and coordinates all program or department evaluation. Other programs coordinate the work of program assessment through a program assessment committee. For very small programs, the work of program assessment is implemented by the nurse administrator and all nursing faculty.

The implementation process involves regular collection of data following methods and time-lines specified by the SPE. The coordinator or committee receives, reviews, analyzes, and interprets the data. The data are compared with the standards identified in the SPE. Committee analysis of the data may result in DeBoor (2023):

- Identification of existing and potential problems
- Identification of new needs
- Demonstration of successes
- Recommendations for program improvement
- Discontinuance of a program or a proposal for a new program

Documentation of action plans for improvement, including people responsible and timeline for completion, is made by the committee or full faculty. Additionally, the committee or coordinator documents a summary of the evaluation, including documentation of success or progress toward achieving implementation of any action plan for improvement. The action plan developed from the analysis of the outcome data is a critical part of quality improvement (Billings & Halstead, 2020).

The implementation of a program assessment plan must include a feedback loop for recommendations and decision making. All faculty must be informed of and participate in any identified plan for improvement. Internal stakeholders (faculty, institutional administration, learners) and external stakeholders (advisory committees, clinical partners) must also receive regular reports of program performance determined by analysis of the SPE and regular updates on progress on action plans for program improvements.

Evaluating the Program Assessment Plan

It is very important that the SPE undergoes regular evaluation for effectiveness. Faculty need to review the SPE to determine any areas in which criteria identified for measurement may have changed. For example, accreditation standards may change, resulting in adjustments to desired ELAs. Changes to PLOs or institutional/program mission statements might alter outcomes to be measured. Faculty must review the SPE at least annually to determine whether the measurements identified provide adequate data to inform decision making. Timelines for data review need to be evaluated and updated. For measures that are performing well, less frequent assessments may be indicated; for measures that are underperforming, increased assessments may be indicated. Ongoing feedback from stakeholders may indicate that the SPE needs to be adjusted. For example, employer feedback may report that graduates are lacking in a particular performance area. The SPE may need adjustment to develop an action plan for additional data collection to further investigate an identified performance problem or an action plan for improvement on this performance area.

CNE®/CNE®n Key Point

Remember: The SPE of the nursing program needs to be viewed as a living document that is ever evolving, capturing the ongoing performance of the curriculum and determining the direction for the program.

References

Accreditation Commission for Education in Nursing (ACEN). (2020). *The 2017 ACEN accreditation manual – Section III: Standards and criteria.* Updated https://www.acenursing.org/acen-accreditation-manual-standards-a/.

American Association of Colleges of Nursing (AACN). (2021). *The essentials: Core competencies for professional nursing education.* https://www.aacnnursing.org/Portals/42/AcademicNursing/pdf/Essentials-2021.pdf.

Billings, D. M., & Halstead, J. A. (2020). *Teaching in nursing: A guide for faculty* (6th ed.). St. Louis: Elsevier.

DeBoor, S. S. (2023). *Keating's curriculum development and evaluation in nursing education* (5th ed.). New York: Springer Publishing.

Healthy People. (2020). *Social determinants of health.* https://www.healthypeople.gov/2020/topics-objectives/topic/social-determinants-of-health.

Ignatavicius, D. (2019). *Teaching and learning in a concept-based nursing curriculum: A how to best practice approach.* Burlington, MA: Jones & Bartlett Learning.

Iwasiw, C. L., Andrusyszyn, M. A., & Goldenberg, D. (2020). *Curriculum development in nursing education* (4th ed.). Burlington, MA: Jones & Bartlett Learning.

National League for Nursing (NLN). (2012). *Outcomes and competencies for graduates of practical/vocational, associate, baccalaureate, master's practice doctorate, and research doctorate in nursing.* New York: National League for Nursing.

Oermann, M. (2017). *A systematic approach to assessment and evaluation in nursing.* Washington DC: National League for Nursing-Wolters Kluwer.

Oermann, M. H., & Gaberson, K. B. (2021). *Evaluation and testing in nursing education.* New York: Springer Publishing.

CHAPTER 5 Practice Questions

1. Which statement best defines a nursing program learning outcome (PLO)?
   A. Specifically describes knowledge, skills, and attitudes learners will demonstrate
   B. Identifies the objectives learners will attain for the nursing courses
   C. Delineates expectations for graduates broadly and in general terms
   D. Describes the philosophy of the nursing program for graduates

2. The nurse educator is working with other members of the curriculum committee to develop PLOs for a nursing program. Which outcome statement would be most appropriate?
   A. Apply the nursing process to provide safe, evidence-based care to meet the diverse needs of patients across the lifespan who have acute and chronic common physical and mental health problems.
   B. Formulate safe and effective clinical judgments guided by the nursing process, clinical reasoning, and evidence-based practice.
   C. Apply knowledge of therapeutic communication in a health history interview for an adult patient.
   D. Develop a teaching plan to promote health and prevent illness appropriate for selected vulnerable populations within a global community.

3. The nurse educator is working with other members of the assessment committee to develop program outcomes (POs) for a nursing program to assess its effectiveness. Which of the following outcomes would be most appropriate for a family nurse practitioner program?
   A. Graduates will function independently as family nurse practitioners in a variety of health care environments.
   B. 85% of graduates will be employed as family nurse practitioners within 3 months of graduation.
   C. 80% of graduates will pass the family nurse practitioner certification examination on their first attempt.
   D. Graduates will attain a passing score on the family nurse practitioner certification practice examination.

4. Which of the following course objectives would be most appropriate for a senior-level nursing student?
   A. Formulate a plan of care that promotes health and safety of the pediatric patient.
   B. Describe interventions that promote health and safety for the older adult.
   C. Perform a health history and health assessment for a pediatric patient.
   D. Use the plan of care to determine effectiveness of promoting health and safety for the older adult.

5. Which statement about course outcomes by the novice nurse educator requires follow-up by the faculty mentor?
   A. "Course outcomes need to be leveled and build across the curriculum."
   B. "Course outcomes should be evaluated for appropriateness of level for the learner."
   C. "The curriculum committee selects and assigns all course outcomes for the curriculum."
   D. "Learners will have multiple opportunities to meet each outcome during the course."

6. Which learning environment is the most appropriate for introducing the following course competency: Demonstrates proper hand hygiene principles?
   A. Capstone clinical experience
   B. Didactic foundations course
   C. Pediatric patient care setting
   D. Foundations' skills laboratory

7. Which statement best represents a SMART course objective in the cognitive learning domain?
   A. Perform a sterile dressing change for a patient with a central line.
   B. Apply knowledge of growth and development to provide age-appropriate care for school-age children.
   C. Summarize an example of two quality initiatives that influenced nursing practice.
   D. Provide leadership in an acute care setting to improve patient care.

8. Which statement by the novice nurse educator indicates a potential need for follow-up by the faculty mentor?
   A. "I will need to adjust these course objectives to align with my learning activities."
   B. "I will select learning activities that help students meet the course objectives."
   C. "I will need to consider the level of student when selecting learning activities."
   D. "I will need to select learning activities that are active and fit with the course context."

9. A faculty mentor is reviewing course objectives developed by a novice nurse educator. Which outcome requires follow-up by the faculty mentor?
   A. Explain the role of the professional nurse in providing patient-centered care within legal and ethical guidelines.
   B. Differentiate the signs and symptoms of common musculoskeletal disorders.
   C. Safely perform pediatric psychomotor skills based on evidence-based standards and policies.
   D. Advance knowledge in health assessment and communication skills.

10. Which learning activity best supports achievement of the following course objective: The learner will discuss ethical considerations when caring for diverse adults in the acute care setting?
    A. Skills demonstration
    B. Journal assignment
    C. Recorded lecture on ethics
    D. Multiple-choice test items

11. Which of the following factors does the nurse educator recognize as the most important when selecting a technologic learning activity?
    A. Cost of the technology activity
    B. Availability of the technology
    C. Support for technology implementation
    D. Technology activity supports course objective

12. Which of the following is most important for the nurse educator to consider when selecting a clinical experience for student learning?
    A. Number of patients available
    B. Distance for learners to travel
    C. Experience supports course outcome
    D. Wide range of patient conditions

13. Which of the following clinical experiences would be appropriate to help learners meet this course outcome: Apply the nursing process to provide safe, evidence-based care to meet the diverse needs of older adult patients who have chronic physical and mental health problems?
    A. Critical care setting
    B. Pediatric practice setting
    C. Postanesthesia care unit
    D. Medical/surgical unit

14. When communicating to learners about clinical experiences, it is most important for the nurse educator to convey which of the following?
    A. Alignment of clinical experience with course outcomes
    B. Course schedule for completion of clinical experiences
    C. Guidelines for time management for the clinical experience
    D. Orientation to all needed technology for the unit

15. Which of the following evaluation strategies would be appropriate for measuring the following course objective: Students will examine the advanced practice registered nursing (APRN) role, its historical background, and associated nursing theory?
    A. Direct observation
    B. Scholarly paper
    C. Case study
    D. Multiple-choice test

16. The nurse educator determines that a concept map assignment will be the best method for evaluating student learning. The educator has selected this method from which learning domain?
    A. Cognitive
    B. Performance
    C. Psychomotor
    D. Affective

17. Which statement is the correct definition for a nursing program mission statement?
    A. Reflects the faculty's beliefs, values, and attitudes about nursing
    B. Describes the purpose of the program in preparing nursing graduates
    C. Delineates the goals of the program and the curriculum for the future
    D. Outlines what the curriculum emphasizes and describes program values

18. Which statement by the novice nurse educator about the nursing program philosophy statements requires follow-up by the faculty mentor?
    A. "I need to review the nursing program's philosophy statements so that I am familiar with the definition of scholarship for this university."
    B. "The nursing program's philosophy statement will help me to understand faculty beliefs, values, and attitudes about nursing and nursing education."
    C. "The nursing program's philosophy statement will need to demonstrate alignment with the university's philosophy."
    D. "I will need to participate in regular review of the program's philosophy statement now that I am a faculty member."

19. Which of the following components is important for nurse educators to incorporate into a nursing program philosophy?
    A. Societal and health care trends related to nursing
    B. Global perspectives on educational trends
    C. External stakeholder feedback on education practices
    D. Faculty beliefs regarding adult learning theory

20. Why should nurse educators include incivility and violence when designing a nursing curriculum?
    A. It should not be included, as it will discourage new nurses from practice.
    B. It helps to prepare graduates for what they may experience as new nurses.
    C. It helps define professional behaviors for the nursing student handbook.
    D. It promotes empathy and understanding for nursing colleagues.

21. Which statement by the novice educator about curriculum design requires follow-up by the faculty mentor?
    A. "Our faculty will need to incorporate use of a simulated electronic health record (EHR) into our curriculum for learners to be prepared for practice."
    B. "Our faculty will need to incorporate opportunities for our learners to participate in interprofessional collaboration into our curriculum."
    C. "Our faculty will need to examine health statistics and issues in our community and incorporate these data into our curriculum."
    D. "Our faculty will need to develop curriculum that has a local focus because learners are not likely to practice outside our area."

22. A novice nurse educator is working with the nursing faculty to determine community priorities for the design of a new curriculum. Which statement by the novice educator requires follow-up by the mentor?
    A. "We should research area infant mortality rates to see if there are critical needs for patient education."
    B. "We should examine which types of chronic conditions most often occur in our community."
    C. "We should examine QSEN Safety Standards to make sure our curriculum incorporates them."
    D. "We should consult local county officials to see if we can find statistics on crime rates and violence."

23. Which of the following learning activities would provide nursing students the opportunity to learn about nursing and health care in a societal context?
    A. Participate in an interprofessional simulation experience.
    B. Complete a case study on breast cancer due to increased rates in the county.
    C. Develop a teaching plan on nutrition for high school students who are pregnant.
    D. Write a research paper discussing access to health care in the United States.

24. The nurse educator is discussing the concept of gas exchange and has reviewed two exemplars with the class, including chronic obstructive pulmonary disease (COPD) and pneumonia. Which type of curriculum model does this teaching/learning approach represent?
    A. Concept-based curriculum
    B. Traditional model
    C. Blocked content model
    D. Adult learning model

25. Which of the following statements by the novice nurse educator requires follow-up by the mentor?
    A. "Concept-based curricular models often overload learners with content."
    B. "I will discuss the two identified exemplars for the concept in my class."
    C. "In a concept-based curriculum, key concepts are embedded throughout the curriculum."
    D. "Traditional models of nursing education block content around focal areas."

26. Which of the following standards would be important for academic nurse educators to review to provide information about regulatory standards for nursing curriculum in the United States?
    A. Quality improvement measures
    B. Scope of practice for the state
    C. Interprofessional standards
    D. Reports from foundations such as Robert Woods Johnson Foundation

27. The nurse educator is providing a simulated learning experience for students with a debriefing session after the experience. This learning activity demonstrates the use of which educational theory?
    A. Adult learning theory
    B. Narrative pedagogy
    C. Experiential learning theory
    D. Constructivism

28. The nurse educator is assigning a journal assignment for learners to record self-reflection on an ethical dilemma experienced during a clinical experience. This learning activity represents the use of which educational theory?
    A. Adult learning theory
    B. Narrative pedagogy
    C. Experiential learning theory
    D. Constructivism

29. Which statement best describes a scrambled classroom?
    A. It is a passive learning method for imparting knowledge.
    B. Learners are scrambled into teams for group activities.
    C. Segments of lecture are interspersed with application activities.
    D. Learners work to solve problems through group interaction.

30. Which learning activity would best simulate a realistic nursing care environment?
    A. In-class activity with role-play of therapeutic communication
    B. Practicing injection skills in the skills laboratory with an injection pad
    C. A written self-reflection on perceptions on immunization practices
    D. Documentation assignment in a simulated electronic health record

31. Which statement by the novice nurse educator requires follow-up by the faculty mentor?
    A. "I will use the learning management system (LMS) to organize my course."
    B. "I would like to customize my course LMS so that it stands out from other program courses."
    C. "I will use my LMS to post learning activities for the students before class so they are prepared."
    D. "It is important that my course LMS is well organized to aid the students' ease of navigation."

32. A nursing program is having difficulty obtaining a clinical site for learners to have opportunities to care for women experiencing labor and delivery. Which is the best solution for the nurse educator to plan?
    A. Additional didactic content centered on the care of the laboring patient
    B. Practice in the skills lab in measuring the fundus and examining fetal heart tone strip samples on a mannequin
    C. Participating in care of a simulated, laboring patient using a high-fidelity obstetric mannequin
    D. Comprehensive concept map assignment centered around care of the laboring patient

33. Which of these methods does the nurse educator recognize as an example of a low-fidelity simulation technology?
    A. Mannequin with heartbeat and lung sounds
    B. Task trainer for IV insertion
    C. Virtual reality experience
    D. Standardized patient

34. Which of the following would be an appropriate leader to facilitate a nursing curricular design?
    A. National nursing education consultant
    B. Newly hired nurse educator
    C. Vice president of academic affairs
    D. Entire faculty of a large department of nursing

35. Which of the following is a major barrier the leader must consider in coordinating nursing curricular design?
    A. Faculty subject matter preferences when assigning coursework for development
    B. Faculty who do not have experience or educational background in curriculum development
    C. Potential reduction in faculty needed after redesigning the curriculum
    D. Learner resistance to changes proposed for the curriculum

36. Which of the following activities would best help novice nurse educators develop curriculum design skills?
    A. Assign them to develop a first-semester course.
    B. Assign them an experienced mentor during the design process.
    C. Provide a nursing education textbook on curriculum design.
    D. Provide an opportunity for a conference on nursing education.

37. After developing the philosophy and mission statement, the curricular course design process begins with the development of program learning outcomes and ends with which of the following?
    A. Course outcomes
    B. Course competencies
    C. Lesson plans
    D. Course calendars

38. Which of the following statements is most important for the nurse educator to consider when selecting learning activities?
    A. Learning activities must align with course objectives.
    B. Learning activities must be varied.
    C. Learning activities must actively engage students.
    D. Learning activities must be described in the lesson plan.

39. Which of these statements by the novice nurse educator about course design requires follow-up by the faculty mentor?
    A. "When designing a new course, I will need to examine what prerequisites students have taken."
    B. "When designing a new course, I will need to examine the level and experience of the student."
    C. "When designing a new course, I will need to examine how my course will prepare students for their next level of learning."
    D. "When designing a new course, I will need to examine my own educational philosophy."

40. Which of the following factors would be most important for a leader of a curricular revision to consider before making curricular changes?
    A. Selecting a change model for the revision process
    B. Identifying key faculty who will support the change
    C. Designing a calendar for implementation of changes
    D. Selecting educational technology for implementation of changes

41. Which of the following common barriers may be experienced by nurse leaders when redesigning curriculum?
    A. The new curriculum will require new clinical sites.
    B. Increased simulation hours may be required for clinical practice.
    C. Many faculty members are inexperienced with curriculum design.
    D. The learners may have a decreased number of clinical hours.

42. Which of the following statements by the novice nurse educator about the old curriculum "teach-out" requires follow-up by the mentor?
    A. "While teaching out the old curriculum, we will need to make sure we have enough faculty during overlap time with the new curriculum."
    B. "While teaching out the old curriculum, we will need to make sure we have enough clinical sites and lab space during overlap time with the new curriculum."
    C. "While teaching out the old curriculum, we will need to make sure that learners have the opportunity to repeat any coursework needed."
    D. "While teaching out the old curriculum, we will need to make sure that all current learners are able to transfer into the new curriculum if desired."

43. Which of the following is an expected result for a nursing program outcome to assess program effectiveness?
   A. Graduates will complete the nursing program within 150% of the degree plan time frame.
   B. Graduates will achieve a 60% on interprofessional collaboration on the program exit exam.
   C. 95% of graduates will achieve a passing score on the final clinical evaluation tool during the preceptorship.
   D. Each graduate cohort will achieve a 75% on the final portfolio project.

44. An update to the AACN *Essentials* document would prompt a nurse educator to take which of the following actions?
   A. Review certification pass rates to determine whether the expected outcome should be adjusted.
   B. Review program learning outcomes to determine whether updates are needed.
   C. Review employment data to see if new expected outcomes should be specified.
   D. Review options for direct and indirect data collection to determine alignment with the AACN *Essentials.*

45. Program learning outcome changes will likely result in needed revision of which of the following?
   A. Course outcomes
   B. Methods for learner evaluation
   C. Textbooks and resources for learners
   D. Revised calendar for review of data

46. Which of the following actions would actively support learners during a curricular revision process?
   A. Providing students with a nursing student handbook
   B. Supplying students with revised course syllabi for the new curriculum
   C. Developing a written handout that describes all changes
   D. Inviting student representatives to attend faculty meetings

47. Which of the following evaluation strategies would be appropriate for measuring the following objective for an advanced physical assessment course: Learners will safely perform culturally competent health histories for adult clients?
   A. Research paper
   B. Direct observation
   C. Case study
   D. Multiple-choice item

48. Which of the following statements provided to learners starting a new curriculum by the novice nurse educator requires follow-up by the mentor?
   A. "We are so excited for you to begin our new curriculum; you will be our test group for determining how successful the program will be."
   B. "We are so excited for you to begin our new curriculum; you will be provided orientation today so that you can be familiar with expectations."

C. "We are so excited for you to begin our new curriculum; faculty are confident that what we have developed will provide you the opportunity for success."
   D. "We are so excited for you to begin our new curriculum; you will receive frequent communications on what to expect throughout your time in the program."

49. A nurse educator is the chairperson for the curriculum committee and desires to assign societal trend areas to research for ensuring currency of the curriculum. Which of the following factors would be important to include?
   A. Use of a simulated electronic health record
   B. Faculty beliefs on prioritization of curricular material
   C. Social media trending topics on the state of nursing
   D. Learner demographics and culture preferences

50. The COVID-19 pandemic is a current example of which type of societal and health care trend that should be reviewed and incorporated into curriculum revision?
   A. Changing population demographics
   B. Global health
   C. Environmental challenge
   D. Natural disaster

51. Which of the following statements is a benefit of incorporating personal devices into classroom activities?
   A. Personal devices can be used in class to simulate what will be expected in practice.
   B. Learners can obtain instant feedback on course assignments and exams.
   C. Personal devices are not a benefit and should be prohibited because of the potential for cheating.
   D. Learners' use of personal devices in class promotes better understanding of course content.

52. A nurse educator participating on the curriculum committee is assigned to learn current practices in postoperative nursing care. Which of the following external stakeholders would be important to survey?
   A. Medical-surgical nursing faculty
   B. Director of nursing program
   C. Recent program alumni
   D. Area clinical preceptors

53. A nurse educator would seek information from which external stakeholder to ensure proposed curricular revisions are compliant with the state scope of practice?
   A. Education specialist with the state board of nursing
   B. Director of nursing program
   C. Staff member from accrediting body
   D. Faculty assigned to the course

54. A nurse educator serving as chair of the curriculum committee assigns which of the following tasks to the program's nursing education consultant?
    A. Developing program learning outcomes
    B. Writing the program's mission and philosophy statements
    C. Reviewing the current state of the curriculum
    D. Leveling course descriptions

55. Which of the following statements should a nurse educator anticipate when implementing a revised curriculum?
    A. Some faculty may have a lack of confidence in the new curriculum.
    B. Clinical sites will be resistant to any curricular changes.
    C. Faculty need autonomy for developing buy-in for curriculum.
    D. Faculty usually have buy-in with evidence-based curricular changes.

56. Which of the following statements would be most important for the nurse educator to consider when implementing a revised curriculum?
    A. Learners are represented during curricular development.
    B. Adjunct faculty are invited to curricular team meetings.
    C. General education faculty are informed of the curricular changes.
    D. The entire faculty must be fully informed of all key curricular elements.

57. Which of the following is the key responsibility for part-time faculty when implementing a revised curriculum?
    A. Part-time faculty should be aware of how their course fits with the general education courses.
    B. Part-time faculty should be aware of how all the curricular components fit together.
    C. Part-time faculty should be aware of how their course fits with the curriculum.
    D. Part-time faculty should be aware of how evidence was selected for curricular decisions.

58. Which of the following statements is true about clinical learning in nursing education?
    A. Laboratory practice of nursing care is ideal for clinical learning.
    B. Active classroom learning activities best promote clinical learning.
    C. Skills practice should be the priority for clinical learning.
    D. Students learn expectations of the practice environment.

59. Which of the following knowledge and skills should be a priority for student learning in a health care agency or facility?
    A. Infusion therapy
    B. Interprofessional collaboration
    C. Assessment skills practice
    D. Professional role behaviors

60. Which of the following statements by the novice nurse educator about clinical learning requires follow-up by the mentor?
    A. "Students need to be in the hospital setting for clinical experiences to learn how to provide patient care."
    B. "Students may need supplemental service-learning activities to enhance their learning related to patient care."
    C. "Students can do a teaching project at a day care center to demonstrate clinical learning."
    D. "Students may spend a day with the nurse at the correctional facility as part of their clinical learning."

61. Which of the following methods is an example of formative evaluation?
    A. Learner portfolio of documents in the final semester
    B. Mid-program standardized exam scores
    C. Scores from standardized exit exam
    D. End-of-program patient assessment

62. Which of the following activities is a program assessment measurement for faculty and prescribed by the institution?
    A. Progress toward tenure
    B. Credentialing
    C. Faculty-to-student ratio
    D. Scores on exit exam

63. Which of the following methods is a direct measure for an expected outcome as part of a program assessment plan?
    A. Scores on standardized exit exam
    B. Survey of student perceptions of learning
    C. Advisory committee report of graduate performance
    D. Program satisfaction surveys by alumni

64. What is the main purpose for a nursing program assessment plan?
    A. Measure learner satisfaction and promotion of a positive program image to the public
    B. Ensure quality improvement and regulations for faculty workload
    C. Provide for adherence to state guidelines and prepare for accreditation visits
    D. Ensure quality improvement and adherence to accreditation standards

65. An academic nurse educator participating on the program assessment committee is developing an expected result for a program learning outcome. Which of the following information is used to determine the desired expectation?
    A. Review of program historical data
    B. Expected outcomes from similar programs
    C. Expected outcomes described in nursing curriculum textbooks
    D. Recommendations by program faculty

66. The feedback loop for program assessment includes gathering data and feedback from which of the following external stakeholders for the data and plan for improvement?
    A. Institutional administration
    B. Advisory committee members
    C. Nursing program faculty
    D. Area program directors

67. The program assessment committee chair is mentoring a novice nurse educator. Which statement indicates the need for follow-up by the mentor?
    A. "All faculty participate in program assessment."
    B. "Program assessment identifies problems with curriculum."
    C. "Program assessment is often led by a program assessment committee."
    D. "Accreditors are only concerned with the data collected."

68. The advisory committee members report that program graduates seem to be lacking skills in interprofessional collaboration (IPC). Which statement regarding program assessment using the systematic plan for evaluation (SPE) is true?
    A. The SPE may need to be adjusted to measure IPC or provide an action plan for improvement.
    B. These are subjective data about graduate skills in IPC and do not affect the SPE.
    C. This information about IPC closes the feedback loop and needs to be re-evaluated at the next advisory committee meeting.
    D. This information is classified as confidential external data and does not affect the SPE.

69. Changes in which of the following factors may indicate the need for evaluation and revision of a nursing program assessment plan?
    A. State requirements for admission
    B. Demographics of student body
    C. Accreditation standard for program completion
    D. Institutional requirements for faculty load

70. Which of the following sources is important for the nursing faculty to consult when designing a curriculum that is current and relevant for practice?
    A. Clinical partners
    B. Area nursing program directors
    C. Institutional administration
    D. General education faculty

71. Which of the following local health care trends would be important to review and incorporate during nursing curriculum design?
    A. HIV rates for the United States
    B. Vaccination rates for polio in African countries
    C. Infant mortality for the Midwest
    D. Incidence of coronary artery disease in the county

72. Which of the following does the nurse educator recognize as an example of a learning activity that is grounded in adult learning theory?
    A. Participation in clinical learning
    B. Completion of a journal assignment discussing an ethical dilemma
    C. Demonstration of foundation nursing skills by instructor
    D. Class discussion related to the circulatory system

73. Which statement by the novice nurse educator about course outcomes requires follow-up by the mentor?
    A. "I will use the course outcomes to guide the development of my lesson plans."
    B. "I will include extra content on cardiac heart rhythms because of my extensive clinical experience in this area."
    C. "I will include course content on the assessment of the pediatric patient, as this is required by the course outcomes."
    D. "I will develop learning activities that align with the course outcomes and lesson plan course objectives."

74. Which of the following outcomes reflect the knowledge, skills, and attitudes that learners are to demonstrate upon program completion?
    A. Course outcomes
    B. Program learning outcomes
    C. Course competencies
    D. Curricular objectives

75. Which of the following statements describes the difference between a traditional and a flipped/scrambled classroom?
    A. The traditional class is a concept-based method for delivering education, whereas a flipped class is not.
    B. There are few differences; both methods require extensive lecture, note taking, and active learning activities.
    C. The flipped/scrambled classroom requires advanced preparation by students, with class time for application of learning.
    D. The traditional class is the preferred, evidence-based method for promoting student learning and retention of content.

Functioning as a Change Agent and a Leader

SUSAN ANDERSEN

LEARNING OUTCOMES

1. Identify factors that affect program and organizational change.
2. Describe effective academic nurse educator leadership styles for facilitating change.
3. Explain the role of academic nurse educators in providing leadership to enhance the visibility of nursing and to address health care and educational needs.
4. Discuss effective methods for creating and sustaining a culture of change within a program, institution, community, or region.
5. Apply evidence-based models of change theory to effectively facilitate change in a nursing program, institution, community, and region.

The academic nurse educator is in a unique and powerful position to act as a positive force for effective change within nursing education and practice by serving as a leader. Through this position of leadership, nurse educators have the ability not only to effect change but also to "create a preferred future for nursing and nursing practice" (Christensen & Simmons, 2020, p. 13). Academic nurse educators impact change in a wide range of areas, including the nursing program, institution, community, and region. Educators must effectively collaborate with a wide range of colleagues and interdisciplinary team members to successfully facilitate change that continually improves nursing education and quality health care. A culture of change that promotes the potential success of achieving and sustaining needed changes should be facilitated and embraced by the educator.

The National League for Nursing (NLN) (2019) identifies eight essential subcompetencies for the nurse educator's role in functioning as a *change agent* and a leader. Table 6.1 provides a list of these required competencies and key points for nurse educators. Nurse educators provide leadership and effect change through their nursing practice, teaching, scholarly activities, research, and service to their institution and community.

Functioning as a Change Agent and a Leader

To enact positive, far-reaching, and long-lasting change, nurse educators need to be informed by research related to leadership and draw on theories and evidence-based methods. Nurse educators demonstrate effective leadership and behavior styles, are future oriented, focus on capacity building, and empower others during periods of change (Iwasiw et al., 2020).

TABLE 6.1	NLN Subcompetencies for Functioning as a Change Agent and a Leader
NLN Subcompetency	**Key Points**
Models cultural sensitivity when advocating for change	Fosters a culturally sensitive environment to promote the acceptance and implementation of desired change.
Integrates a long-term, innovative, and creative perspective into the nurse educator role	Serves as a leader who helps establish a shared vision of values and beliefs for the organization. Works to empower people within their organization to make decisions that support shared goals, values, and vision in a manner that is future focused. Works to create an environment of collegiality that is open to freely sharing ideas and collaboration to promote development of best practices in nursing and nursing education.
Participates in interdisciplinary efforts to address health care and educational needs locally, regionally, nationally, or internationally	Engages in an environmental scan and review of the evidence in health care and nursing education to determine current needs and forecast trends to impart needed change. Designs educational curriculum and learning activities to engage learners in providing leadership and addressing health care needs of the local community and beyond.
Evaluates organizational effectiveness in nursing education	Participates in ongoing comprehensive assessment of the program to determine effectiveness, demonstrate achievement of required standards, and provide for continual program improvement.
Implements strategies for organizational change	Uses change theory models for implementation of organizational change. Provides leadership, role modeling, and mentoring for other faculty and learners to promote a culture of change.
Provides leadership in the parent institution and in the nursing program to enhance the visibility of nursing and its contributions to the academic community	Provides leadership to learners and fellow faculty members at a program level and institutional level through activities in the four areas of Boyer's Model of Scholarship: teaching, application, integration, and discovery to provide leadership to learners. Participates in professional organizations. Obtains certifications that demonstrate excellence in nursing to enhance the visibility of nursing beyond the institution. Provides an informed voice for nursing for health care decision making.
Promotes innovative practices in educational environments	Develops nursing research that informs nursing practice and nursing education. Uses evidence to inform teaching and learning practices. Participates in interdisciplinary collaborative efforts and institutional governance to promote educational practices that are informed by evidence and promote the nursing perspective.
Develops leadership skills to shape and implement change	Develops leadership skills through ongoing continuing education and participation in interdisciplinary collaborative teams to affect positive change for nursing, health care, and higher education.

Data from Christensen, L. S., & Simmons, L. E. (2020). *The scope of practice for academic nurse educators and academic clinical nurse educators* (3rd ed.). Washington, DC: National League for Nursing-Wolters Kluwer.

Modeling Cultural Sensitivity When Advocating for Change

Organizational culture is widely defined as the shared behaviors, beliefs, values, norms, practices, and assumptions of the members. Culture influences all the work and interactions of the organization and can either promote or inhibit the successful implementation of any desired changes. Culture develops over time, influences the social and psychological environment of the organization, and is transmitted to new members through socialization (Iwasiw et al., 2020). Understanding of the organizational culture is paramount when considering change. Cultural knowledge can help inform initiatives and strategies for change. An understanding of current cultural norms, values, and strengths can aid the nurse educator in moving the organization toward the desired change (Iwasiw et al., 2020).

The one constant in health care and education is that they are always changing. The academic nurse educator needs to be prepared to provide leadership for ongoing evaluation of curriculum and implementation of change. The nurse educator must realize that to impact any change, a culturally sensitive environment must be created to foster the acceptance and implementation of the change. It is a vital responsibility of the nurse educator to understand the organizational culture to create a climate that is supportive of the dynamic processes of change the nursing program and institution will undergo (DeBoor, 2023).

The organizational culture provides meaning and stability for its members, and any changes can threaten the values and meanings the members may have about the school, the curriculum, and their position within the organization (Iwasiw et al., 2020). The culture and/or dynamics of an organization can promote or inhibit the implementation of change, whether that change be positive and desired or negative and undesired. Before implementing any changes, the academic nurse educator must understand the individual's and group's beliefs about acceptance of the need for change, commitment to change, and readiness to engage in the work of change. The educator must consider many factors about the organizational culture when proposing change, including (Iwasiw et al., 2020):

- Will the culture be conducive to the change?
- How will the culture affect the work?
- What cultural norms can be built upon?
- What are the values of the culture?
- How will this change affect the culture?
- Who are powerful individuals within the culture, and could they be enlisted as change agents to promote the change?

The educator must anticipate any barriers to change within the culture and be prepared to address any or all of the following (DeBoor, 2023):

- Differing faculty values about nursing education
- Faculty fear of losing control of aspects of the curriculum
- Differing views about curricular priorities
- Lack of support for the need for change
- Uncertainty or inexperience with curricular change
- Incivility among team members
- Faculty feeling that workload and time constraints make the idea of change too overwhelming

The academic nurse educator needs to maintain a culturally sensitive attitude when enacting change to best promote success and sustainability of desired changes. Adoption of change happens at varying rates; some faculty adopt the change right away, some take longer, and some may refuse to ever adopt the desired change. Shared dialogue about the change helps decrease change-related anxiety (Iwasiw et al., 2020).

To maximize the successful implementation of any change, it is important for the educator to maintain an environment that is culturally sensitive for all change discussions and work. Successful implementation of change is enhanced if the educator creates an inclusive environment by (Billings & Halstead, 2020):

- Involving key faculty and faculty leaders
- Setting agreed-upon goals with the group for the change
- Maintaining transparency throughout the change process
- Ensuring openness and respect for all opinions to be shared
- Setting agreed-upon timelines for the change

It is the nurse educator's responsibility to help create a culturally sensitive environment that is inclusive, civil, and respectful and that garners support for a shared vision of excellence and continuous quality improvement. Without this commitment to inclusivity and sensitivity in the organizational cultural environment, it is impossible for the nurse educator to enact change that will keep pace with what will be required to maintain a nursing program that is adaptive to change and reflective of high-quality nursing education.

Evaluating Organizational Effectiveness in Nursing Education

Evaluating organizational effectiveness for continual quality improvement is an important function of the academic nurse educator. All members of the faculty should be involved in the *program assessment* process. The program assessment process involves ongoing and comprehensive evaluation of program data to inform the need for improvement and decision making. The purpose for program assessment (sometimes referred to as *program evaluation*) is to determine the extent a program meets expected outcomes. The program assessment plan, or systematic plan for program evaluation, provides a road map for the direction for program decisions and a plan and documentation method for the evaluative process (Billings & Halstead, 2020). Learning organizations perform best when program decisions are made in a collaborative setting and are supported by accurate operating data (Oermann, 2017). The program assessment plan provides evidence of the organization's response to both internal and external requirements for accountability (Oermann & Gaberson, 2021) Internal requirements for accountability are set by the faculty, learners, and administration of the organization. External demands are set by those regulating the program externally and include state regulators and accreditors.

When developing a comprehensive program assessment plan, it is important to review the literature to design a plan that is evidence-based. Several evidence-based program assessment models that can be used as a framework for determining an assessment plan are described in the literature. Some assessment plans are based on accreditation or state approval standards. Using these standards as a framework ensures the program is meeting all accreditation and state approval requirements for a program. It may not be as comprehensive as use of a model but does ensure state and national standards are met. Some programs do not engage in developing or implementing an assessment plan until time for an accreditation visit, which is an unacceptable practice. Ongoing program evaluation must be continuous for actual improvement to occur (Billings & Halstead, 2020). See Chapter 5 for further information on the program assessment process.

Accreditation is a national voluntary process that assures the public that all standards for the program are met and that the education is the quality expected. Programs are accredited both by a regional accreditor for the institution and a program accreditor for the nursing program. Nursing program accrediting agencies include:

- Accrediting Commission for Education in Nursing (ACEN): Accredits practical, diploma, associate, baccalaureate, master's, and doctoral programs
- National League for Nursing Commission for Nursing Education Accreditation (NLN-CNEA): Accredits practical, diploma, associate, baccalaureate, master's, and doctoral programs
- Commission on Collegiate Nursing Education (CCNE): Accredits baccalaureate and master's degree nursing programs, practice-focused nursing doctoral programs such as the Doctor of Nursing Practice (DNP) degree, postgraduate advanced practice registered nurse (APRN) certificate programs, and entry-to-practice residency programs
- Canadian Association of Schools of Nursing: National accrediting body for registered nurse (RN) education in Canada

The focus of accreditation is on quality improvement and establishing if national standards of excellence are met. It requires documentation of internal assessment through a self-study process and external assessments conducted through site visits by accrediting visitors. State regulation of the nursing program is like accreditation in that it is designed to protect the public's best interest. However, approval is not voluntary; a nursing program cannot operate without approval by either the state board of nursing (prelicensure programs) and/or by state commissions or boards of higher education.

CNE®/CNE®n Key Point

Remember: Approval by a state agency is required and recognizes a program as meeting state nursing education regulations. *Accreditation* is the national voluntary process by nongovernmental agencies that recognize a program as being qualified to provide excellence in nursing education.

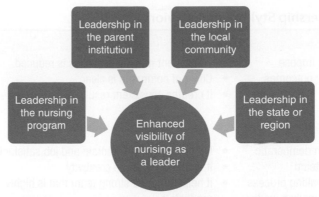

FIG. 6.1 Providing leadership in nursing education and the resultant impact of the enhanced visibility of nursing.

Enhancing the Visibility of Nursing and Its Contributions as a Leader

Through the demonstration of effective leadership skills, the academic nurse educator can serve as a change agent and enhance the visibility of nursing in the institution, community, and beyond. Fig. 6.1 demonstrates the relationship between providing nursing leadership in these areas and the resultant impact of enhancing the visibility of nursing. It is essential for nurse educators to be prepared to provide leadership to advance nursing practice, nursing education, and science (Halstead, 2019). Nurse educators must seek out opportunities to continually develop and enhance leadership skills to teach and role model leadership abilities that, in turn, empower graduates to serve as leaders who will then influence the advancement of nursing and health care. Additionally, nurse educators provide leadership through innovative teaching practices to teach advocacy for both their community and the nursing profession. As a leader in nursing education, the educator participates in and provides leadership for interdisciplinary efforts to collaborate and address the educational and health care needs of the institution, local region, state, and/or nation. The academic nurse educator provides this leadership through teaching, research, practice, service, and interdisciplinary collaborative activities.

Leadership in the Nursing Program

Nursing faculty are unique in that they are leaders who actively participate in a shared decision-making process to determine the work or actions for the nursing program (Iwasiw et al., 2020). All academic nurse educators are leaders because they are expected to participate in and can influence this collective decision-making process. Nursing faculty leadership can occur in a formal role, such as that of an administrator for the nursing program, course coordinator, level coordinator, lead faculty, or program committee chairperson. Informal leadership may include providing leadership through discussions in a faculty meeting or through interactions with fellow faculty and students. Nurse educators should be familiar with effective leadership models to provide leadership to enact change. Depending on the situation, a variety of leadership skills may need to be employed to facilitate a desired change. For example, most situations in nursing education require transformational leaders who inspire their team with a shared vision and then support and empower the team to achieve this vision. Sometimes a participative leadership style is needed to obtain group approval for a particular decision. Occasionally an authoritarian leadership style is required when a particular decision must occur. For example, an accreditation standard for NCLEX® pass rates may require an authoritarian decision by the nurse leadership team to achieve this standard. Table 6.2 summarizes *transformational, transactional, authoritarian, participative,* and *laissez-fair* types of *leadership styles* and behaviors.

Administrators providing leadership in nursing education are expected to be content experts who have extensive knowledge of the nursing profession and possess managerial expertise. Additionally, administrative leaders need to have analytical abilities, skills for building effective

TABLE 6.2	**Leadership Styles and Behaviors**	
Leadership Style	**Advantages**	**Disadvantages**
Authoritarian: Leaders impose expectations and define outcomes.	• Time spent making decisions is reduced. • Chain of command is clear. • It creates consistent results.	• Very strict authoritarian leaders can lead to employee rebellion. • It inhibits group creativity. • It reduces collaboration. • It increases faculty turnover rate.
Participative: Rooted in democratic theory; leader involves team members in decision-making process, although leader will normally have the last word.	• It increases faculty morale and job satisfaction. • It encourages group creativity. • It helps create a strong team that is highly productive.	• Decision-making processes become slow. • Communication failures can sometimes happen. • Security issues can arise from transparency.
Delegative leadership: "Laissez-faire" ("hands off"); focuses on delegating initiative to team members	• Successful if team members are competent and accountable. • Innovation and creativity are highly valued. • It creates a positive work environment. • It evades difficulties.	• Command responsibility is not properly defined. • It can create difficulty in adapting to change. • Disagreements may divide group, leading to poor motivation and low morale.
Transactional leadership: Transactions between a leader and followers—rewards, punishments, and other exchanges to complete work. The leader sets the goals, and team members know how they will be rewarded for meeting them. Concerned with following established routines and procedures rather than making transformational changes.	• Leaders set specific, achievable goals for team. • Team motivation and productivity are increased. • It minimizes confusion in the chain of command. • It is easy for leaders to implement and easy to follow. • It is task focused and power based.	• Innovation and creativity are minimized. • Empathy is not valued. • It creates more followers than leaders among the team.
Transformational leadership: The leader inspires the team with a vision and then supports and empowers the team to achieve that vision. The leader is a role model for the vision.	• It results in low team member turnover rate. • It promotes team satisfaction, organizational commitment, and retention of members. • It places high value on institutional vision. • Emphasis is on capacity building. • Morale of employees is high. • It uses motivation to gain support of team members. • It is not coercive. • It promotes open relationships.	• Leaders can deceive team members. • Consistent motivation with constant feedback may be needed. • It can sometimes lead to the deviation from protocols.

interpersonal relationships, and the ability to create a productive work environment (Iwasiw et al., 2020). Administrators are expected to provide effective leadership to guide the faculty through any major program changes (e.g., curricular change) and need to be able to (Iwasiw et al., 2020):

- Create a vision and moral purpose for any change.
- Remain flexible.
- Build relationships.
- Demonstrate artistry and tact.
- Create and share knowledge.
- Assist others through the process of change while maintaining desired timelines.
- Assist others with understanding the change.

TABLE 6.3	Boyer's Model of Scholarship (1990) Definitions With Examples of Activities That Demonstrate Program and Institutional Leadership for Nurse Educators		
Scholarship	**Definition**	**Examples of Program Leadership Activities**	**Examples of Institutional Leadership Activities**
Teaching	Effectively communicating the knowledge of the profession to the learner	• Developing innovative curriculum and teaching activities • Disseminating teaching knowledge to colleagues within the program	• Participating in nursing or on institutional curriculum committee • Mentoring a faculty member outside of nursing
Discovery	Discovering new knowledge for application and integration into the discipline and for teaching	• Serving as a content expert with learners and colleagues • Seeking out continuing education so that teaching practices are up-to-date • Developing research that contributes to the work of the program	• Participating in interdisciplinary research • Participating on the institutional review board
Integration	Interpreting and incorporating knowledge across disciplines to develop a larger context of knowledge	• Designing learning activities that provide for collaboration across disciplines • Designing learning models that guide learners to apply previous knowledge to the clinical setting	• Serving on an institutional committee to develop faculty policies • Participating in the development of the institutional mission, vision, and philosophy statements
Application	Demonstrating professional nursing practice and service	• Being an active member of a professional nursing organization • Performing service activities in which practice and theory come together to form new knowledge, such as taking a group of clinical students to provide health education in a senior center	• Practicing in the university community health clinic with nursing students • Engaging in an interdisciplinary service activity, such as serving as a university representative in a county-wide mass disaster event

Data from Billings, D. M., & Halstead, J. A. (2020). *Teaching in nursing: A guide for faculty* (6th ed.). St. Louis: Elsevier.

To sustain any desired changes, the formal leader must maintain the energy of the group, have ongoing attention and commitment to the change, and maintain the culture of the change. Administrators are also responsible for the congruence of the program with the organization. They have responsibility for the selection and assignment of faculty to relevant coursework. Finally, administrators have the responsibility for the oversight of the budget and coordination of all physical resources, including obtaining needed lab equipment or clinical experiences for the program.

An important component of leadership for the nurse educator is that of mentor and professional role model for both learners and fellow nurse educators. The mentoring of students includes academic advisement and support, coaching, and guiding learners through the educational process to their professional careers. Nurse educators mentor faculty members through coaching and guiding new educators as they learn their role as faculty. Not only do those new to teaching require mentoring, but experienced teachers who are new to an institution need mentoring as well (see Chapter 7). Program leadership is also provided through modeling of professional behaviors, civility, and communication as nurse educators serve as continual role models of professionalism for their learners and fellow colleagues.

The role of nursing faculty is in teaching, scholarship, and service to the nursing program and to the school. Through the lens of *Boyer's Model of Scholarship* (1990), in which faculty participate in the *Scholarship of Teaching, Application, Integration, and Discovery,* nursing faculty provide leadership to the program and the institution. Table 6.3 reviews descriptions of these four areas of Boyer's Scholarship, with examples of activities that demonstrate leadership for the program and institution in each area of scholarship. Additional information on scholarship for nurse educators and Boyer's model can be found in Chapter 7.

Leadership in the Parent Institution

The academic nurse educator role includes the responsibility for influencing institutional change that enhances student learning by engaging in the governance activities of the parent institution. Institutional leadership requires the nurse educator to participate in department and university committees that focus on academic and workplace issues such as faculty affairs, student affairs, curriculum, program evaluation, and consultation with administration. Participating in *university governance* requires that the nurse educator not only address the issues of the university but also must be responsive to the issues within the community (Billings & Halstead, 2020).

Participation in regional accreditation activities for the institution also provides the nurse educator an opportunity for leadership. Nurse educators are uniquely suited to this role because of their extensive experience with the nursing education accreditation process, which can be an excellent resource for an institution about accreditation. Accreditation activities could include participation in preparation of regional accreditation documentation or serving as a resource for site visitors.

Interdisciplinary (interprofessional) collaboration with departments outside of nursing also provides an opportunity for institutional leadership. The nurse educator can collaborate with general education faculty in a discussion of the mutual relationship between preparatory general education coursework as it relates to the nursing curriculum. Additionally, the experienced nurse educator can provide mentoring in teaching or research to less experienced faculty members in other disciplines.

Leadership in the Local Community

Academic nurse educators are in the unique position to provide leadership in their role to have a direct positive influence on the health of the community in which they serve. Nursing programs may need to define exactly what community of interest the institution serves. For example, some institutions serve communities that are clearly defined by a certain geographic region where the school is located. Other institutions serve communities across the state or nation through provision of online nursing education outside the geographic region of the school (DeBoor, 2023). Once the community served is defined, nurse educators provide leadership that facilitates state-of-the-art nursing education, clinical experiences, and service-learning activities that positively affect the area the learners and/or institution is located. Additionally, the nurse educator helps prepare graduates to be leaders who then provide leadership and quality care in the community.

Health care is shifting away from the acute hospital-based setting to care that is provided in the community and managed through case managers. When developing a nursing curriculum, the nurse educator needs to incorporate education for the learner on providing *community-based care* in which graduates are expected to demonstrate leadership for coordinating collaborative, community-based care or to act as a primary care provider within the community.

Providing leadership within the community also requires the nurse educator to build or participate in interdisciplinary, collaborative partnerships with other organizations, clinical agencies, and health care providers within the community. Through these relationships, the educator can further identify the needs of the community and facilitate clinical experiences or service-learning activities to address these identified needs.

The academic nurse educator can serve as a content expert and provide continuing education to health care facilities or clinical partners. For example, a nurse educator can provide an expert continuing education session to clinical staff who work with learners on a particular topic. Community leadership can also be provided through serving on area clinical or professional organizational boards to provide a nursing education perspective in local decision making.

Leadership in the State or Region

Leaders in nursing education have a strong and informed voice and have the potential to make positive change in health care, yet they are often left out of important health care discussions because of their lack of recognition as leaders in policy change. Academic nurse educators are well-informed on the current state of health care trends and needs. Nurse educators offer an important perspective of managing the competing priorities of the business of health care with improvement of client outcomes (Halstead, 2019).

By participating in interdisciplinary efforts with government, organization, and health care entities, nurse educators can lead policy change that will affect the health of the people in the state and/or region where they live. Nurse educators can provide leadership on governing boards that make health care decisions for the state or region. Educators can participate in analysis of public policy for a governing agency or provide valuable feedback to legislators (Billings & Halstead, 2020).

The nurse educator can also provide leadership at the state or regional level by participating in area collaborations. For example, in Kansas, the administrators for all the practical, associate, and baccalaureate nursing programs in the state meet quarterly to discuss issues in nursing education and issues related to legislation. A representative from the state board of nursing attends these meetings, and an ongoing dialogue occurs in which administrators are informed of potential legislation in nursing education. Conversely, nursing education administrators provide helpful feedback that the state representative then provides to the legislators. The educator can also provide leadership by serving on a state nursing committee or the state board of nursing.

Membership in professional organizations such as the American Nurses Association (ANA) or the NLN provides opportunities for the academic nurse educator to demonstrate leadership and provides a means for enhancing the visibility of nursing at a state or regional level. Active membership in a professional organization provides an opportunity for many similar-minded professionals to join to have a larger voice and provides opportunities for enhanced professional prospective, knowledge development, and the opportunity to create change (Cline et al., 2019). Professional nursing organizations provide development in leadership for nurse members. They provide knowledge to help members maintain currency in nursing and nursing education and stay informed on health care legislation. These organizations provide nursing representatives to attend state and national legislative events so that nursing is represented and has a voice in decision making.

Obtaining *professional nursing certification* in a specialty area is another avenue for demonstrating nursing leadership. Certification demonstrates expert knowledge in a nursing practice area and ensures educators are well informed on current best practices on which to base their teaching. Certification can be obtained in a practice area specialty such as pediatrics or critical care. Additionally, the academic nurse educator can obtain certification as an expert academic nurse educator by obtaining the Certified Nurse Educator credential (CNE®), as an academic clinical nurse educator by obtaining the Certified Academic Clinical Nurse Educator credential (CNE®cl), and/or as an academic novice educator by obtaining the Certified Academic Novice Educator credential (CNE®n). All academic educator certifications are offered through the NLN and demonstrate that the highest standards of excellence, professionalism, and leadership in nursing education are met.

Nursing leadership in academia can extend beyond the borders of the state and region. For example, the academic nurse educator can serve as a host for a visiting scholar. Educators may also facilitate or participate in study abroad programs. Nurse educators participate in national or international interdisciplinary efforts to provide care or conduct research. The findings of these efforts are ultimately disseminated through publications and provide leadership to not only nursing education but to nursing and health care communities as well.

Participating in Interdisciplinary Efforts to Address Health Care and Educational Needs

Nurses working together with interdisciplinary professionals (often referred to as *interprofessionals*) offer each other new perspectives on health care issues and provide a renewed energy to the team (Halstead, 2019). This collaboration to address health care and educational needs can develop a network and partnership that work toward a shared vision to effect change and achieve quality patient care. Interdisciplinary teams that educators can participate in can be varied and include *community partnerships, educational-practice partnerships,* institutional interdepartment partnerships, and nursing program partnerships with other educational institutions.

Interdisciplinary collaboration needs to be part of the nursing curriculum at all program levels. Learners must be educated in the importance of interdisciplinary collaboration and be provided with the skills needed to participate in collaborative teams. The curriculum needs to include content on interdisciplinary communication, unification of priorities between health profession programs, and the role of nursing in collaborative partnerships (Halstead, 2019).

Addressing Needs Within the Institution

The academic nurse educator can provide leadership to improve health and address needs within the campus community. An *environmental scan* can be done to determine the health needs of the learners and faculty and available resources within the organization. Faculty can work with nursing students through service learning to provide health care education, promote awareness of health-related issues such as access to care, and address issues such as access to basic needs such as food (Billings & Halstead, 2020). Many colleges offer food pantries to aid learners due to the increasing numbers who do not have financial resources. Nurse educators can provide leadership to promote awareness and obtain needed resources to affect identified needs. For example, they can help arrange clinical experiences in the campus health clinic where nursing students can provide health promotion education. These experiences provide leadership to the campus community and at the same time provide valuable clinical experience for nursing students. Today's learners are greatly affected by many mental health conditions and often have limited access to needed care. The nurse educator can work with the institutional counseling department and involve nursing students to help with promoting awareness, providing health promotion information, and aid in obtaining any needed resources to support learners struggling with mental health challenges. Additionally, the nurse educator can use this opportunity to work with learners to affect any negative stigma associated with mental illness.

Addressing Local Needs

It is important for nurse educators to provide leadership in interdisciplinary efforts to address health care and educational needs for the community they serve. An environmental scan of the community with environmental data analysis is an important intervention that can identify health needs and trends to target with the curriculum. Forecasting health care needs for the community through regional and national data analysis and review of evidence can be a proactive method for anticipating potential concerns (Billings & Halstead, 2020). For example, when COVID-19 began, interdisciplinary teams in various communities throughout the world began local preparations for managing this pandemic in their local area. Chapter 5 provides further information on developing nursing curriculum to aid in addressing local health care needs within the community. The academic nurse educator can serve as a leader for community health initiatives by providing expertise to the community in health care knowledge and by using educational abilities to effectively provide education to community members as needed.

Practice partnerships between faculty and health care agencies can not only provide care to the clients they serve but can also help prepare learners for future practice as nurse leaders and foster achievement of educational goals (Billings & Halstead, 2020). Some faculty may have a joint appointment to spend part of their time teaching and part of their time as a practitioner in a community health clinic, thus providing leadership in both areas.

In their role as nurse educators, faculty can involve learners in all areas of meeting community needs. Learners can be engaged in community leadership through participating in community-based research projects, area health care initiatives, and service-learning projects. In this way, leadership begins to become instilled in learners, preparing them to begin to serve as leaders and participants in their community upon entry into practice.

Addressing Regional Needs

Nurse educators can address regional and even global health care needs by participating in collaborative efforts to effect positive change. The priority for nurse educators is to improve health and promote health equity with a global focus that transcends boundaries (Billings & Halstead, 2020). Nurses are challenged to work to their full scope of practice and to contribute to the redesign of health care across the region within an interprofessional collaborative team.

Area communities are increasingly diverse and represent countries from around the world. Nurse educators working with learners have the capacity to provide care for and communicate with individuals within the community who come from diverse backgrounds that may differ from that of the educator. This opportunity to work with international populations provides the educator and learners the opportunity to better understand and address a wide range of global health concerns that are present within the community. Additionally, nurse educators can participate in interdisciplinary, global health partnerships to design learning activities that provide care and health leadership to populations abroad. Educators can involve learners in these partnership activities and, in turn, learners gain experience in a different health care system, gain an enlarged worldview, and become aware of global health issues.

Familiarity with social determinants of health can aid the nurse educator in determining priority areas of health care needs for the region. These priorities can guide the educator in determining interventions for creating positive change through curriculum design, selection of learning activities for students, and participation in legislative efforts to promote needed change.

Finally, the nurse educator needs to be familiar with priority needs for nursing education in the region. Current challenges facing nursing education include but are not limited to nursing faculty shortage, aging of current faculty, lack of diversity within nursing faculty, limited resources for providing clinical education, decreased resources for higher education, and rapid expansion of technology.

Implementing Strategies for Change

Some organizations are very successful in implementing change, whereas others are unsuccessful in either enacting or, more importantly, sustaining needed change. Change in the work of the nursing program happens not only within the culture of the organization but also within the individuals working within the organization (Iwasiw et al., 2020).

For successful implementation and maintenance of change to occur, a change agent or leader often needs to begin by considering an evidence-based change model on which to guide change. Selecting the change model allows for a framework for progress of work and can be selected by the group to provide a common frame of reference for the change process. Table 6.4 provides examples of *theoretical change models* that can provide a framework for change and provides an understanding of the process of change. Assessment of readiness for change and preparation for anticipated change involve examining and preparing to address a wide range of attitudes toward change. The classic *Roger's Change Model* (1962) describes five types of adopters of change characteristics. In this model, some group members will be innovators and early adopters of change and will need little intervention to gain support. Others will be late adopters or laggards who will need much more evidence for change and influence to garner their support of needed change. Without addressing group members' readiness for change or gaining buy-in for change, the change cannot be enacted or maintained.

TABLE **6.4**	Examples of Theoretical Change Models
Models of Change	**Key Points**
Lewin's Three-Step Model (1947)	Change involves three steps: 1. Unfreeze the present level. 2. Move to the new level. 3. Freeze the new change.
Lippitt's Seven-Step Change Theory (expansion of Lewin's theory to place emphasis on change agent)	1. Diagnose the problem. 2. Evaluate motivation and capability for change; identify resources. 3. Assess the change agent's motivation and resources. 4. Select progressive change objectives; develop action plans and strategies. 5. Explain the role of the change agent to all involved and clarify expectations. 6. Maintain change by facilitating feedback. 7. Gradually terminate the helping relationship of the change agent.
Roger's (1962) diffusion of innovations	This theory explains how an idea gains momentum and diffuses through a system or population. Adoption of a new idea does not happen simultaneously among the group. It is important to understand the characteristics of adopter categories to understand the desired audience and prepare strategies for helping them adopt the desired change. • **Innovators:** Early adopters, assume risk; requires little intervention to gain support. • **Early adopters:** Embrace change easily, leaders, and are aware of need for change. Strategies to support: Communicate implementation of change. • **Early majority:** Rarely leaders but adopt ideas earlier than average. Strategies to support: Provide success stories and evidence for need for change. • **Late majority:** Skeptical of change, will only adopt if majority of others have tried. Strategies to support: Include information on how many others have adopted the change. • **Laggards:** Bound by tradition, conservative. Very skeptical and hardest to convince. Strategies to support: Provide statistics and gain support of others in the group to help encourage them to support the change.
Social cognitive theory	Learning and change occur in a social context with the reciprocal interaction of the person, environment, and behavior, with an emphasis on social influence and external/internal social reinforcement. Focus is on achieving self-efficacy (an individual's judgment about the ability to carry out a behavior at a certain level), which will aid in sustaining/maintaining desired change.
SWOT analysis	This model determines an organization's readiness for change and examines: **S:** Strengths of the present operation you can draw on to facilitate change **W:** Weaknesses that may hinder change **O:** Opportunities; what future opportunities exist related to the change **T:** Threats; what are the potential threats to the desired change

Change should be evidence-based and data driven. For example, nursing programs should use program assessment plans to analyze curricular performance and drive needed curricular changes. Additionally, the program assessment process aids in creating a sustained group focus for maintaining change. Any proposed changes should align with the goals and mission of the organization. Faculty, administrator, and stakeholder support for the change is critical. All involved in the change will need the knowledge and skills to engage in the change; the change agent will need to be prepared for potential resistance to the desired change. The timing of the change is critical, and attention needs to be given to potential competing priorities (Billings & Halstead, 2020). For example, trying to complete a curricular revision at the same time as an accreditation self-study may result in an overwhelming amount of workload for faculty. Faculty may not have adequate time to properly develop both major works at the same time, which may result in faculty fatigue and lack of buy-in for the desired change. The organization should be capable of the change and be able to obtain any necessary fiscal, physical, or human resources needed for implementation. The change agent will need to assess how this change will be implemented and procure needed resources in advance of implementation.

Changing Within the Nursing Program

Barriers and resistance to any desired changes within the nursing program need to be anticipated, including faculty who are inexperienced with desired change, who have a lack of trust for needed change, or who feel they have a lack of time to implement change. Fear and resistance to change are also major barriers the change agent may face. Continual or frequent changes can result in "change fatigue," which can lead to group members appearing critical, disengaged, apathetic, or ambivalent (DeBoor, 2023).

Changes within the nursing program often require a change in the culture of the program. Faculty readiness for change and the belief in the ability to implement the change need to be examined and addressed. The change agent can create an environment of team readiness and acceptance for desired changes by involving key faculty, having agreed-upon desired outcomes, maintaining a transparent process, providing frequent and ongoing communication, creating a shared timeline, and demonstrating respect for all opinions. Presenting faculty with data or evidence for change can be a powerful motivator for acceptance of change as nursing faculty are firmly grounded in evidence-based practice.

Initiating and maintaining any proposed change often take ongoing intensive efforts by the change agent or leaders of the proposed change. Some strategies that have been effective in implementing change in a nursing program include (Oermann, 2017):

- Developing a unified purpose
- Group creation of the mission/vision/philosophy statements
- Using outside consultation and guidance
- Expressing a unified leadership culture by the formal unit leader
- Gathering/communicating data in a way that all can understand
- Tying the change to external influences, including accreditation standards, state educational boards, and boards of nursing
- Using a timeline and taking small steps toward the desired goal
- Identifying a faculty leader to set agendas and meetings to help guide the change
- Using small groups for tasks that report to a larger group (e.g., task forces)

CNE®/CNE®n Key Point

Remember: Selecting an appropriate change agent for leading and facilitating needed change within the nursing program is an important first step when considering change. The change agent might be a/an:

- Nurse administrator
- External consultant
- Group of key faculty leaders
- Nursing committee
- Clinical education leader

Changing Within the Institution

As experienced nurse leaders who are grounded in knowledge of change theory, nurse educators are in a key position to effect positive change within the institution. Participating on institutional committees provides the nursing faculty the chance to influence processes and policies at the institutional level that will affect the nursing program. Nurse faculty participating in interdisciplinary collaboration on institutional committees can work to create a shared vision for the institution that incorporates the nursing program perspective. Results of environmental scanning done by nurse faculty can be reported to the institutional committees to inform decision making. Participation in institutional governance provides nursing faculty the opportunity to be involved in leadership at the institutional level and to aid in providing direction for the organization while ensuring that nursing has a voice in all decision making (Halstead, 2019). Participation in an institutional committee is a service activity. This service provides an opportunity for the nurse educator to participate in shared institutional governance and provides an opportunity to shape institutional policies and facilitate change that ultimately affects the nursing program.

It is important for the academic nurse educator acting as a change agent to be familiar with the process of change within the institution. Participating in faculty governance will increase knowledge and awareness of the institutional processes of change. Additionally, nursing faculty will become aware of budgetary priorities for the institution and become familiar with the process for requesting needed resources. Any change within the nursing program is also likely to need to go through the approval process of the institution. Faculty familiarity with the institutional change process can aid the program in obtaining needed approvals for desired changes or resource requests in a timely manner. For example, curricular changes are likely to need approvals by division and/or college curriculum committees. Leaders of the desired change will need to prepare supporting evidence and communications to institutional leaders so that the rationale for the desired change can be understood and a shared vision for the change can be created.

Changing Within the Local Community

Nurse educators afford change in the community through their participation on area committees, on advisory boards, and in legislative efforts. Nurse leaders work to create change through interdisciplinary community collaborations and partnerships that facilitate collaboration between nursing education and practice (Halstead, 2019). Additionally, nurse educators can serve as change agents in the community by participating in collaborative practice settings where they can provide leadership to the interdisciplinary care team on best practices.

When implementing change in the community, many of the same principles will need to be considered to effect desired change within the community. The change agent will need to (Oermann, 2017):

- Identify relevant stakeholders.
- Determine the level of interest/influence of each stakeholder.
- Engage the stakeholder as early as possible.
- Communicate desired change frequently through a variety of methods to all involved.
- Solicit feedback from stakeholders.

The academic nurse educator can act as an agent for change in the community through relationships and ongoing discussion with community partners and advisory committee members. Through open dialogue with these external stakeholders, the nurse educator can build relationships that aid in facilitating change both in the nursing program and in the external community environment. These ongoing dialogues can aid the nurse educator in effecting change that positively affects the nursing program, such as clarifying expectations for student learning needs in the clinical site. Conversely, expectations from the community partner can be clearly communicated to the nurse educator. The nurse educator can then serve as a change agent to facilitate changes needed by the community partner to continue to provide clinical education and to create an effective learning environment for students.

Developing Leadership Skills in Others to Shape and Implement Change

The academic nurse educator serves as a leader who helps establish a shared vision of values and beliefs for a community or organization that lays the groundwork for future decisions and work (Iwasiw et al., 2020). Great leaders work to empower people within their community or organization to make decisions that support these shared goals, values, and vision of the community (Fig. 6.2). The leader's role is to inspire and coach members of the organization to fully participate in the work of the community to enact effective, positive change. It is essential for academic nurse educators to first develop themselves as a leader in nursing to be able to teach and role model leadership skills. These skills will ultimately impart leadership ideals and principles to learners, faculty members, their organizations, and beyond. The role of the nurse educator leader includes inspiring and coaching members of the group to be fully participative in the work of the community (Society for Human Resource Management [SHRM], 2021).

The nurse educator works to develop leadership skills in learners in several ways. First and foremost is through the development of the nursing curriculum. Integration of evidence-based leadership competencies into the curriculum such as those found in the NLN excellence in nursing education model (2006) can promote a comprehensive method for developing these abilities for learners. The NLN model describes competencies for curriculum for promoting leadership and preparing for role expectations upon graduation. Inclusion of these competencies in the curriculum will help to ensure that learners are prepared for their role as future nurse leaders. The nurse educator also promotes leadership skills for learners by serving as a role model for leadership within the program, community, state, and nation. Tenure and promotion requirements often require newer faculty to provide leadership at a local and regional level; then with increased promotion, they require leadership at a national and international level (Billings & Halstead, 2020). Other methods for developing leadership abilities in learners could include incorporating

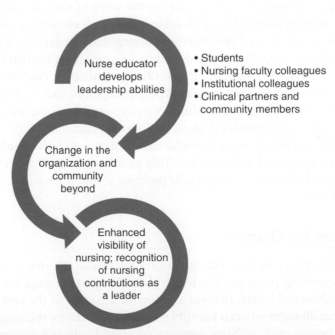

FIG. 6.2 Developing leadership abilities in others through nursing education to enact change and enhance the visibility of nursing.

reflective assignments that examine leadership topics, providing a peer mentor for learners, role-playing scenarios in which leadership is required, and providing periodic feedback to learners on leadership behaviors.

The nurse educator also may serve as a leader by helping to develop leadership skills among the nursing faculty team or by providing leadership to the team on the work of the program and/or curriculum. The work of the faculty team is unique in that all members are called to be leaders who use collective decision making to determine the work of and priorities for the program. This work often involves shared and/or shifting leadership within the group. Because all faculty are required to provide leadership to learners and colleagues within the nursing education unit, it is imperative that all faculty be fully prepared to provide this leadership. Leaders in academia often feel unprepared for this role; often they are unexpectedly thrust into the role of academic leadership without mentoring (Iwasiw et al., 2020). It is important for faculty to be properly developed, supported, and prepared to be able to provide leadership within the nursing educational unit. Methods for providing leadership development for faculty include:

- Assigning an experienced mentor
- Assuming progressively more demanding responsibilities
- Providing support to attend a conference or workshop on leadership
- Encouraging self-appraisal of leadership development
- Providing periodic check-ins with feedback by the leader

Adapting to Changes Created by External Factors

External contextual factors that create the need for change within nursing education are defined as forces or situations that occur outside the nursing educational unit that have the potential to influence curriculum or educational processes. These can originate in the community, region, country, or world (Iwasiw et al., 2020). Faculty must have a clear understanding of these potential forces of change to build a foundation for an effective nursing curriculum. As discussed in Chapter 5, many external societal and stakeholder factors can potentially result in a need for change within the nursing program.

All faculty need to participate in continual external environmental scanning, dialogues with external stakeholders/practice partners, and research of evidence-based sources to aid in informing the educational unit of trends and propose any needed changes. Faculty should involve the broad view of external community stakeholders in the work of the curriculum. External stakeholders need to be engaged in the design, development, implementation, and evaluation of the curriculum to create an educational program for nursing that is reflective of current practice.

To successfully adapt to identified needed changes, faculty must remain flexible and responsive to change. In today's environment of rapid evolving technology, continual change should be an expectation for all faculty. Faculty should expect change not only in health care trends but also in educational practices, including methods of delivering education, methods of instruction, educational technology, and curricular designs (Billings & Halstead, 2020).

Any changes should be led by someone who demonstrates effective leadership abilities (see Table 6.2 for a summary of leadership styles). This process will result in better facilitation and implementation of needed changes, which will promote a smoother adaptation process for the nursing educational unit.

Creating a Culture for Change

Creating a culture for change begins with the leader but is also the shared responsibility for all educators within the nursing program. The leader should begin to engage the team in the work of identifying shared values and beliefs to form a vision for the work of the unit. This action results in a commonality that all members can identify with and that can be referred to should any conflicting views arise (Iwasiw et al., 2020). Creating a successful culture for change is also enhanced by encouraging leadership development of members of the group and providing support for this development. Additionally, a successful culture of change demands an environment of civility and collegiality for any desired work to be completed (Halstead, 2019). Maintaining an environment of civility should be an expectation for all members of the educational unit.

> **CNE®/CNE®n Key Point**
>
> *Remember:* Maintaining an environment of civility and collegiality is the responsibility of all faculty members in the educational unit. A civil environment is a healthy work environment and promotes a culture of support for all members. This in turn provides an environment that will effectively support change.

Certain conditions or external forces, such as failure to achieve a desired program outcome, can help promote a culture of change. This situation can result in increased commitment and sense of urgency by the team to commit to needed change. Six steps to creating a culture for organizational change include (University of Minnesota Libraries, 2010):

1. Creating a sense of urgency, which communicates need for the desired change
2. Changing leaders or other key players
   - Removing anyone who may be a barrier
   - Enlisting a change agent to facilitate needed change
3. Role modeling desired behaviors expected of the members of the unit by leaders
4. Training and support for the team to promote acceptance, understanding of, and sustainability for change
5. Changing the reward system for the team, including rewarding those who embrace the values of the group
6. Creating new rituals, symbols, or habits for the team to replace old ineffective habits

Changing Within the Nursing Program

It is important for the nurse educator to participate in creating and maintaining a culture that is prepared for anticipating and successfully managing change within the nursing program. As previously discussed, it is expected that nursing faculty maintain a nursing program that is current. This is achieved through ongoing environmental scanning and responsiveness to identified needs for change. Nurse educators need to be prepared to be responsive to this ongoing change as well. Persisting in curricular traditions can result in a program that can become stagnant and may eventually experience failure to achieve outcomes that are reflective of current trends in nursing and health care.

Effective leaders for promoting and leading desired change need to be identified. Many faculty leaders are unwillingly thrust into a role of leadership and are not provided adequate development or support to successfully perform their role. It is essential that formal leaders be provided adequate development and support so that they understand the process for implementing change and the importance of creating a shared vision among the organization. Well-prepared leaders are essential to optimizing the long-term success of an organization and creating a culture for change.

Creating a culture of change within the nursing program also requires creating a culture that is collaborative within the organization. Experienced faculty, novice faculty, and learners must participate in creating an effective environment of change. Experienced faculty bring institutional memory, knowledge of curriculum, understanding of policies and resources, and familiarity with approval processes. Novice faculty bring new ideas that are not bound by the traditions of the program, which can help move group thinking forward. Learner involvement informs faculty on their experiences, perspectives, and needs. Involving learners also aids their understanding of the complexity of the program and provides learners a rationale for needed changes (Iwasiw et al., 2020). Additionally, faculty must collaborate outside the organization with institutional faculty, advisory committees, clinical and community partners, and other educational programs so that they can inform and be informed of the nature of change within the program.

Changing Within the Institution

Creating a culture of change within the institution requires that nursing faculty engage in the institutional governance system. Without engagement in the institutional governance system, faculty surrender the right to participate in informed decision making and influence decisions that affect the nursing program (Halstead, 2019). Participation in institutional governance and the creation of a culture of institutional change can ultimately benefit the nursing program further by bringing awareness to the nursing program's priorities and needs.

Faculty experienced in facilitating nursing curriculum can help create a culture of change within the institution through role modeling effective change behaviors. Nursing faculty have extensive experience with quality improvement, accreditation, and program assessment that is data driven. This knowledge can be shared with institutional faculty who may not be as familiar with these areas. Nursing faculty can assume a leadership role in the institution and serve as a guide, cheerleader, source of support, mentor, and agent of change for institutional needs.

Advocating for Nursing, Nursing Education, and Higher Education in the Political Arena

Nurses are widely known to be staunch advocates for their clients and the health of their community. However, they are also reported to have limited engagement in the legislative process and are perceived by some to lack power or knowledge related to policy and politics (Halstead, 2019). Active involvement in professional organizations is an important method for nurse educators to be fully informed of health care issues and engaged in advocacy for policy change. Professional organizations composed of large numbers of nurses provide a larger voice for advocacy and resources for representation of the nursing voice in the political arena. Professional organizations provide ongoing research and information regarding issues relevant to nursing and health care. For example, the NLN (2021) has a web page that provides a Legislative Action Center that provides important and current information on health care policies currently undergoing review. Membership in the ANA (2021) provides advocacy in federal agencies and the White House for nursing and advances the nursing profession across the United States. The ANA works to advocate for nursing at the state level by advocating for nurse practice acts and participating in legislative efforts. The ANA also states that a membership provides the member a chance to advocate for the profession on a grassroots level. Both organizations provide means for the nurse educator to communicate more easily with legislators working on health care and education-related policy. Nurse educators can be involved with policy at an international level by joining an international nursing organization and serving as an international advocate for nursing and health care. The International Council of Nurses (ICN, 2021) provides a wide range of position statements and is accepted into official relations with the World Health Organization (WHO). The ICN ensures nurses have a voice in the development and implementation of international health care policy.

Nurse educators participating in collaborative research that fosters positive patient outcomes and safe and high-quality care can in turn provide advocacy for nursing that can result in policy change (DeBoor, 2023). Nurses who conduct research to improve nursing care promote the importance of evidence-based standards for professional nursing practice. These evidence-based standards then can inform legislation related to nursing practice and nursing education. In this way, nurse researchers provide advocacy for the profession in informing legislation that is based on data and evidence-based standards.

Nurse faculty become advocates in the political arena for nursing education and practice by educating learners to become agents of change who influence legislation and advocate for nursing (Halstead, 2019). This process can occur through classroom instruction on leadership and health care political processes. Nurse faculty also promote learner understanding of advocacy and leadership through role modeling of these behaviors. Incorporation of current issues in health care and social determinants of health into the curriculum can help learners be fully informed of the health care priorities for their community and can encourage learners to become advocates to improve the health of their community. Faculty can accompany learners to legislative events and facilitate dialogue between learners and legislators. Additionally, faculty can introduce learners to joining a professional organization to promote advocacy for the profession by sponsoring a group such as the National Student Nurses Association (NSNA). The academic nurse educator serves as a leader in nursing to advance the profession through advocacy and mentoring. Through this leadership, nurse educators can have current and future impact on the profession that in turn will result in far-reaching, long-lasting, and positive change.

References

Asterisk (*) indicates a classic or definitive work on this subject.

American Nurses Association (ANA). (2021). *ANA membership benefits: Make your voice heard.* https://www.nursingworld.org/membership/member-benefits/.

Billings, D. M., & Halstead, J. A. (2020). *Teaching in nursing: A guide for faculty* (6th ed.). St. Louis: Elsevier.

Christensen, L. S., & Simmons, L. E. (2020). *The scope of practice for academic nurse educators and academic clinical nurse educators* (3rd ed.). Washington, DC: National League for Nursing-Wolters Kluwer.

Cline, D., Curtin, K., & Johnston, P. A. (2019). Professional organization membership: The benefits of increasing nursing participation. *Clinical Journal of Oncology Nursing, 23*(5), 543–546.

DeBoor, S. S. (2023). *Keating's curriculum development and evaluation in nursing education* (5th ed.). New York: Springer.

Halstead, J. A. (2019). *NLN core competencies for nurse educators: A decade of influence.* Philadelphia: Wolters Kluwer.

International Council of Nurses (ICN). (2021). *Who we are.* https://www.icn.ch/who-we-are.

Iwasiw, C. L., Andrusyszyn, M. A., & Goldenberg, D. (2020). *Curriculum development in nursing education.* Burlington, MA: Jones & Bartlett.

*Lewin, K. (1947). *Field theory in social science.* New York: Harper & Row.

National League for Nursing (NLN). (2006). *Excellence in nursing education.* http://www.nln.org/docs/default-source/professional-development-programs/excellence-in-nursing-education-model-(pdf).pdf?sfvrsn=0.

National League for Nursing (NLN). (2019). *Certification in nursing education.* http://www.nln.org/Certification-for-Nurse-Educators.

National League for Nursing (NLN). (2021). *Legislative action center.* http://capwiz.com/nln/home/.

Oermann, M. (2017). *A systematic approach to assessment and evaluation in nursing.* Washington, DC: National League for Nursing-Wolters Kluwer.

Oermann, M. H., & Gaberson, K. B. (2021). *Evaluation and testing in nursing education* (6th ed.). New York: Springer Publishing.

*Rogers, E. M. (1962). *Diffusion of innovations* (4th ed.). New York: The Free Press.

Society for Human Resource Management (SHRM). (2021). *Developing organizational leaders.* https://www.shrm.org/resourcesandtools/tools-and-samples/toolkits/pages/developingorganizationalleaders.aspx.

*University of Minnesota Libraries. (2010). *Organizational behaviors.* https://open.lib.umn.edu/organizationalbehavior/chapter/15-5-creating-culture-change/.

CHAPTER 6 Practice Questions

1. Which activity has the potential for effecting the greatest change for the continual advancement of nursing?
   A. Empowerment of graduates to be leaders
   B. Changing a national health care policy
   C. Creation of nursing research to improve care practices
   D. Providing community leadership on a health care initiative

2. The nurse administrator has developed a professional uniform policy for nursing students without consulting faculty. Which leadership style is the nurse administrator demonstrating?
   A. Participative
   B. Transactional
   C. Delegative
   D. Authoritarian

3. The nurse administrator is developing a policy that provides incentives for faculty to attend committee meetings. Which leadership style is the nurse administrator demonstrating?
   A. Participative
   B. Transactional
   C. Delegative
   D. Authoritarian

4. The nurse administrator has a vision for the nursing education program and wants to empower the team to achieve the vision. Which leadership style is the nurse administrator demonstrating?
   A. Participative
   B. Transactional
   C. Transformational
   D. Authoritarian

5. Which definition best describes organizational culture?
   A. Shared work of the organization
   B. Shared demographics of the organization
   C. Shared beliefs of the organization
   D. Shared abilities of the organization

6. Which intervention by the nurse educator would promote a culturally sensitive organizational climate when facilitating a discussion of a proposed curricular change?
   A. Allowing all faculty at the meeting unlimited time to share opinions
   B. Providing faculty leaders extra time in the meeting to present feedback
   C. Setting parameters to limit the discussion to certain topics
   D. Ensuring openness and respect for all opinions to be shared

7. The nurse educator would like to present information on a desired curricular change to the faculty. Which action demonstrates sensitivity to the culture of the organization and would best promote acceptance of the desired change?
   A. Reassure faculty that they will be provided release time to implement the change.
   B. Involve key faculty and faculty leaders in presenting the change to the group.

C. Limit discussion of the proposed change to experienced faculty.
   D. Set all timelines and deadlines for the change for the group.

8. What is the main difference between program accreditation and program approval by state regulatory agencies?
   A. Program approval is not required but is voluntary.
   B. Accreditation is not required but is voluntary.
   C. Accreditation's purpose is to protect the welfare of the state.
   D. Program assessment is required only for accreditation purposes.

9. The nurse educator is preparing to present a proposal to faculty for a new method of teaching drug calculation. Which intervention would assist the nurse educator to manage any barriers to implementing needed change?
   A. Provide frequent communication of the proposed change using a variety of methods.
   B. Identify potential threats to the proposal and report this to nursing administration.
   C. Notify all faculty that the change will be required by accreditors.
   D. Implement change in the course and demonstrate how easily this can be implemented.

10. Which activity is an external method of evaluation for accreditation and program approval?
    A. Congruence of program mission with institution
    B. Drafting of the self-study
    C. Documenting achievement of program outcomes
    D. Site visit by accrediting agency

11. Which activity demonstrates leadership to learners in promoting civility?
    A. Modeling of professional behaviors in the clinical setting
    B. Serving on a university student affairs committee
    C. Participating in an interdisciplinary faculty discussion on civility
    D. Developing a research tool that measures learner civility

12. Which activity is an example of providing program leadership through the Scholarship of Teaching?
    A. Participating in an institutional search committee
    B. Providing instructional mentoring to an inexperienced faculty
    C. Developing an interactive presentation on asthma for active learning
    D. Presenting information on outcomes of research at a national conference

13. Which activity is an example of providing institutional leadership through the Scholarship of Integration?
    A. Serving on a committee to develop faculty policies for the institution
    B. Serving on the nursing program research committee
    C. Participating in a community health clinic with learners
    D. Mentoring a biology faculty member on a research project

14. The nurse educator is planning a service-learning project as part of a rural nursing course. Which type of scholarly leadership is being demonstrated?
    A. Scholarship of Discovery
    B. Scholarship of Teaching
    C. Scholarship of Application
    D. Scholarship of Integration

15. The nurse educator would like to participate in a leadership activity related to the Scholarship of Discovery at the institutional level. Which example would best demonstrate this type of activity?
    A. Participating in an interdisciplinary research project with the college of pharmacy to promote safety for patients on a ventilator
    B. Participating in a collaborative effort with the math department to create a dimensional analysis teaching activity for nursing students
    C. Participating in a collaborative university service activity with the college of dentistry to promote health in the older adult population in the community
    D. Participating in an interdisciplinary department committee with the school of public health to promote community education on vaccine safety

16. Which statement by the novice nurse educator about institutional leadership would require intervention by the faculty mentor?
    A. "By serving on the committee to revise the institutional mission statement, I will be demonstrating leadership in the scholarly area of integration."
    B. "I need a nurse faculty mentor in order for me to learn more about conducting research at this institution."
    C. "I am taking my learners to spend a clinical day to participate in a bioterrorism event for the community to demonstrate institutional-level leadership."
    D. "As part of the faculty affairs committee for the university, I will be providing leadership that will affect faculty policies related to tenure."

17. Which activity demonstrates nurse educator leadership at the community level?
    A. Coordinating an immunization clinic abroad
    B. Providing continuing education to area clinical partners
    C. Presenting research at a national nursing education conference
    D. Participating in a statewide collaboration to affect legislation

18. Which clinical learning activity would best help develop students' leadership at the community level?
    A. Caring for a pediatric patient in the acute care setting
    B. Clinical postconference discussing community health needs
    C. Creating a nursing care plan to address the needs of the older adult
    D. Having learners work with a case manager who coordinates care

19. Which clinical activity would promote learning about interdisciplinary collaboration for providing leadership at the community level?
    A. Participating with the local health department to provide an immunization clinic
    B. Participating in an international study-abroad event to provide health care services and health promotion
    C. Speaking at the state student nurse association conference as part of a group
    D. Observing the collaboration of the team in an area operating room during a clinical rotation

20. Which activity demonstrates nurse educator leadership at the state level?
    A. Serving as a representative on a professional conference committee
    B. Serving as a representative on the university outreach committee
    C. Serving as a representative on the board of a nursing education committee
    D. Serving as a representative on a professional nursing organization committee

21. Which statement by the novice nurse educator about joining a professional organization requires intervention by the mentor?
    A. "Joining a professional organization is optional and is focused on networking."
    B. "Joining a professional organization gives nursing a larger voice."
    C. "Joining a professional organization is an important manner for providing leadership."
    D. "Joining a professional organization enhances the visibility of nursing."

22. Which statement by the novice nurse educator demonstrates understanding of the importance of obtaining professional certification in nursing education?
    A. "Obtaining a professional certification in nursing education is not as critical as obtaining clinical professional certification."
    B. "Obtaining a professional certification in nursing education does not demonstrate leadership."
    C. "Obtaining a professional certification in nursing education demonstrates standards of excellence have been met."
    D. "Obtaining a professional certification in nursing education demonstrates a higher level of clinical knowledge."

23. Which activity demonstrates the nurse educator addressing health-related needs at an institutional level?
    A. Promoting immunization awareness through an area coalition within the county
    B. Providing a clinical service-learning experience for students at the area food pantry to learn about area food needs
    C. Accompanying students in the student nurses' association to a legislative event to discuss health care policy
    D. Providing a service-learning experience to discourage negative mental health stigma on campus

24. Which activity would be an important first step for the nurse educator to consider when looking to address institutional health-related needs?
    A. Conducting an environmental scan to determine and prioritize institutional health-related needs
    B. Developing health promotion materials that are at an appropriate level for the desired student learner
    C. Creating a service-learning project that addresses a need that aligns with course objectives
    D. Evaluating the effectiveness of a newly implemented campus food pantry

25. The nurse educator is involving clinical students in providing care to other learners with HIV at the campus student health services center. This learning activity is an example of addressing health care needs at which of the following levels?
    A. Program level
    B. Institutional level
    C. Community level
    D. Regional level

26. Which activity will provide an opportunity to address local health care needs through interdisciplinary efforts and provide leadership development for learners?
    A. Clinical education experience providing client care at a county-funded hospital
    B. Clinical education experience providing client care at a practice partnership clinic
    C. Clinical education experience providing education at a day care center
    D. Clinical education experience obtaining vital signs and providing education at a senior adult health fair

27. Which statement best describes the purpose for an environmental scan of the community?
    A. Environmental scanning is required for program accreditation.
    B. Environmental scanning is used to guide selection of clinical sites.
    C. Environmental scanning of the community is used to identify health needs to guide the curriculum.
    D. Environmental scanning is conducted by the institution rather than the nursing faculty.

28. Which activity best describes an evidence-based method for forecasting health care needs for the local community?
    A. Analysis and review of county health statistics
    B. Focus group discussions of health care concerns with area interest groups
    C. Review of the local news reports for the area on health care needs
    D. Review of nursing textbooks on community health

29. Which clinical activity is easily implemented and will best assist students to learn to address global health concerns?
    A. Participating in a study-abroad women's health clinic
    B. Providing care at an international medical mission
    C. Completing a concept map diagramming a major global health issue
    D. Working with international populations within the community

30. Which outcome is of the greatest benefit to learners involved in global health partnership activities?
    A. An enlarged worldview
    B. Experience in a variety of languages
    C. Opportunity to network with health care providers
    D. Increased opportunity for hands-on experience

31. Which source would best aid the nurse educator in developing curriculum that addresses the priority health needs for the region?
    A. QSEN competencies
    B. Essentials for baccalaureate nursing programs
    C. Social determinants of health
    D. Scope of practice statement

32. Which model is founded on unfreezing the present level, moving to a new level, and freezing the new change?
    A. Lewin's model
    B. Lippitt's change theory
    C. Roger's diffusion of innovations
    D. Social cognitive theory

33. The curriculum committee is considering a curricular change and examining the strengths and weaknesses related to the potential change. This activity is an example of which change theory?
    A. Lewin's model
    B. SWOT analysis
    C. Roger's diffusion of innovations
    D. Social cognitive theory

34. The curriculum committee is implementing a curricular change and examining the rate at which the faculty may accept the new change to address potential concerns. This process is an example of implementation of which change theory?
    A. Lewin's model
    B. SWOT analysis
    C. Roger's diffusion of innovations
    D. Social cognitive theory

35. The nurse consultant is assisting a program to implement a curricular change. The consultant selects progressive change objectives, develops an action plan for the change, and explains the consultant's role in the change process. This process is an example of implementation of which change theory?
    A. Lewin's model
    B. Lippitt's change theory
    C. Roger's diffusion of innovations
    D. Social cognitive theory

36. Which activity is an important first step before considering change in a nursing curriculum?
    A. Analysis of faculty behaviors to determine acceptance for change
    B. Review of leadership strategies for change agent
    C. Creation of a timeline for desired change
    D. Selection of a change theory to guide the intended change

37. Which statement by the novice nurse educator indicates an understanding of potential faculty reactions to change?
    A. "Some faculty may have differing views on whether this change should be implemented."
    B. "Faculty will embrace the change easily, as it is forward thinking."
    C. "The curriculum committee recommends this, so it will be eagerly adopted."
    D. "Professor A teaches this course but will support its elimination if it is recommended."

38. Which statement about creating an environment of readiness for change by the novice nurse educator requires intervention by the nurse mentor?
    A. "Key faculty leaders will need to be involved in preparing for the change."
    B. "The nurse administrator needs to create a timeline for implementation of the change."
    C. "The faculty will need to create agreed-upon goals for the change."
    D. "Data will need to be presented to support this change if faculty are going to accept this."

39. Which statement by the novice nurse educator indicates an understanding of the importance of participating in faculty governance?
    A. "Serving on the institutional faculty committee will ensure that nursing has a voice in policy development."
    B. "Serving on an institutional committee is really more about the Scholarship of Discovery."
    C. "Institutional committee work does not directly affect our work in the nursing program."
    D. "Only experienced faculty members should consider serving on an institutional committee."

40. Which statement about creating change at the institutional level by the novice nurse educator requires intervention by the nurse mentor?
    A. "I would like to participate in the institutional student affairs committee so that I can provide the nursing perspective."
    B. "My mentor serves on the institutional curriculum committee as a service activity for the institution."
    C. "Nursing does not need a representative for the institutional assessment committee, as we have our own program assessment plan."
    D. "I will review the duties of each institutional committee to see which would be a good fit for my interests."

41. Which activity would best promote leadership abilities in learners?
    A. Role modeling leadership skills and abilities
    B. Assigning self-reflection writing assignments examining leadership topics
    C. Assigning a peer-mentor for each learner
    D. Developing a curriculum that includes evidence-based leadership competencies

42. Which assignment would best develop leadership abilities in a new nurse faculty member?
    A. Chair of the curriculum committee
    B. Instructor for the nursing leadership course
    C. Creating the research team for a new project
    D. Working with an experienced faculty member to develop a course

43. Which statement by a nurse leader demonstrates an understanding of effectively promoting leadership abilities within faculty members?
    A. "I will need to try to obtain resources for the new faculty to attend the leadership conference this fall."
    B. "I will need to assign the new faculty to a high-level course to provide them the opportunity to demonstrate leadership."
    C. "I will need to meet with the new faculty at the end of the school year to help them reflect on any leadership questions they may have."
    D. "I will need to make sure all new faculty do not work on any parts of the curriculum development we have to do this year."

44. Which statement by a nurse leader demonstrates an understanding of effectively adapting to change created by external factors?
    A. "This curriculum has been successful for the last 10 years. It would be best not to make changes at this time, as everything seems to be working."
    B. "I will need to attend the advisory committee meeting for this fall so we can ask clinical partners for their input on this curricular decision."
    C. "It is the responsibility of the more experienced instructors to participate in environmental scanning for educational and health care trends to determine what should go in the curriculum."
    D. "Nursing faculty are best suited to make all curricular decisions. Those without a nursing education graduate degree really should not be contributing to decisions about curriculum."

45. Which statement by the novice nurse educator indicates a need for intervention by the nurse mentor?
    A. "The nursing faculty will need to continually review accreditation standards for potential changes."
    B. "I would like to attend a conference so that I can learn about any new changes in my field of nursing."
    C. "Nursing faculty should consider joining area professional organizations to learn more about any changes in the community."
    D. "Global health care trends are not as relevant for nursing curriculum, as they may not affect our community."

46. Which nurse educator characteristic would best promote adaptability to change?
    A. Flexibility
    B. Curricular knowledge
    C. Clinical expertise
    D. Advanced degree

47. Which situation often creates a sense of urgency for changing an organizational culture?
    A. Incivility among the team
    B. Failure to achieve a desired outcome
    C. Selection of a new team leader
    D. Disagreement on values and beliefs

48. Which outcome would likely result in commonality among group members and promotion of a culture for change?
    A. Creating shared values and beliefs for the organization
    B. Promoting civility and collegiality
    C. Providing leadership development and support
    D. Providing a reward system for those who embrace the values of the group

49. Which factor is a major barrier to a culture of change?
    A. Incivility among team members
    B. Failure to achieve a desired outcome
    C. Inexperienced leader
    D. External stakeholder views

50. Which statement about change by the novice nurse educator indicates a need for intervention by the nurse mentor?
    A. "This curricular discussion should be limited to faculty who are experienced."
    B. "Learner input should be obtained when considering a program decision."
    C. "Nursing faculty should obtain advisory committee feedback on this curricular change."
    D. "Our organization needs to be collaborative to create a culture of change."

51. Which outcome is a major consequence when nursing faculty fail to participate in institutional governance?
    A. Limited opportunity for promotion and tenure for nursing faculty
    B. Inability to participate in or influence decisions that affect nursing
    C. Loss of budgetary resources to other departments
    D. Lack of opportunities to network with other faculty

52. Which statement by the novice nurse educator indicates an understanding of the best method for advocating for nursing in the political arena?
    A. "I will participate on the state board of nursing education committee."
    B. "I will join a national professional nursing organization."
    C. "I will develop a research project that informs policy on nursing care."
    D. "I will teach my learners health care policy and political processes."

Pursuing Continuous Quality Improvement in the Nurse Educator Role

LINDA KAYE WALTERS

LEARNING OUTCOMES

1. Summarize components of a formal orientation and mentoring for the nurse educator.
2. Identify activities that promote socialization to the nurse educator role.
3. Describe the role of the nurse educator as a lifelong learner.
4. Differentiate the four areas of Boyer's Model of Scholarship as a role for the nurse educator.
5. Describe how the nurse educator uses feedback and self-reflection to increase role effectiveness.
6. State examples of legal and ethical standards relevant to nursing and higher education.
7. Explain how nurse educators can manage their teaching, scholarship, and service demands.

Nurse educators are responsible for self-development in their role. Once they are socialized, nurse educators are accountable for pursuing continuous quality improvement in teaching, scholarship, and service.

Engaging in Activities That Promote Socialization to the Nurse Educator Role

Academic nurse educators should be oriented to their role on initial hire and then mentored as they progress in their career.

Orientation to the Nurse Educator Role

Socialization as a nurse educator begins as an introduction to the academic environment for new faculty as part of orientation (Billings & Halstead, 2020). A standardized institutional and nursing program orientation to the role is essential for all newly hired faculty members. For example, as part of general orientation, all faculty need to be informed of their job benefits, take a campus or school tour, and understand the organizational structure and culture.

Then, based on the background and experience of the new faculty, the remaining time in orientation should be tailored to fit the educator's individual needs and experience. Each faculty's orientation process should then be documented to meet nursing accreditation and state board of nursing requirements. The major elements of orientation to the nursing program or department include but are not limited to:

- Physical resources, including classrooms, skills practice labs, simulation labs, and computer labs
- Clinical facility where faculty will supervise learners
- Nursing program curriculum and course syllabi
- Contact personnel/key resources within the nursing department or college of nursing

- Contact personnel/key resources within the academic institution
- Job benefits overview
- Nursing faculty and administrative support staff
- Learning and student support resources in the nursing department and institution

An essential part of orientation for the new nurse educator is to become very familiar with institutional and nursing faculty handbooks. These vital resources outline the faculty policies and procedures that should be followed while the educator is employed in the academic setting. These handbooks also illustrate departmental and institutional organizational charts and provide information on faculty support services, administrative and faculty governance structures and processes, and promotion and tenure expectations, if applicable.

Promotion and Tenure

Most public and private universities and colleges offer educator ranking and tenure systems. Faculty in these institutions must apply for promotion and tenure using well-developed portfolios to present their accomplishments. *Portfolios,* also referred to as *dossiers,* present a collection of scholarly documents to demonstrate the educator's ability to meet the requirements for promotion to a higher rank or achievement of tenure. The purpose of the portfolio is stated at the beginning of the collection and typically includes a *curriculum vitae (CV).* A CV is a document used to outline current and previous professional activities associated with the nurse educator's career, including employment history, educational history, scholarship activities, awards and honors, and professional memberships. This document is extensive and describes the course of the nurse educator's entire career (Christenbery, 2014).

Table 7.1 displays examples of rank, typical promotion and tenure requirements, and common educator activities for each rank. The new nurse educator needs to be aware of these teaching, scholarship, and service expectations during orientation.

TABLE 7.1   **Ranking and/or Promotion and Tenure Based on Scholarship Activities**

Ranking/Promotion and Tenure	Requirements	Scholarship Activities
Instructor: Either multiyear, clinical, adjunct, or lecturer for clinical or nontenure track (not considered a rank for the tenure track)	Teaching	• Facilitating learning • Using best practices to be an effective nursing educator
Assistant professor: Probationary period during which faculty members progress according to institutional standards in teaching, scholarship, and service (tenure track)	Teaching, scholarship, and service	• Facilitating learning • Using best practices to be an effective nursing educator • Actively applying oneself in the nursing education profession
Associate professor: Usually achieved by the sixth year	Teaching, scholarship, and service	• Facilitating learning • Using best practices to be an effective nursing educator • Integrating interprofessional research, presentations, publications, and effective teaching methodologies through discovery and creativity and modes of delivery • Actively applying oneself in the nursing education profession • Actively researching or discovering new knowledge
Full professor: Usually achieved by the tenth year	Teaching, scholarship, and service	• Facilitating learning • Using best practices to be an effective nursing educator • Integrating interprofessional research, presentations, publications, and effective teaching methodologies through discovery and creativity and modes of delivery • Actively applying oneself in the nursing education profession • Actively researching or discovering new knowledge • Functioning as a role model for educators at lower ranks

In addition to the tenure track that provides job security within the institution, colleges and universities offer other appointment tracks for educators who do not desire a tenure position. Table 7.2 delineates nontenure educator roles commonly offered in large institutions.

Many vocational/career educational centers, public community colleges, and proprietary colleges do not have a tenure or ranking system. For example, vocational/career centers or proprietary colleges often do not offer tenure, and educators may maintain the title of instructor or other title during their entire employment.

Faculty Mentorship

Faculty mentoring is one of the many responsibilities of the nurse educator. The mentoring process helps faculty grow as they advance in their new academic role. Each newly hired nurse educator should be assigned to a faculty mentor for assistance with teaching and scholarship development. Ultimately, the mentor and mentee should share similar schedules; the mentor should be both mentally and physically available.

Novice nurse educators typically lack confidence and knowledge about teaching. An integrative review by Dahike et al. (2021) found that a formal mentorship program is essential to enhance the transition of novice educators to the academic setting and role. The time frame for the initial formal mentorship is typically 6 to 12 months, depending on the experience of the nurse educator. According to the National League for Nursing (NLN) (2006), faculty mentoring should occur through a nurse educator's entire career through three stages: early career, mid-career, and late career, as described in Table 7.3.

The role of the *faculty mentor* for the novice nurse educator is to advise and support both new and experienced educators beginning with their first day of employment. The mentor should be well-informed of where the starting point is for each newly hired employee to assist in his or her development as both educator and scholar (Billings & Halstead, 2020). Positive mentoring styles that promote success also provide new faculty empowerment and growth. Part of this mentoring process includes addressing questions or concerns and providing expert coaching; however, mentors typically do not evaluate or supervise new faculty. Another important role of the mentor

TABLE 7.2	Examples of Nontenure Positions and Roles
Example of Nontenure Position	**Role of the Nontenure Academic Position**
Clinical track faculty	Educator who has an advanced practice role; does not engage primarily in research, but may be promoted through a clinical ranking system
Research scientist	Academic role dedicated to conducting funded research and dissemination of findings through publications and presentations
Visiting position	Educator of any rank who has a limited appointment, often 1–2 years
Lecturer	Prerank position similar to instructor in which the educator does not have the credentials for the tenure track
Adjunct/part-time faculty	Part-time educator who often works with learners in the clinical setting but may teach in the classroom or online
Professor emeritus	Title of honor confirmed for retired faculty who may have special benefits such as access to the college or university learning resource center, computer support, and/or office space
Teaching assistant	Graduate student who helps faculty part-time with teaching responsibilities

[a]Adapted from Billings, D. M., & Halstead, J. A. (2020). *Teaching in nursing: A guide for faculty* (6th ed.). St. Louis: Elsevier.

TABLE 7.3	Mentoring Stages and Activities During the Nurse Educator's Career
Mentoring Stages	**Mentoring Activities**
Early career: New to both educator role and institution	• Educate about faculty role • Answer questions • Provide guidance regarding teaching and evaluation activities • Provide information about knowledge, skills, behaviors, and values needed throughout the educator's career • Be supportive
Midcareer: Better understanding of pedagogies, able to work through problems with own solutions; evolving scholar at all levels	• Mentee drives activities • Reciprocal sharing, learning, and growth • Varied mentorships based on needs (e.g., grant writing, publications, and/or leadership responsibilities)
Late career: Mentor–mentee relationship with ongoing growth, networking, and continued contributions to the profession	• Foster a sense of belonging for all faculty • Collaborate in all areas of teaching, service, scholarship, and engagement • Identify and foster growth of leadership qualities

Data from National League for Nursing (NLN). (2006). Position-statement: Mentoring of nurse faculty. *Nursing Education Perspectives, 27*(2), 110–113.

is to assist novice faculty in navigating the political and administrative aspects of the academic setting. Mentoring new faculty should include:

• Introductions to other faculty and staff
• Review of available physical and learning resources
• Job benefits
• Governance structure
• Overview of organizational and academic culture
• Review of courses and content that the mentee will be teaching
• Review of expectations for teaching, research, and service

Socialization into the role of the nurse educator is evident by the educator's behaviors and activities. For example, using the faculty handbook to support decisions regarding learners illustrates the reliance on established policies and procedures. Faculty socialization is also illustrated when the educator seeks opportunities to become an integral part of the institution, such as volunteering for membership on a nursing program/department committee or task force. Some academic institutions require or recommend that faculty be involved in one or more institutional committees or task groups to achieve promotion and/or tenure. Clarification will be needed for individual institutions determining what the overall expectation of service is. According to Halstead and Frank (2011), by the second year of a faculty appointment, the nurse educator should be on at least one departmental committee; by the third year, the educator should seek membership on an institutional committee. Nurse educators should align service opportunities with the mission and vision of their institution in addition to the time investment needed to serve on committees, the duties that are required, if it is elected or nominated, and how it fits into one's personal goals or expertise. Table 7.4 displays examples of service opportunities.

CNE®/CNE®n Key Point

Remember: Socialization into the new nurse educator role should start with a standardized institution and nursing program/department orientation and then be shaped to the needs and experience of each individual. Novice educators should be assigned to *faculty mentors* to assist them with teaching and scholarship development.

TABLE 7.4	Examples of Academic Service Opportunities
Program-Level Service	Curriculum committee Assessment committee Student affairs committee Faculty affairs committee Steering or department committee Grievance committee
Institutional-Level Service	Faculty executive committee Faculty senate Arts endowment committee Graduate council committee Grievance committee

Adapted from Halstead, J. A., & Frank, B. (2011). *Pathways to a nursing education career. Educating the next generation of nurses.* New York: Spring Publishing.

Maintaining Membership in Professional Organizations

Many national and international professional organizations are available for the nurse educator to join as a member and can be divided into two major categories: (1) those organizations that represent nursing practice or clinical specialties, such as the American Nurses Association (ANA), Academy of Medical-Surgical Nurses (AMSN), and Association of Women's Health, Obstetric and Neonatal Nurses (AWHONN); and (2) those organizations that represent nursing education, such as the Organization of Associate Degree Nursing (OADN), American Association of Colleges of Nursing (AACN), and NLN. Nurse educators often join organizations in both categories to continue growth and develop expertise in clinical and educational best practices.

Membership in professional nursing organizations has many benefits for the nurse educator. For example, some organizations publish a peer-reviewed professional journal and/or informational newsletter that is part of the membership fee. OADN publishes *Teaching and Learning in Nursing*; the NLN publishes a nursing research journal called *Nursing Education Perspectives*. In addition to these journals, most professional organizations offer one or more conferences and workshops for continuing education each year. Members often attend at a discounted registration fee.

Some organizations offer certifications in a nursing practice area or education. For instance, the ANA offers multiple clinical specialty certifications at the basic and advanced practice levels. The NLN provides the opportunity to achieve the Certified Nurse Educator® (CNE®), Certified Academic Clinical Educator (CNE®cl), and Certified Academic Novice Nurse Educator (CNE®n) credentials. Achieving certification in any practice or education area validates the nurse educator's expertise and demonstrates proficiency in practice.

As noted by these examples, nursing organizational memberships can advance and validate the educator's knowledge, provide interactions with other nurses, and promote professional and personal growth. Involvement in professional organizations can also provide opportunities for educators to shape health and educational policies through leadership experiences. Maintaining and increasing competence helps nurse educators gain expertise in their nursing specialties in addition to offering guidance in other areas of teaching, scholarship, and service.

Participating Actively in Professional Organizations Through Leadership and Committee Roles

Being a member of a professional organization is not the same as participating *actively* in that organization. Nurse educators are often members of multiple nursing organizations but do not become involved in any of the organization's activities at local, state, or national levels.

Nurse educators in academic settings are expected to demonstrate leadership within their institution and contribute to the nursing profession outside the institution. Opportunities for leadership in professional organizations include being an editor or reviewer for organizational publications, working on a committee or task force, becoming a member of the organization's board or officer, and contributing to special projects, such as updating standards of practice or developing a white paper. Some organizations also solicit members to help support the passage of health care legislation on a local, state, and/or national level.

Active participation in professional organizations at the local, state, or national/international level allows the nurse educator to have a voice in achieving the work and growth of the profession and to satisfy service requirements. Most professional organizations have standing committees and special committees or task forces to achieve the goals of the organization. These subgroups usually report to the organization's board of directors and share their work with the full membership after board approval.

Another leadership opportunity for the nurse educator is to run for office or other positions on the organization's board of directors. These leadership roles are more time consuming than that of committees or special project work but can be very satisfying while shaping the direction of the professional organization and contributing to nursing outside the academic setting. Chapter 6 describes the role of the nurse educator as a leader within the nursing profession in more detail.

> ### CNE®/CNE®n Key Point
>
> **Remember:** Nursing organizational memberships can advance and validate the nurse educator's knowledge, provide interactions with other nurses, and promote professional and personal growth.

Demonstrating Commitment to Lifelong Learning

Nursing programs of every type and level emphasize the need for learners to be committed to lifelong learning. That same commitment applies to nurse educators! Professional development begins with orientation to the academic setting and the nursing program. After orientation is completed, the nurse educator should have administrative and financial support for continuing learning and professional development.

Ongoing changes in health care and the nursing profession demand that nurse educators maintain competency in one's specialty area of practice. Additionally, new educational practices and factors affecting teaching-learning practices require that the nurse educator continue learning through professional development. Nursing students have changing needs as learners. For example, the recent addition of Generation Z learners to nursing classrooms and the online environment presents a new challenge for educators who may not be technologically savvy. Professional development activities can help prepare educators for the needs of increasingly diverse learners. Some of these development activities include:

- Advising
- Classroom management
- Informatics
- Teaching strategies
- Curriculum development and/or revision
- Assisting with accreditation and evaluating the outcomes
- Cultural awareness
- Learning about incivility among faculty and in the classroom

Examples of participation in continuing education activities include reading and writing journal articles; attending webinars; attending nursing program/department workshops; and attending local, state, and national conferences and conventions. Most of these activities provide nursing contact hours that can be applied to nursing licensure and certification renewal. The nurse educator should check the requirements for renewals and plan which qualifying continuing education activities are needed.

Continuing one's formal education to achieve an advanced degree is also part of lifelong learning. A terminal degree (doctorate) is required in many universities and colleges to qualify for promotion and tenure. Many academic institutions provide financial support for faculty to pursue advanced degrees.

Participating in Professional Development That Increases Role Effectiveness

Nurse educators teach in practical/vocational, associate degree, baccalaureate, master's, and doctoral nursing programs. The role of nurse educators varies depending on the level of nursing program and type of educational institution (Oermann et al., 2018). In any nursing program, the primary role of the nurse educator is to facilitate student learning to meet curricular outcomes. Therefore faculty need professional development in educational best practices, both in general higher education and nursing education. As described in Chapter 2, nurse educators no longer rely only on lecture supported by multiple slides to help students learn course content. Various generations of students, diverse learning styles, an increase in online learning, and the availability of high-fidelity technology have all changed the way educators teach and students learn. To maintain currency in best educational practices based on these changes, the nurse educator needs to seek opportunities for faculty development to become as effective as possible in the teaching-learning role.

Managing the Teaching, Scholarship, and Service Demands of the Institution

Scholarship is commonly defined as nurse educator activities that advance the teaching, research, and practice of nursing through a spirit of inquiry. Nurse educators in many colleges and universities are expected to conduct research, obtain grants, write for publication, and engage in service activities. In addition to support and guidance from faculty mentors, educators functioning in these roles need professional development in these areas to be effective.

Boyer's Model of Scholarship (1990) is the most common tool used for evaluating faculty scholarship, faculty performance, and eligibility for promotion and tenure. This model may also be used to help faculty organize a professional portfolio.

According to Boyer, scholarship includes four areas: Discovery, Teaching, Application, and Integration. Table 7.5 outlines these four areas with examples of each one and their general relationship to ranking criteria. Specific ranking and tenure criteria vary from institution to institution. Some educational institutions have no ranking or tenure policies. Nurse educators need to be aware of what is expected for the institution where they are employed.

The Scholarship of Discovery can include primary empirical research, analysis of large data sets, theory development, and methodologic studies. Discovery can be considered as the basis for the other three scholarship areas in that research provides the evidence needed for teaching, application, and integration. Even if not employed by a research institution, all faculty should at a minimum use best current evidence as a basis for their clinical and educational practice.

Engaging in the Scholarship of Teaching is an expectation of all faculty regardless of their institution or program type and requires that the nurse educator demonstrate effective evidence-based teaching-learning expertise. This area of scholarship provides faculty with the opportunity to be innovative and creative in multiple learning environments, including the classroom, online, and clinical settings. Examples of innovative or creative scholarship activities include use of new curricular models, application of technology to facilitate learning, and strategic methods to meet the diverse needs of learners.

The Scholarship of Application focuses on service to the nursing profession at a local community, regional, national, or international level. Service obligations can also occur at the program, department, college, or university level, depending on the organization. Departmental or program-level service examples include serving as a faculty mentor, being a member or leader of a committee or task force, and developing a service-learning project. Local community service

TABLE 7.5	Boyer's Model of Scholarship		
Scholarship Types/Categories	**Key Words**	**Description**	**Specific Example**
Teaching	Learning	• Facilitating learning • Using best practices to be an effective nursing educator	Attend a conference about Kahoot; implement the use of Kahoot into the next class.
Integration	Interprofessional	• Integrating interprofessional research, presentations, publications, and effective teaching methodologies through discovery and creativity and modes of delivery	Social work, nursing, and respiratory therapy students collaborate for a simulation in a hospital setting. Pretest and posttest administered. Results presented to faculty in all departments about lack of understanding of roles in the health care field.
Application	Professional practice and service	• Actively applying oneself in the nursing and nursing education profession	Achieve professional development by attending professional education conferences, participating in committees or task forces, setting up faculty-run clinics, applying research to the profession, and developing and implementing service learning projects.
Discovery	Research	• Actively researching or discovering new knowledge	Research the effectiveness of standardized testing on learner outcomes; publish the research and results.

examples include assisting in vaccination clinics and local church food banks. Professional nursing service could include being a member of an editorial board, journal peer reviewer, grant reviewer, or committee or board member.

Service learning is an educational experience in which learners participate in a "hands-on" activity to meet the health needs of a particular population and to promote civic engagement. This experience is typically either part of an existing nursing program course or a separate course in the curriculum. Learners are trained before performing the service-learning experience so that they are well-prepared for their roles. Service learning is not a replacement for clinical practice, but rather an additional learning experience for both students and faculty.

Benefits of service learning for the student include (Billings & Halstead, 2020):
- Provides an opportunity for collaborative learning and teamwork
- Encourages self-directed learning
- Facilitates leadership skill development
- Develops advocacy and caring skills
- Develops cultural awareness and competence
- Increases insight into self-understanding
- Facilitates academic inquiry
- Allows learners to meet course objectives

The nurse educator and institution can also benefit from service learning experiences. Because service learning is an example of the Scholarship of Application, the nurse educator can document outcomes of the experience and include them as part of the portfolio for promotion and tenure. Having learners use reflective tools such as journaling is an excellent way for the nurse educator to evaluate the effectiveness of the experience and to help validate that outcomes have indeed been met. Service learning can also help create a sense of community on the college or university campus and increase learner recruitment and retention. When service-learning activities are made known publicly, the college or university may gain increased recognition and donations (Billings & Halstead, 2020).

Boyer's Scholarship of Integration requires the nurse educator to collaborate with interprofessional health care team members to interpret and synthesize knowledge to create new models of care or teaching. An example of the Scholarship of Integration is conducting and publishing research on interprofessional simulation.

Managing the educational institution's demands for teaching, scholarship, and service can be challenging for the nurse educator unless a stepwise plan is developed. For example, the novice educator may be completing a master's or doctoral degree while holding the rank of instructor. If the college or university has a ranking and tenure system, the educator at the assistant professor level may focus on the Scholarship of Teaching and Application. When promoted to associate professor, the educator might then focus on the Scholarship of Discovery and Integration. The full professor functions as a role model for other faculty at lower ranks.

CNE®/CNE®n Key Point

Remember: Scholarship is commonly defined as nurse educator activities that advance the teaching, research, and practice of nursing through a spirit of inquiry. According to Boyer, scholarship includes four areas: Discovery, Teaching, Application, and Integration. Engaging in the Scholarship of Teaching is an expectation of all faculty regardless of their institution or program type.

Using Feedback Gained From Self, Peer, Learner, and Administrative Evaluation to Improve Role Effectiveness

Feedback from various evaluations helps the nurse educator gain a sense of role effectiveness. This feedback helps to guide teaching, research, and faculty socialization. One form of evaluation is *self-reflection*. Self-reflection can be used to document educator performance based on previously developed goals for the academic year. Nurse educators need to incorporate thoughts, emotions, decisions, and behaviors related to these goals to better plan for future development in their role. One method of reflection is to document several paragraphs outlining what worked and was accomplished and what did not work or was not accomplished over the past year. Another way to self-reflect is on an ongoing basis, perhaps weekly or monthly, or possibly during specific positive or negative experiences. Self-reflection data may be shared with the faculty mentor for feedback. This feedback should consist of direct and indirect guidance to help interpret the findings and provide support and guidance, while helping to enhance the professional development and skills of the mentee.

Peer faculty evaluations, both formative and summative, can be used to provide feedback on nurse educator performance. A peer may observe a lecture or review an online class as part of the performance evaluation. Desired educator attributes during those teaching activities include organization, content clarity, and learner engagement. Summative evaluation may include a yearly review of all required criteria for an educator's promotion and/or tenure. Many colleges and universities no longer require or encourage peer evaluations.

In most academic institutions, *student or learner evaluations* are thought to be the hallmark of determining the nurse educator's teaching effectiveness. Most universities and/or colleges have a standard course evaluation tool that is given directly to the learners, bypassing the faculty member being evaluated to ensure confidentiality and decreasing fear of faculty retribution based on learner responses. This evaluation tool requires learners to assess various course components and identify the strengths and weakness of the nurse educator who taught the course. The major pitfall of this type of evaluation is that some results may be skewed by personal feelings of one or more learners with disregard to how effective educators actually functioned in their role.

Administrative evaluations are used to ensure establishment and maintenance of professional performance goals, with identification of the nurse educator's strengths and any areas needing improvement. These evaluations may be completed by the chair, director, and/or dean of nursing or health sciences.

Practice Within Legal and Ethical Standards Relevant to Nursing and Higher Education

Functioning within the nurse educator role requires awareness of the legal standards and ethical principles that apply in academia. Many of the same principles that guide nurse–patient relationships guide learner–faculty interactions, ranging from mandated policies by legislative and regulatory agencies to ethical issues that can occur within the program (Billings & Halstead, 2020).

Student Rights

The federal Family Educational Rights and Privacy Act (FERPA) was established to protect student privacy and confidentiality. The nurse educator needs to be familiar with student rights that are delineated within this law, which include the right to:

- Have access to education records
- Request education records amended as needed
- Have control over disclosure of personally identifiable information in learner records
- File a complaint with the U.S. Department of Education if rights are violated

The institution is obligated to keep all learner records confidential. The law covers learners 18 years of age and older. Parents or guardians must have written permission from the learner, even if the parents or guardians are paying for the tuition. If records are in a paper format, they should be kept in a locked cabinet with limited access to key personnel. Paperless records should be password protected with limited access.

Learners' rights are also protected by federal law if they volunteer as research subjects. Before conducting research involving learners, nurse educators must apply to the *institutional review board* (IRB). The purpose of an IRB is to ensure that the rights, welfare, and well-being of people participating in research activities are protected in accordance with federal regulations known as the *1991 Common Rule (Protection of Human Subjects)*. Areas of legal/ethical concern when conducting research on human subjects include confidentiality and informed consent, including delineation of potential risks to participants. Any legal, emotional, economic, psychological, and physical risks must be identified with methods to mitigate them.

CNE®/CNE®n Key Point

Remember: The federal Family Educational Rights and Privacy Act (FERPA) was established to protect student privacy and confidentiality. The nurse educator needs to be familiar with the protection of student rights.

Learner Fairness

Once admitted to the program, learners have a right to fair treatment by outlining all program expectations. Program information and expectations should be specified in the nursing student handbook and reviewed during program orientation. This handbook sets forth the learner requirements and responsibilities in meeting the program outcomes set forth by the faculty. Many institutions require that learners sign a document stating that they have read and understand the policies and expectations in the handbook.

In addition, all program changes that occur during a learner's nursing education should be communicated to learners in a timely manner using a variety of methods such as email, learning management system post, and face-to-face disclosure. Less significant program or course changes may be communicated weeks before implementation. Changes that have a larger impact should be communicated months in advance of their implementation. A curriculum revision that could affect a learner's program of study or course requirements is an example of a major change that should be discussed and communicated in writing to all learners, preferably 6 months to a year in advance before it is initiated. Learners may be required to acknowledge awareness of all program or course changes in writing.

Faculty also discuss learner expectations during orientation to each course, including a review of the course syllabus. A course syllabus may be considered a legal contract between learners and faculty. If changes are made to the course syllabus, the updated version must be dated and sent directly to the learners, with the updated information highlighted in the email. During each course, the nurse educator is obligated to keep learners informed about their progress. Proper notification of failing to progress needs to be provided in a timely manner, including the formal identification of the learner's deficiencies and the plan needed for learner improvement to pass the course. If the learner fails at the end of the course, proper notification of the failing grade needs to be provided in a timely manner, allowing time for a face-to-face meeting if possible. Any type of formal documentation used should be signed by both faculty and learner. The educator should keep all didactic work, clinical assignments, and tests for each learner until the course is completed and learners receive their course grades.

Another issue related to fair treatment of learners is the practice of *just culture* during their course clinical practicum. The Joint Commission (TJC) requires that hospitals and other TJC-accredited clinical agencies need to create a just culture for improving the incidence of errors and near-misses. A just culture avoids blame and uses errors as learning opportunities for quality improvement.

In nursing education, just culture includes:

- Accepting that mistakes are part of the learning process
- Holding learners and faculty accountable for creating a safe learning environment
- Avoiding blame when addressing learner errors
- Limiting any disciplinary action to those learners who are reckless in their practice

Nursing program faculty generally have not widely used this approach for learner errors. A multisite study by Walker et al. (2020) found that learners are expected to avoid errors during clinical practice. This expectation becomes increasingly emphasized as prelicensure learners continue in their nursing program. The study also noted that many nurse educators are not aware of the National Council of Boards of Nursing (NCSBN) national data repository for voluntary reporting of learner errors and near-misses using the Safe Student Reporting tool. These data can help educators focus on common errors and plan strategies to help learners prevent them in a safe learning environment.

Other Relevant Legal/Ethical Issues

Examples of other legal/ethical issues that face today's nurse educators include academic integrity, use of social media, incivility, and high-stakes testing. Cheating across the curriculum is the most common violation of *academic integrity*. Cheating on tests and plagiarizing papers are common examples. In some instances, learners do not realize they are cheating, especially if they do not understand plagiarism. Other learners deliberately cheat by purchasing online textbook test banks. This issue needs to be discussed and enforced for learners to understand what is and what is not considered academic dishonesty. An up-front conversation with examples can possibly deter this problem. Some programs require learners to sign an "honor" statement before each exam to remind them not to cheat and the penalty for cheating if they do.

Most learners rely heavily on *social media* to communicate. However, some learners may not recognize that using social media to post negative comments about faculty, administration, or other learners; sharing photos of patients or clinical agencies; and/or providing course test items is unethical and unprofessional. These types of social media postings are confidentiality and privacy violations that can result in dismissal from school; civil and criminal sanctions may also be imposed.

Social media also provides a platform for learner-to-learner *incivility* and bullying. In some nursing programs, faculty are uncivil to learners or other faculty and learners are uncivil to faculty or other learners. None of these situations are acceptable, and all of them demonstrate unprofessional behavior. Learners need to display professional behaviors in all settings. Faculty are role models for learners and need to act in a professional manner at all times. Some programs have established a zero-tolerance policy for incivility. These policies may include statements such as ". . . this serves as your official warning . . . ," allowing for faculty to dismiss learners upon the first offense. The nurse educator should be aware of learner conduct expectations by reviewing the associated policies. The language could then be placed into syllabi and reviewed on the first day of class, verifying that learners are aware of the institution's already established policies and procedures and the implications for learners.

Another fairness issue that the nurse educator may face is the use of *high-stakes testing*. Most prelicensure programs use commercial standardized exams to help their learners identify content strengths and weaknesses. However, some programs use these tests as an evaluation tool to determine whether the learner passes or fails a course or can graduate on time as expected. The NLN and most state boards of nursing support implementing standardized test requirements. However, they discourage the use of these tests for high-stakes purposes and advise that more than one type of assessment tool be used to evaluate student learning.

CNE®/CNE®n Key Point

Remember: Functioning within the nurse educator role requires awareness of the legal standards and ethical principles that apply in academia. Many of the same principles that guide nurse–patient relationships guide learner–faculty interactions to maintain learner confidentiality and privacy.

References

Asterisk (*) indicates a classic or definitive work on this subject.

Billings, D. M., & Halstead, J. A. (2020). *Teaching in nursing: A guide for faculty* (6th ed.). St. Louis: Elsevier.

*Boyer, E. L. (1990). *Scholarship reconsidered: Priorities of the professoriate*. Princeton, NJ: Carnegie Foundation for the Advancement of Teaching.

*Christenbery, T. (2014). The curriculum vitae: Gateway to academia. *Nurse Educator*, 39(6), 267–268.

Dahike, S., Raymond, C., Penconek, T., & Swaboda, N. (2021). An integrative review of mentoring novice faculty to teach. *Journal of Nursing Education*, 60(4), 203–208.

*Halstead, J. A., & Frank, B. (2011). *Pathways to a nursing education career. Educating the next generation of nurses*. New York: Springer Publishing.

*National League for Nursing (NLN). (2006). Position-statement: Mentoring of nurse faculty. *Nursing Education Perspectives*, 27(2), 110–113.

Oermann, M. H., DeGagne, J. C., & Phillips, B. C. (2018). *Teaching in nursing and the role of the educator* (2nd ed.). New York: Springer Publishing.

Walker, D., Altmiller, G., Hromadik, L., Barkell, N., Barker, N., Boyd, T., et al. (2020). Nursing students' perception of just culture in nursing programs. *Nurse Educator*, 45(3), 133–138.

CHAPTER 7 Practice Questions

1. A nurse educator demonstrates socialization into the academic role when the educator does which one of the following?
   A. Prepares a class lesson plan
   B. Asks to be a nursing committee member
   C. Meets with learners during office hours
   D. Attends a professional development workshop

2. Orientation to the nurse educator role is dependent on which one of the following important factors?
   A. The individual nurse educator's experience and needs
   B. The time when the formal orientation process begins
   C. The number of employees who participate in the orientation
   D. The nurse educator's experience working as a clinical nurse

3. Which of the following activities would not be included in a formal orientation for the nurse educator?
   A. Meeting department faculty and staff
   B. Attending departmental meetings
   C. Developing a new curriculum
   D. Reading the departmental handbooks

4. Which nontenure academic role is a prerank position in which the nurse educator does not have the credentials for the tenure track?
   A. Visiting professor
   B. Teaching assistant
   C. Professor emeritus
   D. Lecturer

5. Early-career nurse educators need mentorship in which one of the following areas?
   A. Identifying active teaching strategies
   B. Identifying professional development for writing grants
   C. Identifying academic leadership positions
   D. Identifying national opportunities for scholarly presentations

6. Nurse educators should either observe or serve on how many committees in the first year?
   A. None
   B. One
   C. Two
   D. Three or more

7. One of the most important commitments to education for the nurse educator is to take which of the following actions?
   A. Taking at least 10 continuing education classes a year
   B. Engaging in lifelong learning experiences
   C. Increasing knowledge in the area of clinical expertise
   D. Meeting yearly certification requirements

8. Which of the following would be considered an element of professional service?
   A. Facilitating an online nursing course
   B. Giving a presentation at a state-level nursing conference
   C. Publishing an article in a peer-reviewed nursing journal
   D. Serving as a member of a board of national nursing organization

9. One of the areas of the nurse educator's expertise is mentoring. Which activity by the nurse educator demonstrates Boyer's Scholarship of Discovery?
   A. Serves as a member of a national nursing mentoring program
   B. Conducts research about the characteristics of a mentor
   C. Collaborates with other department faculty to plan a presentation on mentorship
   D. Publishes in a peer-reviewed journal about the effects of positive mentorship

10. Because of inexperience, it is taking more time than planned for the novice educator to answer questions and to assist with the details during simulations. Which of the following would be the best solution?
    A. Tell the experienced nurse educator to write questions down to be discussed later.
    B. Advise the novice nurse educator to take additional training classes on simulation.
    C. Discuss the situation with the chair or director of the program.
    D. Ask the novice nurse educator to not assist with simulations in the future.

11. Which areas of Boyer's Model of Scholarship should the educator focus on when appointed to the rank of associate professor?
    A. Teaching and Application
    B. Discovery and Integration
    C. Application and Integration
    D. Discovery and Teaching

12. Which activity by the nurse educator best demonstrates Boyer's Scholarship of Integration?
    A. Researching student learning outcomes related to a service-learning project in a course
    B. Becoming an expert in service-learning implementation and acting as a consultant
    C. Reviewing literature about service learning and developing a multidisciplinary service-learning project in a course
    D. Planning and implementing a service-learning project in a current nursing course

13. Which statement by the novice nurse educator requires follow-up by the nurse mentor?
    A. "I am going to apply for the department chair position next week."
    B. "I am excited to sit on the review panel for our curriculum committee."
    C. "I am going to review the faculty testing policy before I develop my exam."
    D. "I am going to attend a professional development workshop on active learning."

14. Mentoring a midcareer faculty member may include which of the following activities?
    A. Support the faculty member in identifying and using innovative pedagogies.
    B. Provide guidance in transitioning the faculty member into an academic leadership position.
    C. Guide the faculty member in socialization to the role of the nurse educator.
    D. Answer questions about the role of the nurse educator.

15. The nurse educator is pursuing a PhD, serving on several committees within and outside the university, and was recently assigned as a mentor to a new faculty member. The educator is feeling exhausted and overwhelmed. Which of the following would be the best action at this time?
    A. Prioritize activities and then complete them in that order.
    B. Report feelings and concerns to the department chair.
    C. Stop all activities except those related to teaching.
    D. Seek counseling to assist in coping with these responsibilities.

16. Which statement by a novice nurse educator indicates understanding of the need to be an active member of one or more professional organizations?
    A. "I am planning to join the American Nurses Association so I can be involved in political activism."
    B. "Joining a professional organization allows me to deduct that expense from my taxes."
    C. "Professional organization involvement will help me grow professionally and personally."
    D. "Being a member of a professional organization will look good on my curriculum vitae."

17. Which of the following activities is an example of the nurse educator's commitment to lifelong learning?
    A. Volunteering to be an advisor for the school's student nurses association
    B. Applying for a position on the board of directors of a nursing professional organization
    C. Agreeing to be a faculty mentor for new nurse educators
    D. Completing a doctoral degree to be eligible for promotion and tenure

18. Which of the following activities by the nurse educator demonstrates Boyer's Scholarship of Integration?
    A. Using an innovative learning strategy that employs virtual reality technology
    B. Organizing a service-learning experience for undergraduate students
    C. Presenting the results of collaborative interprofessional research at a national conference
    D. Designing a new online nursing course on health equity and inclusivity

19. Which activity by the nurse educator demonstrates Boyer's Scholarship of Application?
    A. Obtaining and maintaining the Certified Nurse Educator® credential
    B. Developing a portfolio for institution promotion and tenure
    C. Conducting research on effective teaching/learning strategies
    D. Assisting with revision of the doctoral nursing curriculum

20. Which of the following federal laws was created to protect the privacy of students and their educational records and reports?
    A. FERPA
    B. IDEA
    C. HIPAA
    D. PEG

21. Which of the following is an example of a service-learning experience for undergraduate nursing students?
    A. Providing prenatal care for women in Appalachia
    B. Traveling to Mexico to shop for pottery
    C. Writing a paper about Canada's health care system
    D. Answering five questions about Ireland culture on an exam

22. Which of the following hospital activities will provide the best opportunity for students to complete service learning opportunities?
    A. Planning several health education classes for community members
    B. Completing podcasts about a variety of health topics for community members
    C. Managing a hospital booth at the annual university job fair
    D. Conducting health and blood pressure screenings for senior citizens

23. Which of the following is a benefit of service learning for students?
    A. Helps increase the learners' GPA
    B. Develops cultural awareness
    C. Enhances individual learning
    D. Provides an opportunity to travel

24. What is a collection of documents that summarizes an individual's work and experiences as the nurse educator?
    A. Portfolio
    B. Resume
    C. Concept map
    D. Curriculum vitae

25. When reviewing a portfolio of a nurse educator, which one of the following activities would be included in the scholarship section?
    A. Volunteering at a church or synagogue food bank
    B. Publishing an article in a peer-reviewed journal
    C. Serving on an institutional search committee
    D. Serving on the curriculum committee

26. Which statement by the novice nurse educator demonstrates understanding of the importance of feedback to improve role effectiveness?
    A. "Self-reflection is the best source of feedback to help me improve as a nurse educator."
    B. "I can choose whether to have one or more of my peers evaluate me in the classroom."
    C. "I need to pay close attention to the summary of learner evaluations of my course to decide how to improve."
    D. "I don't really need feedback about my performance because I've been teaching for many years."

27. Which of the following learner rights is protected by the Family Educational Rights and Privacy Act (FERPA)?
    A. Have access to own education records
    B. Miss a designated amount of class and clinical time
    C. Remediate course content that has not been mastered
    D. Request a change in course faculty

28. Which statement by the novice nurse educator indicates understanding of creating a *just culture* in the students' clinical practicum?
    A. "I can fail students clinically if they make a medication error."
    B. "Students who make an error in clinical should be placed on a warning."
    C. "Students are expected to make errors because they are learners."
    D. "A serious clinical error can result in an immediate student failure."

29. Nursing faculty are planning to implement a revised curriculum for the baccalaureate program. Which faculty action is necessary for learners regarding this change?
    A. Notify current and future learners 6 to 12 months before the change.
    B. Ensure that learners can successfully pass the revised curriculum.
    C. Ask learners for their input about the curriculum revision.
    D. Have the learners meet the external consultant who assisted with the change.

30. Which of the following information should not be included on the nurse educator's curriculum vitae?
    A. Educational history, including all degrees
    B. Employment history
    C. Professional awards and honors
    D. Hobbies and special interests

31. Which of the following legal/ethical issues may be avoided or minimized if faculty act as professional role models?
    A. Learner incivility
    B. Inappropriate social media use
    C. Academic integrity violations
    D. High-stakes testing

32. Learners use a variety of social media tools. Which of the following would be most appropriate for a nursing professional?
    A. Twitter
    B. Facebook
    C. LinkedIn
    D. Pinterest

33. Which of the following statements is true regarding standardized exams?
    A. Standardized tests are predictive for passing the licensure or certification exam.
    B. Standardized tests should have high benchmarks.
    C. Standardized tests should be used for assessment purposes only.
    D. Standardized test benchmarks should be met before passing a course.

CHAPTER 8

Engaging in Scholarship of Teaching

SOMER NOURSE | KAILEE BURDICK

LEARNING OUTCOMES

1. Describe the characteristics and qualities of nursing scholars in the academic setting.
2. Summarize evidence-based resources to support and improve teaching.
3. Identify methods of contributing to research on nursing education.
4. Discuss methods for sharing teaching expertise with nurse educators and other health care professionals.

The roots of scholarship in nursing trace back to Florence Nightingale, who exhibited a spirit of inquiry and was a catalyst for change that ultimately led to the development of evidence-based practice in nursing. Scholarship in nursing is currently defined as those activities that "systematically advance the teaching, research, and practice of nursing through rigorous inquiry that (1) is significant to the profession, (2) is creative, (3) can be documented, (4) can be replicated or elaborated, and (5) can be peer-reviewed through various methods" (American Association of Colleges of Nursing [AACN], 2021). The role of the scholar, then, is to develop, disseminate, and implement evidence for best practice in nursing. Engaging in the Scholarship of Teaching in nursing requires educators to exhibit a spirit of inquiry, demonstrate integrity as a scholar, and participate in research activities to further the development of nursing education.

Exhibiting a Spirit of Inquiry

Aristotle viewed teaching as the highest form of understanding. Although nurse educators are often experts in their clinical fields, an essential component of being an educator requires life-long learning. Educators should be constantly examining and analyzing current practices for evidence-based support while also creating new and innovative methods for teaching and learning. The role of a nurse educator is to exhibit a spirit of inquiry about teaching and learning, learner development, and evaluation methods.

Nurse educators working in schools of nursing are expected to engage in teaching, scholarship, and service. Criteria for promotion and tenure of nurse educators are dependent on evidence of achievement in each of these three areas. Faculty have a responsibility to use scholarship to advance the profession of nursing and nursing education. Examples of scholarly roles of the nurse educator may include:

- Conducting original research
- Disseminating research findings
- Identifying gaps in the current research

- Critiquing research for practice
- Using evidence-based teaching and learning practices
- Actively serving in professional organizations

Review of Boyer's Model of Scholarship

Boyer's (1990) Model of Scholarship is the foundation for the development and advancement of the science of nursing education. The concept of a scholar has evolved from one who solely conducts and publishes research to one who also applies research and communicates knowledge to learners. Boyer distinguished the four types of scholarship used by academic nurse educators to demonstrate effective teaching and learning as the Scholarship of *Discovery, Integration, Application*, and *Teaching* (see Chapter 7).

The *Scholarship of Teaching* involves using evidence-based practices to facilitate learning. Educators perform the Scholarship of Teaching by transferring discipline-specific knowledge to learners, developing innovative teaching and evaluation methods, conducting program development and learning outcome evaluation, and providing professional role modeling. Educators may use peer-reviewed publications of research, case studies, or theory development related to teaching as evidence of the Scholarship of Teaching. Writing accreditation and program evaluation reports, innovative use of technology in the classroom, textbook publications, presentations, and grant awards supporting teaching and learning can be used by educators to document evidence of the Scholarship of Teaching.

Nurse educators are required to demonstrate aspects of teaching, service, and scholarship as part of the promotion and tenure process. Boyer's Model of Scholarship lends credibility to all roles of the educator by proposing that scholarship can include both teaching and service and not just the generation of new knowledge through original research.

> ### CNE®/CNE®n Key Point
>
> *Remember:* The *Scholarship of Teaching* involves using evidence-based practices to facilitate learning. Publishing evidence of an innovative teaching strategy is an example of Boyer's Scholarship of Teaching.

Characteristics and Attributes of a Scholar

Scholars are naturally inquisitive about the world around them. Scholars are typically receptive to change and consider self-reflection and peer review important components of the scholarly process. Conard and Pape (2014) describe nursing scholars as having the following characteristics and attributes:

- *Problem solvers and thinkers:* Nurse scholars should be independent thinkers who engage in scholarly activities that advance all aspects of nursing.
- *Collegiality:* Nurse scholars demonstrate the ability to communicate well in both written and verbal forms and develop meaningful connections with nursing colleagues and those in other disciplines.
- *Honesty and integrity:* Nursing as a profession is consistently recognized as being ranked high in honesty. Nurse scholars demonstrate that same level of honesty and integrity through ethical research practices and disseminating accurate and trustworthy research findings.

Nurse educators who demonstrate the characteristics and attributes of a scholar reflect on their own educational practices while also being creative and receptive to new ideas (Oermann et al., 2022). Engaging in regular conversations about teaching/learning practices with peers and colleagues can help the nurse educator further develop as a scholar. Becoming a scholar in nursing education takes time and practice, and nurse educators must consider their current skills as a scholar and reflect upon which skills need further development. Stockhausen and Turale (2011) suggest nurse educators progress toward becoming a scholar in nursing education by first completing a self-assessment of one's own scholarly attributes, identifying an area of scholarship to focus on, becoming an expert in that area of education, and then disseminating products of that scholarship.

Weston and McAlpine (2001) suggest a three-phase approach of progression toward the Scholarship of Teaching. In phase one the educator exhibits growth by intentionally developing personal knowledge about one's own teaching. Phase two involves engaging in dialogue with colleagues about teaching and learning. Phase three involves growth in the Scholarship of Teaching, where the educator continues to develop knowledge about teaching/learning and begins to make a significant impact on nursing education. See Table 8.1 for a list of behaviors and activities through which the educator progresses during the continuum of growth toward the Scholarship of Teaching. It is important to note that the Scholarship of Teaching cannot occur in isolation. True Scholarship of Teaching requires dialogue with learners and colleagues within and across disciplines, mentoring others, and dissemination of findings to affect nursing education.

Using Evidence-Based Resources to Improve and Support Teaching

The National League for Nursing's (NLN's) Scope of Practice for Academic Nurse Educators acknowledges that engaging in the process of scholarship requires educators to "draw on extant literature to design evidence-based teaching and evaluation practices" (Christensen & Simmons, 2020, p. 14). Educators must integrate research from nursing education, higher education, psychology, and other health disciplines to improve and support teaching practices. The Scholarship of Teaching must be supported by theory. Evidence-based teaching can be defined as the "dynamic and holistic system using educational principles validated by evidence to support, maintain, and promote a new level of knowledge for a learner in a variety of settings" (Cannon & Boswell, 2016, p. 9). Evidence-based teaching can take place in a variety of classroom, online, and clinical settings, whereas evidence-based practice occurs only in the clinical setting. Chapter 2 provides examples of evidence-based teaching and learning activities in nursing education.

Using evidence-based teaching involves understanding a current need and creating a question for investigation. Using the PSCOT format can help nurse educators formulate a question that addresses the educational process (Cannon & Boswell, 2016). PSCOT is used to describe:

- P = Population
- S = Strategy
- C = Comparison
- O = Outcome
- T = Time period

TABLE 8.1 Continuum of Growth Toward the Scholarship of Teaching		
Phase One: Growth in Own Teaching	**Phase Two: Dialogue With Colleagues About Teaching and Learning**	**Phase Three: Growth in Scholarship of Teaching**
Develop personal knowledge about own teaching.	Exchange knowledge about teaching/learning practices with colleagues.	Develop significant scholarly knowledge about teaching and learning.
• Reflect on teaching. • Engage in innovative teaching. • Engage in nursing education literature. • Understand principles of teaching and learning. • Conduct self-assessments of effectiveness of teaching, and seek out peer evaluation.	• Engage in dialogue with colleagues about teaching and learning. • Become a mentor for other educators. • Provide leadership in teaching at the disciplinary and/or university level. • Engage with disciplinary and multidisciplinary teaching associations. • Expand understanding of educational theories and concepts.	• Use nursing education literature and research to inform teaching. • Conduct research on teaching and learning. • Present and publish about teaching strategies and own research on teaching/learning. • Mentor others conducting educational research. • Become an expert in an area of nursing education.

Data from Weston, C., & McAlpine, L. (2001). Making explicit the development toward the scholarship of teaching. *New Directions for Teaching and Learning, 86,* 89–97.

The population can be anyone involved in the educational process, such as learners, educators, preceptors, administrators, specific cohorts, or individuals. The strategy is the intervention that will affect the population. The C allows for comparison of the strategy to another educational strategy. Educators identify the expected outcome of the strategy and the time period of its use. The following is an example using PSCOT to format an educational question for investigation:

- P = undergraduate nursing students
- S = international service learning experience
- C = domestic service learning experience
- O = increased cultural awareness
- T = after the first year of practice

Combining the components of the PSCOT would result in: Do undergraduate nursing students who participate in an international service learning experience have increased cultural awareness after the first year of practice compared with students who participated in a domestic service learning experience? Once the research question has been formulated, the educator can begin the process of searching for evidence related to the educational practices in question. A clear and well-developed PSCOT question will help the educator identify keywords and concepts to use in the literature search. Once the literature search has been performed and evidence has been analyzed, the nurse educator must then consider all academic, financial, and resource boundaries when making decisions about implementation of best practices (Cannon & Boswell, 2016).

There are distinct differences between *good teaching, scholarly teaching,* and *the Scholarship of Teaching and Learning. Good teaching* often involves using a variety of effective teaching-learning practices and is characterized by educators receiving positive learner evaluations of teaching and high learner satisfaction. Good teaching involves use of Chickering and Gamson's (1987) seven principles for good practice in undergraduate education. These principles include:

- Encouraging frequent contact between learners and faculty
- Developing reciprocity and cooperation among learners
- Encouraging active learning
- Giving prompt feedback
- Emphasizing time on task
- Communicating high expectations
- Respecting diverse talents and ways of learning

Scholarly teaching involves consulting the literature, using evidence-informed approaches to teaching, reflecting on teaching, attending conferences and workshops on teaching and learning, and consulting with colleagues (Vajoczki et al., 2011). The *Scholarship of Teaching* builds on principles of good teaching/learning and scholarly teaching with the distinction that the knowledge must be disseminated to influence teaching beyond the local context. The Scholarship of Teaching and Learning often involves applying for teaching/learning grants, presenting at workshops and conferences, publishing on teaching and learning, conducting pre-/post-tests on learners' knowledge and skills, and assessing newly implemented approaches to teaching and learning (Vajoczki et al., 2011).

CNE®/CNE®n Key Point

Remember: Use PSCOT (Population, Strategy, Comparison, Outcome, Time period) to formulate a question when investigating evidence-based teaching practices.

Participating in Research in Nursing Education

To further the development of the nursing profession and to effectively engage in scholarship, nurse educators are tasked with designing and implementing scholarly activities in an established area of expertise (Christensen & Simmons, 2020). Participating in nursing research involves defining problems, designing studies, disseminating findings, and using other published findings in practice. Creating new knowledge and evidence for publication in nursing education means that it is likely that the educator will need to obtain institutional review board (IRB) approval to ensure ethical protection of human subjects (Marzinsky & Smith-Miller, 2019). Participating in research while teaching can be challenging to accomplish and maintain. Lack of time, knowledge, mentoring, and confidence are commonly identified barriers to participating in nursing education research. Educators may have difficulty securing funding for research in nursing education. Sources of grant money for nursing education research may include organizations such as the NLN, Sigma Theta Tau International (STTI), and the American Nurses Association (ANA). Educators may attempt to secure federal grant money within the U.S. Health Resources and Services Administration (HRSA).

To advance the science and support the body of knowledge that guides nursing education, the NLN released a position on nursing education research priorities. The following are the NLN's (2016) recommendations for nursing education programs:

- Provide resources to support nursing education–focused research.
- Support faculty to evaluate and use evidence-based teaching practices.
- Advocate for funding to support nursing education research that is linked to practice outcomes.
- Promote interprofessional partnerships to bridge the practice/education gap.
- Use the science of learning research to implement and evaluate effective teaching/learning practices.
- Foster a research environment for faculty, learners, and nurse scientists that embraces both practice and educational research.
- Foster the development of collaborative programs of research across disciplines and institutions.

Educators, academic institutions, and nursing organizations must prioritize nursing education research to further advance the science of nursing education. As more and more nurses will be needed to support the nursing workforce, educators must ensure that the education being provided to new nurses is evidence-based and linked to positive clinical practice outcomes.

Sharing Teaching Expertise With Colleagues and Others

Teaching and learning is the primary responsibility of the academic nurse educator. Nurse educators, regardless of level of education, should use best practices in teaching and share practices within their area of expertise. In nursing education, evidence-based teaching must consider both what is best practice for didactic teaching and clinical practice (Cannon & Boswell, 2016). Just as nursing embraces lifelong learning, so does the practice of nursing education. Nurse educators should have a strong foundation of evidence to support the practices and methods used and should understand their effectiveness with learners. Nurse educators should not rely simply on the way they were taught but instead add to the body of knowledge about best practices in nursing education. As part of this obligation, dissemination of best practices in teaching with colleagues, other health professionals, and educators is fundamental to growth.

Collaboration is one of the first steps for the nurse educator to share expertise in teaching and learning. Just as nurses at the bedside work as a team, nurse educators should also work together to collaborate, develop, and share teaching expertise. Working together as a team when making decisions about courses, programs, or curriculum within a school of nursing allows for sharing of teaching expertise. Sharing expertise in a team setting can happen informally as educators discuss teaching strategies and concerns. More formal ways of sharing expertise can also be implemented. Setting aside time during meetings for programs or curriculum is one method that can be used to allow nurse educators to share teaching practices being used and the outcomes. This allows educators to have a resource and promotes collaboration. Often, sharing of ideas among colleagues can spark relationships and promote collaboration to engage in scholarly work surrounding teaching.

The development of new knowledge about teaching is an important aspect of the academic nurse educator role and can be enhanced through active collaboration. Nurse educators often develop new methods for teaching and assessing learners that can be greatly expanded upon by engaging with other interested educators. Developing novel ways of teaching and learning in the following ways can engage the nurse educator in scholarship (Oermann, 2022):

- New courses
- Course/lecture materials
- Interactive tools
- Assessment methods
- Clinical evaluation methods
- Clinical learning tools

Tracking and evaluating outcomes from any new development is a critical element to add to the body of knowledge about nursing education. As the nurse educator creates original educational tools/materials, dissemination of these tools and their outcomes is critical.

Disseminating scholarly work is imperative to share with peers and encourage critiques of the work. Sharing scholarly work through publications is one of the more common methods to disseminate knowledge (Oermann et al., 2022). With most submissions being in an online format, nurse educators have access to a variety of nursing and interprofessional health care journals, which allows best practices and research to be shared widely. Access to journals can be widely gained in an online format. Use of the library resources within the academic setting can allow for opportunities to have access to journals without nurse educators having to accrue high costs personally. Each journal has a different focus and accepts differing types of scholarly work. Some journals have a strong focus on primary research. Some examples of such journals include *Nurse Education Today, Nursing Outlook, Journal of Nursing Education,* and *Journal of Nursing Scholarship.* Other nursing education–related journals are more open to articles that demonstrate the application of nursing education research and include *Nurse Educator* and *Nurse Education in Practice.* Nurse educators have forums available that allow for sharing of best practices and innovative ideas in nursing education through such journals. Seeking out opportunities to share either original research or application of teaching practices and outcomes can be one opportunity to share knowledge.

Conferences are another opportunity for nurse educators to share teaching expertise through networking, which can often lead to connections with other faculty and promote future collaboration. Another benefit of conference attendance is the ability to listen to speakers present best teaching practices and educational research. This information can generate new ideas and allow educators to share best teaching practices with their own program faculty. Nurse educators also have opportunities to submit an abstract to present a podium or poster presentation at local, state, national, or international conferences.

Although sharing teaching expertise with other nurse educators is essential to advance the practice of nursing education, it is important to engage in developing teaching practices that enhance interprofessional collaboration among learners. Attending conferences that engage different health professionals, working in the academic setting with other health professions on campus, and reaching out to health professions on other local campuses in the area are examples of ways to collaborate. Disseminating knowledge about teaching expertise can often affect multiple health disciplines, and engagement across professions can promote health care as whole. Nurse educators should be open to learning about teaching expertise in other health disciplines to expand their focus and have a greater impact on teaching future nurses.

Technology can also provide many different avenues for sharing teaching expertise. Webinars can be accessed in online formats and can be on demand for easier access for the nurse educator. Seeking out opportunities to share expertise in these virtual formats can allow more broad access to audiences for the nurse educator.

Social media is another important tool to consider for sharing teaching expertise. Facebook, Twitter, and Instagram are examples of social media platforms where nurse educators can share this information. Many scholarly articles focus on the use of social media with nursing students. Nurse educators should consider the implications of maintaining professionalism online while promoting the profession of nursing. Social media platforms can be used to engage other nurse educators in information being disseminated via articles, webinars, or conferences. In a more informal manner, nurse educators can also use accounts on social media to share teaching expertise. Although this format is not often recognized in a scholarly sense, it can provide a community of educators to collaborate with and share practices affecting nursing education.

> **CNE®/CNE®n Key Point**
>
> *Remember:* Teaching expertise in nursing education can be shared via publications, conferences, professional organizations, and social media.

Demonstrating Qualities of a Scholar

As nurse educators engage in scholarly activities and work to disseminate knowledge about teaching, they have an obligation to demonstrate integrity, courage, perseverance, vitality, and creativity. Merriam-Webster (n.d.) defines integrity as "the quality of being honest and fair." Engaging in scholarly work makes it important for the nurse educator to consider the ways that fairness and honesty are upheld and demonstrated. Having the courage to stand up for new ideas and ideas in the face of adversity sparks a creative mindset to allow for growth in nursing education. These qualities align with the NLN's scope and competencies for nurse educators (Christensen & Simmons, 2020). It is up to nurse educators to consciously consider their own behaviors surrounding scholarly work. The qualities demonstrated by the nurse educator help set the example for learners who are observing and learning in addition to colleagues who may be influenced.

The nurse educator must engage in regular training to participate in scholarly work. The Collaborative Institutional Training Initiative (CITI) Program (n.d.) is one way the nurse educator can complete up-to-date education regarding conducting research and working with human subjects. This training is often required when nurses attend graduate school and should be updated on a regular basis to conduct research. Understanding the ethics around research and regularly engaging in the content and any updates can help the nurse educator conduct fair research involving human subjects in the academic or clinical setting. Staying up to date on ethical practices is necessary to engage in work as a nurse scholar and to conduct rigorous research that is safe.

Another consideration for demonstrating integrity as a scholar is the use of the IRB. An IRB provides an independent review of plans for research to ensure ethical responsibility and protection of research participants (Grady, 2015). Most higher education institutions have an IRB, and if nurse educators are also engaging in research involving a clinical agency, the health care system where the research will be conducted also would likely have an IRB process. It is imperative for nurse educators to understand and go through the rigorous review of IRB to conduct sound research. This also allows nurse educators to publish or present their findings and demonstrate that the ethical responsibility of IRB review was upheld. The IRB can provide different levels of review depending on the type of research being proposed and the inherent risk to participants of such research (Grady, 2015). Understanding the role of the IRB and going through the process when proposing research ensure that the nurse educator is upholding integrity in scholarly duties.

Just as the role of the IRB is to keep participants safe from harm, the nurse educator should also consider the ethical obligation of working specifically with learners. Any research involving learners should undergo the IRB process; however, the nurse educator must also understand that learners may be considered a vulnerable population. Nurse educators have a great influence over learners and can affect things such as grades, progression, and graduation. Learners should never be used for research without their consent and understanding of the risks and benefits. Also, the ability to consent or deny should be conducted by someone outside of the scope of influence of the learner and be done anonymously. Although there is much information to be gleaned from teaching and working with learners, nurse educators must uphold their responsibility to learners first and foremost.

Role modeling appropriate ethical behaviors is important for learners and colleagues. Nurses are held to high ethical standards that translate to nursing education. Nurse educators set the example and standards for students who are learning and growing and for colleagues who look up to them or whom they mentor. Learners should be engaged in research starting at an early level of nursing education to foster the spirit of inquiry and grow future nurse educators and researchers.

Demonstrating integrity, courage, perseverance, vitality, and creativity as a scholar is a personal responsibility for each nurse educator. The values of the nursing profession apply directly to the approach needed to conduct scholarship that demonstrates it is ethically sound. Conducting scholarly work as a nurse educator can be challenging and requires demonstration of courage, perseverance, and vitality to forge ahead with adding to the body of knowledge for nursing education. Demonstrating failure and persisting ahead despite adversity are important in the role of nurse scholar. These qualities are important for future nurse professionals to witness and observe so they can adapt and take those qualities into their own practice. All nurse educators need to understand the principles behind sound research, ethical review, and obligations that are required when working with learners and other vulnerable populations. Integrity is always at the center of the work of the nurse educator. Engaging as a scholar requires high standards by the nurse educator to develop and influence the next generation of nurses to practice with a mindset of inquiry.

CNE®/CNE®n Key Point

Remember: The academic nurse educator can demonstrate integrity as a scholar by going through the appropriate ethical review channels when proposing and conducting research.

References

American Association of Colleges of Nursing (AACN). (2021). *Defining scholarship for the discipline of nursing.* https://www.aacnnursing.org/news-information/position-statements-white-papers/defining-scholarship.

*Boyer, E. (1990). *Scholarship reconsidered: Priorities of the professoriate.* Lawrenceville, NJ: Princeton University Press.

Cannon, S., & Boswell, C. (2016). *Evidence-based teaching in nursing: A foundation for educators* (2nd ed.). Burlington, MA: Jones & Bartlett Learning.

*Chickering, A., & Gamson, Z. (1987). Seven principles for good practice in undergraduate education. *The Wingspread Journal, 9*(2), 1–5. https://files.eric.ed.gov/fulltext/ED282491.pdf.

Christensen, L. S., & Simmons, L. E. (2020). *The scope of practice for academic nurse educators and academic clinical nurse educators* (3rd ed.). Washington, DC: National League for Nursing.

Collaborative. (Institutional Training Initiative (CITI) Program. (n.d.). Get to know CITI Program. Retrieved September 10, 2021 from https://about.citiprogram.org/get-to-know-citi-program/.

*Conard, P., & Pape, T. (2014). Roles and responsibilities of the nursing scholar. *Pediatric Nursing, 40*(2), 87–90.

*Grady, C. (2015). Institutional review boards: Purpose and challenges. *Chest, 148*(5), 1148–1155. https://doi.org/10.1378/chest.15-0706.

Marzinsky, A., & Smith-Miller, C. (2019). *Nurse research and the institutional review board.* American Nurse. https://www.myamericannurse.com/nurse-research-and-the-institutional-review-board/.

Merriam-Webster. (n.d.). Integrity. In Merriam-Webster.com dictionary. Retrieved September 10, 2021, from https://www.merriam-webster.com/dictionary/integrity

National League for Nursing (NLN). (2016). NLN releases a vision for advancing the science of nursing education: The NLN nursing education research priorities (2016-2019). *Nursing Education Perspectives, 37*(4), 236.

Oermann, M., De Gagne, J., & Phillips, B. (2022). *Teaching in nursing and the role of the educator: The complete guide to best practice in teaching, evaluation, and curriculum development* (3rd ed.). New York, NY: Springer Publishing.

*Stockhausen, L., & Turale, S. (2011). An explorative study of Australian nursing scholars and contemporary scholarship. *Journal of Nursing Scholarship, 43*(1), 89 96.

*Vajoczki, S., Savage, P., Martin, L., Borin, P., & Kustra, E. (2011). Good teachers, scholarly teachers and teachers engaged in the scholarship of teaching and learning: A case study from McMaster University, Hamilton, Canada. *The Canadian Journal for the Scholarship of Teaching and Learning, 2*(1), 2. https://doi.org/10.5206/CJSOTL-RCACEA.2011.1.2.

*Weston, C., & McAlpine, L. (2001). Making explicit the development toward the scholarship of teaching. *New Directions for Teaching and Learning, 86*, 89–97.

CHAPTER 8 Practice Questions

1. Nursing programs use Boyer's Model of Scholarship as a guide for making which of the following decisions?
   A. Awarding promotion and tenure to faculty
   B. Assigning courses for faculty to teach
   C. Awarding grant money to applicants
   D. Identifying student learning needs

2. The nurse educator wants to conduct a survey of campus nursing students' perceptions of online learning during the COVID-19 quarantine for possible publication. What should the nurse educator do first?
   A. Administer a pretest to determine current level of knowledge of online learning.
   B. Apply for a grant to fund the study.
   C. Obtain institutional review board approval for the study.
   D. Consult with a statistician to assist with data analysis.

3. What activity is appropriate for a new nurse educator who wants to develop a professional portfolio that demonstrates evidence of the Scholarship of Teaching?
   A. Serve on a faculty governance committee.
   B. Publish findings of use of an innovative classroom learning activity.
   C. Conduct a study on the use of pet therapy for geriatric clients.
   D. Apply for an interdisciplinary grant for service-learning student travel.

4. The novice nurse educator wants to know which type of teaching/learning strategy is most effective for first-semester nursing students learning how to insert an indwelling urinary catheter. What is the best method for determining which type of strategy to use?
   A. Ask other colleagues who teach first-semester students what they are using.
   B. Formulate a PSCOT question and begin a literature review.
   C. Continue the same teaching strategies used by the previous instructor.
   D. Conduct a literature search on proper indwelling urinary catheter insertion technique.

5. A new nurse educator developed a PSCOT question for investigation. What is the nurse educator's next step?
   A. Survey the learners about their satisfaction using the new teaching method.
   B. Use two methods of teaching to uncover which practice is most effective.
   C. Use the PSCOT to help identify gaps in learner knowledge.
   D. Use the PSCOT to identify keywords and concepts when searching the literature.

6. The nurse educator is preparing to apply for promotion and tenure at the university. Which of the following items in the educator's professional portfolio would demonstrate Boyer's Scholarship of Teaching?
   A. Creating and implementing an interprofessional simulation with nursing and social work students
   B. Academic advising and mentoring of first-generation college students entering the nursing program
   C. Submitting consistently high learner evaluations of teaching in the educator's course
   D. Publishing two peer-reviewed articles on implementation of innovative teaching methods

7. The nurse educator who regularly reflects on teaching practices, uses evidence-based teaching methods, attends conferences, reads nursing literature, and disseminates scholarship in peer-reviewed publications is demonstrating which of the following principles?
   A. Good teaching
   B. Scholarly teaching
   C. Scholarship of Integration
   D. Scholarship of Teaching

8. Which of the following demonstrates recognition of the Scholarship of Teaching for the nurse educator?
   A. Serving on a department committee
   B. Receiving a grant award supporting teaching and learning
   C. Reviewing a new textbook to use in a nursing course
   D. Volunteering at a local food bank

9. Which of the following scenarios demonstrates integrity as a scholar by the nurse educator?
   A. Gains consent for research on learners by asking them during class
   B. Undergoes the institutional review board process for a research study
   C. Conducts analysis on test scores for research but does not tell the learners
   D. Shares data collected in learner clinical evaluations for a colleague's research

10. The nurse educator is testing a new method for teaching about a medical-surgical nursing–related topic. How should the nurse educator share this experience?
    A. Meet with other medical-surgical nursing faculty to discuss the method and findings.
    B. Publish the findings as a replication study in a nursing education journal.
    C. Do not share the experience with colleagues because of academic freedom.
    D. Present the findings at a national conference about nursing education.

11. A nurse educator wants to investigate the correlation between grades in the first semester of nursing school and success on the NCLEX®. Which of the following steps should the nurse educator take to begin conducting this scholarly work?
    A. Start collecting data to make a case for the scholarly work.
    B. Ask the program director for grades and NCLEX® statistics on predetermined learners.
    C. Investigate journals in which the research and data can be published.
    D. Write a proposal to be reviewed by the institutional review board.

12. A novice nurse educator has developed a new method to conduct clinical evaluations. The nurse educator believes the responses by learners would be appropriate to present at a regional conference on nursing clinical education. What should the nurse educator take as the next step to present the data?
    A. Develop a proposal for review to retroactively study the data collected.
    B. Remove all identifying data before submitting an abstract to the conference.
    C. Contact the learners to ask for consent.
    D. Nothing needs to be done to present the findings by the nurse educator.

13. A nurse educator wants to engage in best practices for simulation debriefing. To gain more knowledge and to conduct a study on simulation debriefing, the nurse educator should consider which of the following?
    A. Forget the idea because there is a shortage of funds.
    B. Go to the simulation director to ask for funding.
    C. Ask the dean to fund to the project.
    D. Apply for a grant to obtain funding.

14. The nurse educator is working with graduate students regarding the development of evidence-based practice and ethical research. Which of the following assignments would be most appropriate to engage students in learning about ethical practices for conducting research?
    A. Develop a slide presentation that covers all ethical concerns about research.
    B. Require the students to complete the CITI Program training.
    C. Develop an assignment in which students must analyze an unethical research proposal.
    D. Remind students to use their best nursing judgment when engaging in research.

15. The novice nurse educator is developing a portfolio for an annual review process. Which of the following is an example of evidence-based teaching?
    A. Teaching using only lecture because that is how the nurse educator was taught
    B. Using all the course content from a colleague who shared the course material
    C. Developing a collaborative assignment to be used based on a review of current nursing education literature
    D. Engaging learners to develop a course assignment based on their perceived needs

16. A nurse educator has completed a study on mentoring in graduate students. Which of the following is an appropriate method to disseminate the findings of this research study to a broad audience?
    A. Publish the findings in the department newsletter.
    B. Present the findings at the nursing department meeting.
    C. Informally present the findings to colleagues in passing.
    D. Present at a national conference for nursing education.

CHAPTER 9

Functioning Within the Educational Environment

DONNA D. IGNATAVICIUS

LEARNING OUTCOMES

1. Identify the influence of social, economic, political, and institutional forces on nursing and higher education.

2. Summarize the impact of historical and current trends on decision making in higher education.

3. Explain how respect, collegiality, professionalism, and caring can help build a supportive organizational climate.

4. Describe the role of the nurse educator in the governance of the institution and the nursing program or college of nursing.

Academic nurse educators must have knowledge about how to function within the academic educational setting and recognize the factors that influence their role within their program and the institution. Historical perspectives and current trends and issues in higher education help to shape the organizational climate within which nurse educators affect change and model professionalism and collegiality.

Identifying the Influence of Social, Economic, Political, and Institutional Forces on Nursing and Higher Education

Forces that influence the role of the nurse educator can be categorized as social, economic, political, or institutional. These internal and external factors also affect the nursing profession, nursing education, and higher education.

Social Forces Influencing Nursing and Higher Education

Many external social forces and issues affect nursing and nursing education. Examples include but are not limited to:

- Health care reform
- Health equity issues
- Aging population
- Community and public health
- Increasing natural disasters and violence
- Globalization and global health

A major legislative bill known as the *Patient Protection and Affordable Care Act* (PPACA) was passed and signed into law in 2010 in which all U.S. citizens have access to affordable health insurance. This *health care reform* initiative also included amendments for nursing workforce development programs under Title VIII that are appropriated annually by the U.S. Congress. These programs primarily benefit nursing in rural and underserved areas, which ultimately increases workforce diversity. However, health equity issues continue to exist today.

The COVID-19 pandemic accentuated many of these issues and caused unanticipated health problems, including increased substance use and suicides. *Health equity issues* have also been highlighted, as the number of COVID hospitalizations and deaths is higher in people of color and those with comorbidities such as diabetes mellitus, obesity, and cardiovascular disease.

Individuals over 65 years of age have been particularly affected by the recent pandemic. The fastest-growing segment of the U.S. population is people over 65 years of age. Individuals in this *aging population* have multiple health needs that affect their daily lives and require specialized knowledge to manage. Many of these individuals reside in the community, including senior citizen centers, assisted living facilities, and long-term care agencies.

For some time, health care has begun to move more from acute care to community and public health. Increased *natural disasters and violent incidents* in the United States and throughout the world continue to strain acute care and public health resources. The recent pandemic has taxed acute care hospitals and, at times, created confusion related to public health policies regarding infection transmission and protection.

For more than 10 years, nursing and other health care professions have recognized the need to include *global health* in their curricula. Nurses and other health care team members encounter many patients and their families from all over the world. Therefore nurses need to learn how to incorporate the patient's health beliefs and practices into the plan of care to be patient-centered. Some colleges and universities offer service-learning experiences that are often international (see Chapter 7).

Nurse educators should be knowledgeable about the impact of each of these societal factors and integrate them when developing or revising curriculum, planning learning experiences, and developing program policies. Closely aligned with social factors influencing nursing and higher education are economic forces that often drive institutional or program decision making.

CNE®/CNE®n Key Point

Remember: Nurse educators should be knowledgeable about the impact of major social factors and integrate them when developing or revising curriculum, planning learning experiences, and developing program policies.

Economic Forces Influencing Nursing and Higher Education

One of the biggest concerns for higher education is financial constraints caused by the cost of education and shrinking state budgets. The tuition and fees from learners are only a portion of an academic institution's budget. These costs to learners have markedly increased, causing high learner debt as graduates enter the workforce. Increasing calls for more affordability, accountability, and transparency of schools, colleges, and universities resulted in publication of institution outcomes such as graduation rates and graduate employment rates.

As a result of the lack of financial resources, salaries for faculty lag behind those in industry and other sectors. Nurses who decide to leave their clinical positions to teach in an academic institution often have a $20,000 to $30,000 annual decrease in salary when compared with the salary they earned in a clinical agency. Consequently, they may need to work part-time in a second job or work during the summer when they are not on a 9- or 10-month academic contract. Proprietary schools usually pay nurse educators at a similar rate to what they earn in a clinical position. Knowledge of a potential salary difference can help nurse educators decide where they want to teach and plan accordingly to meet their personal budget.

Decreasing financial resources also result in lack of or inadequate learning resources, such as upgraded technology including classroom media and equipment. For example, nursing programs are increasing their use of simulation as part of clinical learning experiences; however, the cost of high-fidelity mannequins is sometimes prohibitive. Many programs apply for grants or request foundation monies to help update or expand their simulation centers and equipment.

A number of colleges and universities are experiencing decreasing learner enrollments, and others are decreasing their enrollments due to cuts in financial resources. Nursing program learner applications in most schools have continued to increase. However, some nurse administrators have chosen to limit enrollment due to faculty shortage, limited agencies for clinical experiences, and lack of preceptors (Halstead, 2019).

For schools that have adequate financial resources, nursing programs may expand to generate additional revenue gained from requiring prenursing students to take general education courses. This revenue, combined with funding sources such as grants and foundations, can help acquire new learning resources that would be needed for additional learners. Physical space must be allocated to accommodate additional learners unless learners take online courses. However, recruiting adequate faculty can be challenging due to poor academic salaries and a shortage of nurses who have formal graduate preparation in nursing education.

As a result of financial constraints, some colleges and universities are combining resources, creating partnerships or consortia, or merging organizations such that learners can continue their education. In other cases, small private colleges or career schools have closed, particularly proprietary schools that need to make a profit to continue operating.

Political Forces Influencing Nursing and Higher Education

Nurse educators need to be aware of the political forces that affect both nursing education and higher education in general. Some institutions have a strong legislative and political presence, especially large public universities that receive state funding and community colleges that receive local funding. Changes in political party prominence can alter the amount of funding schools receive.

Nursing and nursing education are usually supported by elected political parties and state and local government representatives. Recently there has been a growing concern by the general public, though, about nursing shortages and access to health care when and where it is needed (Iwasiw et al., 2020). The pandemic has further exacerbated the nursing shortage and limited access to hospital and nursing home beds due to lack of staff.

Some nursing education programs place an emphasis on health policy and expect faculty to model political advocacy and recruit learner involvement. For other programs, health policy is not a major part of the nursing curriculum, often due to lack of faculty knowledge (Halstead, 2019).

Institutional Forces Influencing Nursing and Higher Education

Although all higher education institutions aim to focus on knowledge acquisition, the purposes of academic learning environments differ. For example, some colleges and universities are public and others are private. *Public institutions* are funded primarily by learner tuition and state governments and are usually nonprofit. *Private institutions* are funded by learner tuition, fees, alumni, and endowments. They may be either nonprofit or for profit. Both public and private institutions attract learners from all over the country. Larger universities often attract learners from other countries to help promote a global learning environment.

The majority of public and private colleges and universities are overseen by an institutional governing board; tenured faculty usually participate in self-governance and institutional strategic planning. Examples of faculty governance activities include:
- Developing program and institutional policies
- Creating faculty promotion and tenure guidelines

- Partnering with administration to manage institutional and program issues
- Serving on a variety of program and institutional committees

To reduce costs and increase financial flexibility, many colleges and universities employ part-time/adjunct and nontenured faculty. As a result, fewer tenured faculty are available to participate in self-governance (Halstead, 2019). Table 9.1 reviews common faculty positions and their responsibilities for most 4-year colleges and universities.

Both public and private institutions provide information about their academic focus. For instance, some universities are research intensive, whereas others are not. Nurse educators need to select the educational environment that best fits with their career goals and values (Billings & Halstead, 2020).

Whereas 4-year colleges and universities prepare learners for baccalaureate and advanced degrees, public *community colleges* offer 1-year certifications and 2-year associate degrees in a variety of professional and technical specialty areas. Community colleges are designed to "serve" the community in which they are located and offer educational programs that prepare the area workforce. For example, rural community colleges may offer courses in agriculture, and urban colleges may offer urban planning courses. Many learners who attend these colleges usually live in the local community and attend the college as "commuters." Tuitions and fees are lower than 4-year schools because these colleges are partially funded by local governments.

By contrast, *for-profit academic institutions* typically follow a business or organizational model in which decisions are made by a corporation or other entity with input from stakeholders, including faculty. In the past 20 years the number of proprietary educational institutions has markedly increased. Academic educators are often paid at a higher salary than those working in public academic institutions, but there is often no system for promotion and tenure. Unfortunately, some proprietary systems encounter financial challenges and close abruptly without ensuring that learners can transfer to other institutions to complete their education.

Another difference among academic settings is the *mission* of the organization. As discussed earlier in this book, an organizational mission is a statement about the purpose of the institution. This statement directs the strategic goals, values, and curricula of the institution. For example, faith-based colleges and universities may require all learners to complete one or more courses related to the designated faith and underlying beliefs.

Nurse educators need to be aware of the major differences among academic institutions to ensure that their own values and goals are consistent with the educational environment (Billings & Halstead, 2020). For instance, in some faith-based colleges and universities, educators and other employees must be members of the designated religious faith. Educators who want to actively participate in self-governance should seek employment in public colleges and universities. Those who do not want to conduct research may seek employment in a community college, where teaching and learning expertise is more valued.

TABLE 9.1	Common Faculty Positions With Descriptions for Colleges and Universities
Faculty Position	**Description of Position Responsibilities**
Adjunct	Part-time role; faculty can be assigned to clinical or didactic experiences; no scholarship or service required
Clinical track	Full-time; faculty may only teach clinical courses; no scholarship or service required
Instructor	Full-time; faculty can be assigned to clinical or didactic experiences; usually no scholarship or service required
Tenure track	Full-time; probationary period working toward tenure; faculty teaches in the clinical and/or didactic learning environment; scholarship and service required
Tenure	Full-time; faculty teaches in the clinical and/or didactic learning environment; considered a permanent position or appointment

CNE®/CNE®n Key Point

Remember: Nurse educators need to be aware of the major differences among academic institutions to ensure that their own values and goals are consistent with the educational environment.

Regardless of institution type and mission, all schools, colleges, and universities have the same requirements for higher education *accreditation* by a nationally recognized regional accrediting body, such as the Higher Learning Commission and Middle States Commission on Higher Education. The purpose of regional or national accreditation is to ensure that institutions of higher education are meeting predefined criteria or standards for quality.

Nursing programs may be voluntarily accredited by one of several nursing accrediting bodies. Depending on the accrediting organization, this voluntary process includes the development of a program self-study by faculty, a visit by a team of peers, and a decision on whether the program earns initial or continuing accreditation for a designated period. Achieving nursing program accreditation validates excellence in meeting nationally established educational practices.

Because of the increased cost of higher education and lack of qualified faculty, some colleges and universities have increased their enrollments by offering flexible off-campus courses through distance education. *Distance education* is most often delivered online as a course or entire program. Most graduate degree programs in nursing are offered completely in an online format except for the clinical practicum. Most prelicensure nursing programs are provided in a traditional classroom (except during the COVID-19 pandemic) but may use a hybrid format that combines in-classroom learning with online learning. Nursing faculty teaching these courses need to have expertise in online learning and ensure that learners have access to the necessary electronic hardware and high-speed Internet before they enroll in distance education.

Educational delivery in institutions of higher learning today also includes an increased emphasis on other *emerging technologies*. For example, in nursing education, the use of high-fidelity mannequins to create and implement quality clinical simulations allows students to learn how to provide nursing care to complex patients. The use of apps like Kahoot! and Socrative for audience response and review of nursing content has enabled learners to practice knowledge retrieval, a prerequisite for making safe, appropriate clinical judgments.

CNE®/CNE®n Key Point

Remember: Distance education is most often delivered online as a course or entire program. Nursing faculty teaching these courses need to ensure that learners have access to the necessary electronic hardware and high-speed Internet before they enroll in distance education.

Making Decisions Based on Historical and Current Trends and Issues in Higher Education

Higher education institutions have existed since colonial times, when educators were experts who taught and shared their own knowledge. Since that time, the knowledge explosion has led to a proliferation of learning resources, and each major field of study has become increasingly specialized.

Exploring an institution's history can reveal the founding values and goals of the school and the successes and challenges that the institution experienced. For example, monies from public land grant sales were allocated to establish colleges of agriculture in the mid-19th century when farming was the predominant occupation. Most of these colleges have now been transformed into larger universities, but they continue to have a department or college of agriculture.

Another example of unique higher education history was the creation of historically black colleges and universities (HBCUs). These schools were established after the U.S. Civil War when Blacks were restricted from seeking higher education. In response to this restriction, the United

States funded designated institutions to give opportunities to Blacks, especially in the southern part of the country.

Every higher education institution has a history that can affect the way that current decisions are made. Iwasiw et al. (2020) suggest exploring the answers to questions such as:

- When was the higher education institution founded and why?
- Have the institution's mission and vision changed over time? If so, why?
- What programs are offered in the college or university?
- Were programs created for a niche market in the community?

Nursing education also has a unique history that influences current decision making and has contributed to current trends. The same questions for exploring an institution's history can be applied to colleges or departments of nursing.

Nursing education began as hospital-based programs to ensure that hospitals could "train" and supervise learners to prepare them for hospital employment. Graduates received a diploma provided by the hospital and took 2 days of licensure examinations ("boards") to become a registered nurse (RN).

Today most prelicensure programs preparing learners to become entry-level RNs or graduate programs preparing advanced practice nurses (APNs) are located on a college, school, or university campus. Nursing faculty employed in these higher education institutions must meet the teaching, scholarship, and/or service requirements that all college or university faculty are expected to achieve. These additional expectations may cause novice nurse educators to feel this workload is unachievable and must decide if the academic role is the best professional role fit or if another work setting is more desirable (Halstead, 2019). The priority for all academic nurse educators is to develop and maintain teaching and clinical expertise. Additional academic expectations can be gradually pursued with the guidance of the faculty mentor or nurse administrator. Scholarship and service expectations are described in detail in Chapter 7.

Adding to the complexity and time commitment associated with the academic nurse educator role is the lack of nursing faculty due to aging and retirements. APNs are often employed to replace retired faculty. Although APNs are expert clinicians, they are not formally educated as nurse educators. Therefore funding for professional development in best educational practices should be allocated to help develop these clinically focused faculty.

Many nursing programs have a small number of full-time tenured faculty. As a result, they may decide to employ large numbers of part-time or adjunct faculty to teach either in the classroom or online or, more commonly, teach learners in the clinical setting. These faculty typically have full-time jobs in other organizations and therefore do not have time to attend faculty or course meetings or provide input into program policies. The result of this faculty "mix" is often miscommunication and lack of consistency, a major concern and source of anxiety and frustration for nursing students.

Integrating Respect, Collegiality, Professionalism, and Caring to Build a Supportive Organizational Climate

Every organization, including higher education institutions, has its own culture that is learned by each new employee. Organizational culture is a "way of being" in that it embodies the shared values, expectations, and attitudes within the institution. According to Iwasiw et al. (2020), organizational climate overlaps with culture and focuses on shared perceptions of processes, including policies and procedures. The climate of higher education institutions also includes identification of employee behaviors that are supported and expected.

Nurse educators can help build a supportive academic climate by demonstrating professionalism and professional behaviors, including respect, caring, and collegiality. Inherent in the role of the nurse is the desire to behave in a professional manner while displaying a sense of caring in the learning environment. For example, nurse educators should provide frequent and timely constructive feedback to learners regarding their performance. This action shows caring and respect for learners. Learners deserve and demand mutual respect from faculty.

A positive organizational climate in which people are appreciated promotes high productivity, innovation, and satisfaction and positive faculty and learner socialization. Disrespect, incivility, and aggression can cause decreased productivity and dissatisfaction, liability, decreased faculty and learner retention, and psychological distress (Iwasiw et al., 2020).

Disrespect and incivility may be demonstrated by learners against other learners or by learners against faculty, especially if they are angry about performing poorly or failing. Conversely, some faculty may be uncivil to their peers, learners, or nurse administrator. Examples of uncivil faculty behaviors include (Billings & Halstead, 2020):

- Setting learners up to fail
- Encouraging learners to leave the program or transfer to another role or field
- Verbal abuse, such as yelling, name calling, and belittling
- Targeting learners to "weed them out"

Billings and Halstead (2020) describe a continuum of learner misconduct that ranges from annoying acts to administrative violations and criminal conduct (Table 9.2). Some behaviors could be categorized in two of these types of misconduct, such as verbal or physical abuse.

Incivility is not a professional behavior and can create major challenges in achieving a collegial academic environment (Halstead, 2019). Nurse educators are expected to role model positive professional behaviors in the academic and clinical environments.

Incivility and other negative behaviors should be discouraged through faculty and learner policies or institutional and nursing codes of conduct. Nursing programs have an obligation to support healthy workplaces. The National League for Nursing (NLN, 2018) published the Healthful Work Environment Tool Kit to help nursing faculty examine their work settings and develop an action plan to create a supportive work environment. Examples of questions that should be addressed during the assessment of the work environment include (NLN, 2018):

- To what extent do the faculty and administrators value a culture of civility in the learning environment?
- Are expectations for civil behavior by learners, staff, faculty, and administrators made explicit?
- Do faculty role model civil, collegial behavior to learners?
- Is civil, collegial behavior linked to faculty performance evaluation?
- Is civil, collegial behavior included in assessment of learner performance?
- Is an effective communication system in place, including one to address conflict?
- How is a sense of community and collegiality promoted and developed among faculty?

TABLE 9.2	Types of Learner Misconduct With Description and Examples

Type of Misconduct	Description	Examples
Annoying acts	Behaviors that may not be desirable but do not violate the institutional/program code of conduct	• Talking disruptively in class • Texting during class • Sleeping in class • Arriving late to class or clinical setting
Administrative violations	Behaviors that violate the institutional/program code of conduct	• Cheating on tests • Dishonesty • Plagiarism
Criminal conduct	Behaviors that violate local, state, or federal criminal law; also violate institutional/program code of conduct	• Verbal or physical abuse • Stealing • Threats of violence • Obscene behaviors • Substance possession or sale

Data from Billings, D. M., & Halstead, J. A. (2020). *Teaching in nursing: A guide for faculty* (6th ed.). St. Louis: Elsevier.

Considering Nursing Program Goals and Institutional Mission When Proposing Change or Managing Issues

One of the many roles of the academic nurse educator is to facilitate change by being a change agent or acting as a champion for change. To function effectively in the change process, the educator must determine whether the proposed change or issue is aligned with the values and mission of the institution. For instance, if the faculty of a nursing department want to offer a part-time nursing program because learners enrolled in a community college often need to work full-time, the institutional mission should be reviewed. Community colleges include access and responsiveness to community needs as part of their mission. If learners and other community stakeholders identify the need for a part-time program option, the faculty need to explore whether the option can be developed given possible resource limitations and other factors.

Any type of proposed change must also be aligned with the goals of the nursing program. If the faculty and nursing administration have adequate resources and desire to grow by increasing enrollment, for example, an additional program option might be feasible. However, if resources are limited and faculty shortages exist, the change may not be appropriate. Facilitating change in a nursing program or within a higher education institution is described in detail in Chapter 6. The mission of the higher education institution and nursing program should also be carefully considered when issues arise that need to be managed.

Participating in Institutional and Departmental Committees

Nurse educators should be engaged in institutional and nursing program governance to have the opportunity to participate in decision making. Participating in institutional and/or department committees is part of the service role of the academic nurse educator and is an example of Boyer's Scholarship of Application (see Chapter 7). Many faculty enjoy being part of institutional governance through their faculty senate, institutional committees, or task forces. Other faculty are less enthusiastic about participating in institutional governance or have limited time to devote to committee work. Some institutions, especially for-profit or proprietary organizations, do not provide opportunities for faculty to participate in institutional governance.

Most nurse educators do participate in the governance of a program, department, or college of nursing if they are provided the option to do so. Programs with small faculties may not have a separate committee structure; rather, they function as a committee of the whole involving the entire faculty. Larger faculties usually have standing committees that include the curriculum committee and program evaluation committee. Other programs create committees based on accreditation standards. All faculty belong to the full nursing faculty organization (NFO), which typically meets once or twice a month. Committee work is summarized at the NFO meetings, and recommendations for action are shared to make program decisions.

References

Billings, D. M., & Halstead, J. A. (2020). *Teaching in nursing: A guide for faculty* (6th ed.). St. Louis: Elsevier.

Halstead, J. A. (Ed.). (2019). *NLN core competencies for nurse educators: A decade of influence*. Philadelphia: Wolters Kluwer.

Iwasiw, C. L., Andrusyszyn, M-A, & Goldenberg, D. (2020). *Curriculum development in nursing education* (4th ed.). Burlington, MA: Jones & Bartlett Learning.

National League for Nursing (NLN). (2018). *Healthful work environment toolkit*. http://www.nln.org/docs/default-source/professional-development-programs/healthful-work-environment-toolkit.pdf?sfvrsn=20.

CHAPTER 9 Practice Questions

1. The nurse educator is leading a task group to revise the nursing curriculum. Which statement by the educator demonstrates consideration of social forces that affect nursing education?
   A. "Our decreasing admission of nursing students may cause us to lose faculty."
   B. "We need to be consistent with the mission and philosophy of our institution."
   C. "Content on caring for patients with infections should be increased in the curriculum."
   D. "We need a better policy on how to manage incivility in our program."

2. The nursing curriculum committee is planning to recommend changes based on the results of the COVID-19 pandemic. Which recommendation is most important?
   A. Need to address health equity issues and the role of the professional nurse
   B. Need to include more statistics about the incidence and prevalence of infection
   C. Need more time to practice how to use personal protective equipment
   D. Need to include more opportunities to practice sterile technique

3. Which statement by a nurse educator helping to plan clinical experiences for a new nursing program requires follow-up by the mentor?
   A. "We may need to increase our simulation hours due to clinical placement shortages."
   B. "We should increase our maternal–infant clinical hours because more babies are being born now."
   C. "We have to train our clinical preceptors to ensure they know what our expectations are."
   D. "We need more clinical hours for learners to care for aging adults in all types of settings."

4. Which statement by a nurse educator demonstrates understanding of how economic forces influence nursing education?
   A. "Nursing faculty are often paid more than nurses in clinical practice."
   B. "Most nursing students do not have high learner debt when they graduate."
   C. "Most colleges are experiencing increased learner enrollments."
   D. "Some small colleges and universities have closed or merged in recent years."

5. Which of the following characteristics applies to most proprietary schools?
   A. Funded by local and state governments
   B. For-profit institutions
   C. Governed by an institutional board
   D. Poor-quality faculty

6. Which of the following expectations is part of any nurse educator's academic role?
   A. Modeling political advocacy
   B. Submitting grant applications
   C. Obtaining a doctorate for tenure
   D. Mentoring new faculty

7. Which of these faculty positions is typically a part-time role with didactic or clinical assignments?
   A. Adjunct
   B. Instructor
   C. Clinical track
   D. Tenure track

8. The nurse recalls that which of the following is the primary purpose for community colleges?
   A. Offer low-tuition courses and programs
   B. Conduct research in education
   C. Offer certificates and associate degrees
   D. Serve the workforce of the community

9. A nurse educator is seeking employment in an educational institution to participate in self-governance. Which type of institution would most likely be consistent with the nurse educator's goals?
   A. Private career school
   B. Private liberal arts college
   C. Public vocational-technical school
   D. Public university

10. A nurse educator recognizes that the primary purpose of regional college accreditation is which of the following?
    A. To demonstrate the ability to meet quality educational standards
    B. To be able to award master's and doctoral degrees
    C. To apply for funding from foundations and grant sources
    D. To better compete with other local colleges

11. A nurse educator is planning an online course. Which requirement is most important for the course to be successful?
    A. Providing the course for beginning learners
    B. Years of experience as a nurse educator
    C. Type of nursing program in which the educator is employed
    D. Access to necessary hardware and Internet for learners

12. A novice nurse educator reports a concern to the mentor about the multiple expectations required in the academic role. What is the best response by the mentor?
    A. "I can help you with planning to get everything accomplished."
    B. "It's a lot to do, but at least you have the summer off."
    C. "Your main responsibility now is to gain expertise in teaching."
    D. "If you want, I can help cover one of your classes."

13. Which statement by the nurse educator requires follow-up by the mentor regarding the expansion of a nursing program?
    A. "The college will be able to give the nursing faculty a raise in their salaries."
    B. "Prenursing students take general education courses, which increases revenue."
    C. "There is a high demand for nurses in our community workforce."
    D. "Having a stronger nursing program helps our reputation in the community."

14. A nursing education administrator wants to expand a nursing program. Which factor would most likely limit that expansion?
    A. Lack of learner interest in nursing
    B. Lack of adequate nursing faculty
    C. Lack of learning resources
    D. Lack of classroom space

15. A nurse education administrator recently hired three master's-prepared advanced practice nurses. What is the priority for these newly hired faculty?
    A. Applying for doctoral study
    B. Becoming committee members
    C. Participating in professional development
    D. Planning clinical research projects

16. Which phrase accurately defines institutional culture?
    A. Shared values, expectations, and attitudes
    B. Policies and procedures
    C. Acceptable learner behaviors
    D. Decision-making approaches

17. Which action by a nurse educator best demonstrates building a supportive academic climate?
    A. Engaging learners in active learning
    B. Celebrating the end of semester with a learner luncheon
    C. Providing timely constructive feedback to learners
    D. Ensuring that learners follow the dress code

18. Which outcome is most likely within a positive institutional climate?
    A. Psychological distress
    B. Uncivil faculty and learner behaviors
    C. Increased faculty salaries
    D. High productivity and satisfaction

19. Which of the following behaviors demonstrates faculty incivility?
    A. Meeting with learners after class to review class notes
    B. Encouraging a learner to transfer to a program in another role
    C. Setting up an appointment to meet with a learner during office hours
    D. Failing a learner for unsafe clinical performance

20. Which of the following learner behaviors demonstrates criminal conduct?
    A. Cheating on a unit examination
    B. Plagiarizing a scholarly paper
    C. Abusing an assigned patient
    D. Disrupting an in-class session

21. Which statement by the novice nurse educator about learner performance requires follow-up by the mentor?
    A. "I plan to use the clinical evaluation tool to determine if learners meet expectations."
    B. "I will calculate learner course grades as outlined on the course syllabus."
    C. "I provided constructive feedback to learners after their simulation experience."
    D. "I plan to weed out those learners who should not become nurses."

22. The nursing faculty are planning ways to help students learn about avoiding uncivil behaviors. Which learning strategy would likely be most successful to meet this goal?
    A. Unfolding case study
    B. Role modeling by faculty
    C. Lecture with discussion
    D. Concept map

23. Which factor is most important for the nurse educator to consider when planning a major curriculum change?
    A. Budgetary constraints
    B. Learning resources
    C. Mission and values
    D. Physical space

CHAPTER 10

Planning for Success on the Certified Nurse Educator (CNE®) and Certified Nurse Educator Novice (CNE®n) Exams

DEANNE A. BLACH | DONNA D. IGNATAVICIUS

LEARNING OUTCOMES

1. List essential study resources needed for success on the CNE® and CNE®n examinations.
2. Describe how to design an individualized study plan to take the CNE® or CNE®n examination.
3. Identify tips for how to be successful when preparing and taking the CNE® or CNE®n examination.

Nursing education takes place in a variety of settings, including technical and career schools, hospitals, 2-year colleges, 4-year colleges, and universities. The academic nurse educator certification was developed to establish nursing education as a specialty area of practice and create a means for nurse educators to demonstrate their expertise in the role. Barbe and Kimble (2018) found that nurse educators felt personal accomplishment, personal satisfaction, and validation of knowledge when they passed the Certified Nurse Educator (CNE®) examination.

From 2005 through 2010 the CNE® examination pass rates were 80% or higher but gradually decreased with scores between 50% and 60% in 2018 and 2019 (Lundeen, 2018). According to the National League for Nursing (NLN, 2021), the pass rate for the CNE® exam in 2020 increased to 69%. When the examination was first offered, experienced nurse educators were the first to take it. Having experience in curriculum development or revision and/or going through a nursing program accreditation process is very useful when taking the CNE® examination.

New nurse educators can apply to take the CNE® examination if they obtain at least a master's degree in nursing education and have an active, unencumbered registered nurse (RN) license. These minimal requirements mean that examination candidates may not have adequate experience teaching in a nursing program. Even though nurse educators coming out of graduate school meet eligibility criteria, the exam was not developed to measure graduate program outcomes.

A study by Fitzgerald et al. (2020) found that graduate programs offering a focus on or degrees in nursing education typically only address four of the eight core competencies used as the basis for the CNE® examination, which may help explain the earlier decline in pass rates. Less than 50% of 529 master's in nursing education programs included in the study addressed these academic nurse educator core competencies:

- Competency II: Facilitate learner development and socialization
- Competency V: Function as a change agent and leader
- Competency VII: Engage in scholarship
- Competency VIII: Function within the educational environment

As a result of this research and the lower CNE® examination pass rates for *new* academic nurse educators, the NLN developed another certification credential for novice educators with less than 3 years of academic experience. This exam was piloted in 2022. New educators can choose to take the Certified Nurse Educator Novice (CNE®n) exam instead of or in addition to the CNE® exam.

As described in Chapter 1, the same eight core competencies used as a basis for the CNE® examination are also used for the CNE®n exam, but the percentage of questions for each competency differs.

Another factor that has influenced CNE® examination pass rates is the type of institution in which the nurse educator works; pass rates are the highest for nurse educators teaching in bachelor's of science in nursing (BSN), master's, and doctoral nursing programs (Lundeen, 2018). The explanation for this finding may be that these educators are employed by institutions that focus on scholarship, service, and leadership—a major emphasis on the CNE® examination. The focus of nurse educators who teach in practical, diploma, and associate degree nursing programs is excellence in teaching/learning rather than scholarship. This type of educator typically has less experience in the full scope of the academic nurse educator role, which may decrease the chance of success on the CNE® examination (Lundeen, 2018; Ortelli, 2016).

It is important to keep in mind that the content on both certification exams applies to all educators, regardless of the type of nursing program or institution in which they are employed. Each educator candidate planning to take these examinations will have strengths and areas where focused study and review are needed.

Once the nurse educator is approved by the NLN to take an exam, it must be scheduled within 90 days. During the time between being approved and when the exam is scheduled, the educator should access needed study resources, design an individualized study plan, and take a quality review course. It is not recommended to take the CNE® or CNE®n exam without a focused study plan.

CNE®/CNE®n Key Point

Reminder: Each candidate planning to take the CNE® or CNE®n examination will have strengths and areas where focused study and review are needed. It is not recommended to take these exams without a focused study plan.

Identifying and Accessing Essential Study Resources

The NLN now offers three different certification examinations for nurse educators:
- Certified Nurse Educator (CNE®)
- Certified Academic Clinical Nurse Educator (CNE®cl)
- Certified Novice Educator (CNE®n)

Each of these examinations has its own candidate handbook. Nurse educators should be sure to access the version that corresponds with the exam they intend to take.

The *Certified Nurse Educator Candidate Handbook* provides the topical outline for content tested on the CNE® examination. The *Certified Nurse Educator Novice Candidate Handbook* provides the topical content tested on the CNE®n examination. These test plans delineate the percentage of each content topic represented on the examinations based on the eight core competencies for academic nurse educators (see Chapter 1). In addition to the test plan, the *Handbooks* provide a comprehensive list of study resources recommended by the NLN. It is not necessary for the educator to purchase every resource or try to review every resource. Instead, it is best if the educator selects one or two resources from each major content area, such as curriculum and assessment. School libraries or peer faculty may own these resources or can obtain access to them. Accessing the most current edition of each resource is essential, though.

Newly graduated educators may already be familiar with some of the recommended study resources because they used them as textbooks in their graduate programs. One of the most commonly used textbooks in graduate programs focused on nursing education is *Teaching in Nursing: A Guide for Faculty* (Billings & Halstead, 2020). This comprehensive book includes content on all of the academic nurse educator competencies and should be part of every nurse educator's personal library.

The NLN *Scope of Practice for Academic Nurse Educators* is another essential resource for nurse educators planning to take either of the certified nurse educator examinations. This small paperback book can be purchased separately or as a resource combined with the competencies for the academic clinical nurse educator (Christensen & Simmons, 2020). Both references present the history and development of the core competencies, including definitions and related subcompetencies.

Another essential study resource for preparing to take these examinations is Halstead's (2019) *NLN Core Competencies for Nurse Educators: A Decade of Influence.* In this book each core competency is explored in its own chapter, starting with a literature review to identify themes for each competency and ending with the gaps that need to be addressed in the future.

CNE®/CNE®n Key Point

Remember: The *Certified Nurse Educator Candidate Handbook* and *Certified Nurse Educator Novice Candidate Handbook* provide a comprehensive list of study resources recommended by the NLN. It is not necessary for the educator to purchase every resource or try to review every resource. Instead, it is best if the educator selects one or two resources from each major content area, such as curriculum and assessment.

CNE® Exam Evolution

The initial CNE® examination was based on an analysis of academic nurse educator survey data in 2005. This practice analysis was repeated in 2011 and in 2017 to continue to validate the eight core competencies (Halstead, 2019). Early test takers of the exam and speakers who conducted the first CNE review courses emphasized the need for test candidates to focus on educational and change theories as part of their study plan. Certified nurse educators described their exams as being very theoretical and difficult. Some described the certification examination as the most difficult test they had ever taken, especially the interpretation of test statistics. The editor of this review book took the CNE® examination for the first time in 2016 and found that it included questions that tested educational theories, change theories, and interpretation of test statistics. However, these items did not make up the majority of the exam as anticipated, perhaps indicating a less theoretical emphasis.

In 2021 this book's editor recertified by taking the CNE® examination for a second time. She did not qualify to recertify using the point system because she is not employed in an academic institution as nursing faculty. The editor noted the following overall positive changes in the more current exam. Other nurse educators who have recently taken the CNE® examination noted the same trends.

- Minimal number of exam questions testing the application of educational and change theories
- Minimal and less difficult questions on interpretation of test statistics
- More practical questions with clearer and more concrete choices
- Shorter test item stems and choices (which allowed the editor to complete the exam in a shorter time frame when compared with the previous exam)

When compared with the 2016 exam and as expected, there were more exam questions on current topics and national trends in nursing education and society. There was also a lower cut score required for passing when compared with the previous exam. Keeping these positive trends and changes in mind is important when preparing to take the CNE® examination and should help the nurse educator decrease cognitive testing anxiety.

Designing an Individualized Study Plan

When planning where to focus one's time to study for the CNE® or CNE®n examination, the nurse educator should consider the previously discussed factors that affect success and the type of exam the educator plans to take. For example, if the educator has no or minimal teaching experience and decides to take the CNE®n examination, the focus of review and study should be on those competencies that make up the majority of the exam, such as Facilitate Learning (Competency I), which comprises 39% of that exam. For educators employed in a practical, diploma, or associate degree nursing program, the focus of review and study should be those competencies that are not within their current role. For example, none of these types of academic institutions require scholarship as part of the nurse educator's role. Once these factors are considered, the educator is ready to refine the plan of study.

The most important step in developing an individualized study plan is to identify content areas where the nurse educator feels confident and those areas where the educator feels more review is needed. For example, from this book editor's experience, many educators identify their "weak" content areas to be:

- Educational and adult learning theories
- Change theories
- Testing statistics
- Boyer's Model of Scholarship

To help refine the study plan, nurse educators should use study aids and resources that best meet their own learning preferences. For example, for an auditory learner, having access to recorded webinars that are part of a certified nurse educator review course may be the most useful. The read/write learner usually writes notes, keeps note cards, and highlights key information.

All nurse educators should also access the two CNE® or CNE®n self-assessment exams (SAE Form A and SAE Form B) by purchasing them on the NLN website for a 90-day period. These practice exams are 65 items each and provide the educator with experience of how the test will look in an online format, the type of questions to expect, and the tested content similar to what is on the actual exam. The NLN cautions these practice exams are not predictive of passing the official exam.

The self-assessment exams can be completed in multiple sessions, but once submitted for scoring, the exam is no longer accessible to retake. Each test item has the correct answer with the rationale available after the test has been submitted for scoring to analyze why a question was missed and why.

As a suggestion, SAE Form A can be used as a pretest to help determine what content areas need further review for the educator's study plan. Form B can be taken as a posttest after a period of study to determine which content areas have improved and which ones may still need review and study.

As part of an individualized study plan, the nurse educator may take a CNE®/CNE®n review course. Whether or not to take a review course is a personal choice. Some nurse educators take a course well in advance of the actual exam to help identify areas of strength and areas that need review and more study. Others take the review course closer to the time the examination is scheduled so that the content review is recent.

For educators who have minimal or no teaching experience, a CNE®/CNE®n review course is highly recommended. Nurse educators teaching in practical, diploma, or associate degree nursing programs should also consider taking a quality review course.

Not all review courses are the same length or have the same scope. The best review courses tend to be 1 to 2 days in length, target specific areas of content that reflect the CNE®/CNE®n test plans, and provide multiple opportunities for attendees to take practice questions with feedback from the instructor. A good review course should clarify the most relevant content to study and be facilitated by a certified nurse educator who has taken the CNE® or CNE®n examination within the past few years.

> **CNE®/CNE®n Key Point**
>
> *Remember:* For educators who have minimal or no teaching experience, a certified nurse educator review course is highly recommended. Nurse educators teaching in practical, diploma, or associate degree nursing programs should also consider taking a quality review course.

Use of Review Books

The NLN has endorsed only one CNE® examination review book written by a former member of their board of governors. This book is included in the list of recommended study resources in the NLN candidate handbooks. A brief content review for each of the eight core competencies for the academic nurse educator (one chapter for each competency) is presented, followed by 10 to 20 practice questions at the end of each chapter. Answers and rationales for chapter questions are provided at the end of the book, but there is no comprehensive practice test that simulates the official exam.

This newly published review book edited by Donna D. Ignatavicius was written to help nurse educators planning to take either the CNE® or CNE®n examination. The main focus of this book is on practice questions to best prepare the test candidate. Eight of the book's 10 chapters present a robust content review corresponding with the test plan for each of the eight core competencies, which is then followed by 25 to 70 CNE®/CNE®n–type practice questions at the end of each chapter. An additional comprehensive examination of over 150 test items is available for practice at the end of the 10 chapters. The answers, rationales for both the correct and incorrect responses, and references for test items in both the chapter practice tests and comprehensive exam are provided at the end of this book.

Nurse educators planning to take either the CNE® or CNE®n examination should be cautious in their purchase of review books. A number of companies that publish review books for multiple certification and licensure exams in a variety of disciplines offer CNE® review books. Many are written by individuals who are not experts or are not well known in nursing education.

Managing Cognitive Test Anxiety

Many individuals have high anxiety when preparing to take a test, often referred to as cognitive test anxiety. Certification examinations are not as high-stakes as licensure exams which, if failed, prohibit the testing candidates from starting their careers. However, the CNE® and CNE®n exams cost a significant amount of money, require time for study, and require time to complete. Candidates who fail either the CNE® or CNE®n examination have to wait 90 days to reapply to take it and pay the same amount as they did the first time.

To reduce test anxiety, nurse educators need to implement self-management and stress-reduction strategies such as those listed in Table 10.1. In addition, the exam candidate needs to practice multiple review questions to become familiar with question formats, how questions are stated, and at what cognitive level the questions are asked.

As stated in the *Certified Nurse Educator Candidate Handbook* and *Certified Nurse Educator Novice Candidate Handbook*, each exam consists of 150 four-option multiple choice questions (only 130 questions are scored) that are presented at one of these three cognitive levels:
- *Recall:* The ability to recall or recognize specific information
- *Application:* The ability to comprehend, relate, or apply knowledge to new or changing situations
- *Analysis:* The ability to analyze and synthesize information, determine solutions, and/or evaluate the usefulness of a solution

TABLE 10.1	Strategies to Decrease Cognitive Test Anxiety	
Self-Management Strategies	**Stress-Reduction Strategies**	
Be sure to get at least 8 hours of sleep the night before the exam.	Practice mindfulness before leaving for the testing center; use apps such as Calm to assist.	
Avoid consuming alcohol before sleep the night before the test.	Practice deep breathing exercises with your eyes closed before starting the exam at the testing center.	
Be sure to eat a light meal before leaving for the testing center.	Perform stretching exercises or take a walk before leaving for the testing center.	
Drink adequate liquids, including water, before taking the exam to prevent dehydration.	Use imagery techniques, meditation, and/or prayer before starting the test.	
Avoid drinking too many caffeinated beverages the evening and morning before leaving for the testing center.	Be sure to check that your transportation to the testing center is secure, such as checking the vehicle gas tank, reconfirming arrangements with the individual taking you to the center, and so forth.	

Examples of questions at each of these three cognitive levels are presented in the following box.

Examples of CNE®/CNE®n Examination-Style Test Items

Recall Example: The nurse educator is leading a task group to revise the nursing curriculum. What component of the current curriculum would the educator suggest to review first?
A. Program learning outcomes
B. Degree plan
C. Philosophy
D. Program plan for evaluation
   Answer: C

Application Example: The nurse educator plans methods for assessment of learning in a clinical nursing course. Which of the following assessments best measures learning in the affective domain?
A. Clinical evaluation tool
B. Concept mapping
C. Learner interview of clinical nursing leaders
D. Reflective journaling
   Answer: D

Analysis Example: The KR-20 of a nursing unit exam is 0.56. What is the nurse educator's best action if the exam is used for learners next semester?
A. Increase the length of the exam.
B. Allow more time for learners to take the exam.
C. Make the exam more difficult.
D. Change at least half of the test items.
   Answer: A

Practicing questions that are aligned with all eight core competencies of the academic nurse educator should be a major part of CNE® or CNE® examination preparation.

Interpreting and Answering Test Items

Interpreting and answering test items can be challenging, especially for nurse educators who have not taken any type of test for many years. Whether the nurse educator practices test items like the ones in this review book or takes one of the official NLN certification examinations, each item needs to be approached in a systematic manner using these strategies and tips:

- First, read the entire test item stem (information and question) very carefully looking for key words and terms. Be sure you can determine what the question is asking.

- Recall that the core competencies for the academic nurse educator consist of minimal content related to clinical learning when compared with the core competencies for the academic clinical nurse educator (CNE®cl).
- Keep in mind that the term "learner" is used in the CNE® and CNE®n exam items most often instead of "student."
- Pay special attention to words like "best" or "most important" in the question. For example, if a question asks for the *best* answer, it is likely that all choices may be feasible, but one is the best. Unlike other exams, key words are not bolded.
- Although the CNE® and CNE®n examinations avoid negative terms like "not" and "except" in the test stems, a few questions include the phrase "requires follow-up by the mentor." An example of a test item including this phrase is presented in the following box.

Example of CNE®/CNE®n Examination-Style Test Item

Which statement by the nurse educator regarding collaborative testing requires follow-up by the mentor?
A. "I will divide my students into small groups for the collaborative test."
B. "I plan to give a few points to students for their work on the collaborative test."
C. "Students will be able to learn from each other using collaborative testing."
D. "Students can use their resources to find the answers for the collaborative test."
Answer: D

In this question, three of the choices (Choices A, B, and C) would be accurate and not require follow-up. Choice D is *not* accurate, thus requiring follow-up by the mentor, and is the correct answer to the test item.

- Read and consider all choices in a given item, even if the answer seems obvious. Keep in mind that all of the choices may be somewhat correct if an item is asking for the best answer.
- Remember that CNE® and CNE®n examination items vary in their level of difficulty from relatively easy to more difficult. If an item seems too easy, it is probably intended to be easy.
- The educator may struggle to select the correct answer either because the test item seems confusing or vague, none of the choices seem to be the correct response, or the educator does not have the knowledge to answer the item. In this situation, try to eliminate two choices that you know are not correct. That leaves only two choices from which to choose. Selecting an answer by guessing is appropriate in this situation and is not penalized.
- Keep in mind that most test items are generic in scope and not program-type specific.
- Brand names or vendors are not included in the CNE® or CNE®n examination. For example, a specific type of audience response system or app name likely would not be included.

CNE®/CNE®n Key Point

Remember: CNE® and CNE®n examination items vary in their level of difficulty from relatively easy to more difficult.

Taking the CNE® or CNE®n Exam

In addition to using strategies for managing cognitive test anxiety (see Table 10.1), these tips for preparing for the testing day can help promote success on either of the certified nurse educator examinations:

- Schedule your exam for the time of the day in which you are more alert. Some educators choose to test early in the morning, whereas others prefer to take the exam later in the day.
- Be sure to get at least 8 hours of sleep the night before your test date and enter the testing area well hydrated and fed. Food and drink are not allowed in the testing area.
- Dress comfortably and in layers that can be removed or replaced depending on the room temperature in the testing center.

- Plan to take minimal personal belongings to the testing center, but be sure to bring your personal ID with your name as it appeared on your exam application. These items will be secured in an assigned locker before you enter the computer testing area.
- Although seemingly obvious, be sure to go to the restroom before signing in and securing your personal belongings.

Once you are settled at a computer to take the exam, consider these additional tips:

- Start by taking a few deep breaths to relax; adjust the chair to be as comfortable as possible.
- Don't skip the practice time to get used to the computer, mouse, and item formats, even if you are tech savvy. This activity can help you become less anxious and get set for the exam. The 3-hour time limit does not begin until you click on the box indicating to start the actual test.
- As you are answering the exam questions, write down the number of any test item that you would want to revisit *after* responding to all the items.
- Exam candidates have 3 hours to take 150 items and can revisit any item during that time. Although you are not allowed to have your cell phone or watch in the testing area, a countdown clock is shown on the computer screen for the entire exam. Plan on taking at least 50 to 60 items each hour such that you will have time to revisit any items. Don't spend too much time on any one item.

Common mistakes that nurse educators *can avoid* include:

- *Rushing through a question and missing key words in the stem or in the choices:* To prevent this mistake, read each question stem at least twice. Take each answer back to the stem and reflect on the answer of "Is this the best choice to answer the question?" "Is the choice the most relevant?" "Am I missing something?"
- *Changing your test answers too often:* To prevent this mistake, be sure not to list too many test items you want to revisit at the end of the test. Try to limit the number to 10 to 15 items if possible.
- *Having difficulty recalling knowledge needed to answer the test item correctly:* To prevent this problem, don't randomly guess. Instead, delete as many choices as possible that you know are not the correct response(s). Then re-read the remaining choices and ask, "Is this choice logical or feasible?" "Could this choice work in our program or institution?"

CNE®/CNE®n Key Point

Remember: Plan on taking at least 50 to 60 items each hour so that you will have time to revisit any items. Don't spend too much time on any one item.

References

Barbe, T., & Kimble, L. P. (2018). What is the value of nurse educator certification? A comparison study of certified and noncertified nurse educators. *Nursing Education Perspectives, 39*(2), 66–71.

Billings, D. M., & Halstead, J. A. (2020). *Teaching in nursing: A guide for faculty* (6th ed.). St. Louis: Elsevier.

Christensen, L. S., & Simmons, L. E. (2020). *The scope of practice for academic nurse educators and academic clinical nurse educators.* Washington, DC: National League for Nursing.

Fitzgerald, A., McNelis, A. M., & Billings, D. (2020). NLN core competencies for academic nurse educators: Are they present in the course descriptions of academic nurse educator programs? *Nursing Education Perspectives, 41*(9), 4–9.

Halstead, J. A. (Ed.). (2019). *NLN core competencies for nurse educators: A decade of influence.* Philadelphia: Wolters Kluwer.

Lundeen, J. D. (2018). Analysis of first-time unsuccessful attempts on the certified nurse educator examination. *Nursing Education Perspectives, 39*(2), 72–79.

National League for Nursing (NLN). (2021). *Certified nurse educator (CNE®) 2021 candidate handbook.* http://www.nln.org/docs/default-source/default-document-library/cne-handbook-2021.pdf?sfvrsn=2.

Ortelli, T. H. (2016). Candidates' first-time performance on the certified nurse educator examination. *Nursing Education Perspectives, 37*(4), 189–193.

PART 2

Assessing Readiness for the CNE® and CNE®n Exams

Comprehensive Practice Exam

ANGELA SILVESTRI-ELMORE

1. Which characteristic does the nurse educator recognize as similar for both Generation X and Generation Y learners?
   A. Prefer face-to-face learning when possible
   B. Need frequent feedback from instructors
   C. Are technologically proficient
   D. Like to work individually for learning

2. Which action by the nurse educator is the most important for promoting motivation for adult learning?
   A. Provide positive feedback and reinforcement.
   B. Use lecture as the most common teaching strategy.
   C. Conduct a survey of adult learning styles.
   D. Assign pertinent readings from the course textbook.

3. If a small group of learners becomes disruptive during class, which strategy is the most helpful for the nurse educator to use?
   A. Tell the disruptive learners to leave the classroom.
   B. Randomly assign seats to break up the disruptive group.
   C. Ask the disruptive learners to share their comments with the class.
   D. Advise the learners that their grades will be affected by their behavior.

4. The nurse educator should be aware of which characteristic when teaching nontraditional learners?
   A. These learners tend to identify with and model their peers.
   B. Family and work responsibilities can be stressors.
   C. Intrinsic motivation is more evident in these learners.
   D. These learners have limited life experiences to inform their studies.

5. Which action would the nurse educator take to best incorporate more technology into the classroom?
   A. Ensuring adequate institutional technology support
   B. Conducting faculty development focused on technology use
   C. Obtaining funding to provide mobile devices for learners and faculty
   D. Employing nurse educators who are technology experts

6. Which evaluation method could be used to formatively assess a learner's competence in performing urinary catheter insertion?
   A. Assess the learner's understanding of safe urinary catheter insertion on a written examination.
   B. Use a skills checklist to observe the learner performing the skill and provide constructive feedback.
   C. Observe the learner's ability to safely perform the skill in the clinical setting and document in the final clinical evaluation.
   D. Assign a written case study on urinary catheter insertion and grade based on a grading rubric.

7. Which strategy would the nurse educator use to best promote learner development and foster a productive learning environment?
   A. Emphasize that uncertainty is acceptable in learning.
   B. Divert attention away from tense or uncomfortable topics.
   C. Select learners to answer questions during class.
   D. Ask individuals to speak on the behalf of the class.

8. What should the nurse educator primarily consider to determine whether a teaching-learning activity is a good fit for student learning?
   A. Learning outcomes
   B. Learner preferences
   C. Available resources
   D. Administrative support

9. The nurse educator teaching an online course understands that best practice centers on which essential factor?
   A. Use of passive learning
   B. Emphasis on task completion
   C. Clear faculty evaluation of learner work
   D. Communication between learners and faculty

10. Which activity by the nurse educator best promotes the faculty–learner relationship?
    A. Discussing grades and course progression
    B. Engaging learners in mentored research projects
    C. Giving prompt constructive feedback on learner work
    D. Discussing ideas from class during open office hours

11. Which statement does the nurse educator recognize as the most accurate regarding learners with documented disabilities?
    A. Learners with disabilities need to navigate barriers independently.
    B. It is the responsibility of the learner with a disability to seek needed resources.
    C. Learners with disabilities usually have documented evidence of the disability before starting their education.
    D. Learners with disabilities may perform well in certain areas and may not perform well in other areas.

12. Which statement made by the nurse educator demonstrates a desirable attribute of an academic advisor when a learner reports dissatisfaction on a grade received on a class assignment?
    A. "Other than talking to me, how have you addressed this concern so far?"
    B. "Your instructor is an expert, so the evaluation of your work is correct."
    C. "You can follow the grievance policy to attempt having the grade changed."
    D. "We can review your assignment together and see where improvement can be made."

13. Which domain of learning is addressed when the nurse educator asks learners to complete a self-assessment as a part of their clinical evaluation?
    A. Social
    B. Cognitive
    C. Affective
    D. Psychomotor

14. The nurse educator planning activities to address the cognitive domain of learning would use which teaching-learning activity?
    A. Writing a personal health improvement plan
    B. Transferring a patient from the bed to the chair safely
    C. Analyzing laboratory results for a patient case scenario
    D. Listening to a patient's experience at end of life

15. Which teaching-learning strategy would the nurse educator select to use with a class of mostly visual learners?
    A. Traditional lecture
    B. Technical skill practice
    C. Reflective journal
    D. Graphic images

16. Which statement does the nurse educator recognize as incorrect about adult learners?
    A. Adults are not responsible for their own learning.
    B. Adults are self-directed as they chronically age.
    C. Adults prefer assignments that help them meet learning outcomes.
    D. Adults are goal-oriented to achieve their careers.

17. Which statement by a nurse educator about learner diversity requires follow-up by the mentor?
    A. "I asked my learners what activities and strategies they prefer in the classroom."
    B. "I asked my learners to volunteer for a diversity committee to manage any problems."
    C. "I asked learners to volunteer to share information about their diversity."
    D. "I try to be very respectful and role model respect for all of my learners."

18. A nursing program has an admitting class with a larger number of veterans than in past years. Which characteristic of this group should influence the nurse educator's selection of teaching-learning activities?
    A. Veterans tend to work as individuals when engaging in a learning experience.
    B. Veterans work very well in groups or teams to meet the desired outcome.
    C. Veterans have a high incidence of physical and mental disabilities.
    D. Veterans are at high risk for failure because they tend to be first-generation college learners.

19. What does the nurse educator recognize as the most important purpose of policies regarding incivility in the nursing program?
    A. To help promote learner success in the program
    B. To provide a way to increase affective learning
    C. To socialize learners into the professional role
    D. To create a welcoming environment

20. Which of the following teaching-learning activities fosters learner development in the affective domain?
    A. Answering an unfolding case study
    B. Taking a history of a standardized patient
    C. Developing a clinical concept map
    D. Completing a reflective journal

21. Which statement by a nurse educator about professional development of learners requires follow-up by the mentor?
    A. "I shared how I have developed professionally with my learners yesterday."
    B. "I have a lot of respect for all of my learners and try to role model that respect."
    C. "I don't let learners attend professional development conferences because they will miss class."
    D. "I told learners about campus organizations to help them develop as potential leaders."

22. Which teaching-learning activity by the nurse educator would best help students learn how to practice civil behaviors?
    A. Role modeling of civil behaviors by nurse educator
    B. Writing a scholarly paper on how to use civil behaviors
    C. Analyzing a case study that focuses on inclusivity
    D. Keeping a diary of students' own behaviors

23. A learner reports long-term hearing loss and requests to use an amplified stethoscope in the skills laboratory. What is the nurse educator's best response?
    A. "I will need to check with the lab coordinator about whether we have one of those devices."
    B. "I will be sure we have that device for you before you come to lab for practice."
    C. "We are not allowed to have those devices for learners because they cost a lot."
    D. "I will need documentation on exactly how bad your hearing loss is now."

24. Which learning activity would be most effective in assisting learners to apply principles of ethical behavior?
    A. Role modeling ethical behavior in the clinical setting
    B. Using case studies that incorporate ethical principles in decision making
    C. Providing safe environments in which learners can discuss ethical principles
    D. Using learner discussion groups to talk about personal experiences involving ethics

25. What is the best approach for nurse educators to find mentors to help them achieve their goals?
    A. Look for experienced mentors.
    B. Seek mentors from the nursing field.
    C. Find a mentor from a different institution.
    D. Pursue mentors who align with career goals.

26. Which of the following is most important when evaluating learner support services?
    A. Guidance for financial aid is available to learners.
    B. Transcript evaluation processes are accurate and timely.
    C. Learners receive an adequate orientation to the program.
    D. Support for achieving learning is adequate and accessible.

27. Which factor is most important for the novice nurse educator when engaging in teaching, service, and scholarship?
    A. Manageable workload
    B. Ongoing self-evaluation
    C. Administrative support
    D. Teaching relevance and competence

28. Which activity demonstrates the ability of nurse educators to disseminate scholarly work?
    A. Engaging in interprofessional activities
    B. Working as an advisor on a doctoral committee
    C. Sharing teaching innovations in a public forum
    D. Serving as a manuscript reviewer for a peer-reviewed journal

29. Which types of scholarship would be most appropriate for the nurse educator who is an assistant professor?
    A. Teaching and Discovery
    B. Application and Integration
    C. Discovery and Integration
    D. Teaching and Application

30. What statement does the novice nurse educator recognize as the most accurate statement regarding institutional scholarship requirements?
    A. Scholarship is required if faculty are appointed for the tenure track.
    B. Scholarship is an expectation of all faculty regardless of experience.
    C. Scholarship is not a requirement for novice nurse educators because teaching is their focus.
    D. Scholarship productivity is required for faculty working at teaching-intensive institutions.

31. Which activity could the nurse educator pursue to satisfy service requirements?
    A. Substituting as a guest lecturer in a nursing class
    B. Presenting at a local nursing education conference
    C. Serving on a nursing program progression committee
    D. Meeting with learner advisees on an ongoing basis

32. Which general description best characterizes the Scholarship of Teaching?
    A. It is achieved through data-driven research.
    B. It centers on the discovery of new knowledge with other disciplines.
    C. It involves inquiry about teaching and learning.
    D. It includes engaging in service-learning opportunities.

33. The novice nurse educator is demonstrating successful socialization to the role by engaging in which activity?
    A. Obtaining a terminal degree in nursing
    B. Networking at professional nursing conferences
    C. Becoming certified in a clinical specialty area in nursing
    D. Maintaining a portfolio documenting the quality of teaching

34. Which statement about pursuing professional development is essential for the nurse educator to understand?
    A. Professional development opportunities should be approved by a mentor.
    B. The need for professional development changes as experience is gained in the role.
    C. Professional development activities should be broad and varied.
    D. The educator can expect to pay for all professional development experiences.

35. Which of the following best describes the role of a faculty mentor for a novice nurse educator?
    A. Provides advice and support for the educator
    B. Evaluates educator's role performance
    C. Reports on educator's progress to administration
    D. Assists with educator's teaching responsibilities

36. A learner's parents ask the nurse educator to discuss the learner's grades. What is the educator's best response?
    A. "I will be glad to discuss the learner's grades during my office hours this afternoon."
    B. "I will need to check with my dean to see if I am allowed to discuss the learner's grades."

C. "You can meet with our administrative assistant who keeps all of the grades for our learners."

D. "I will need permission from the learner before I can discuss the learner's grades with you."

37. Which of the following activities by the nurse educator is an example of Boyer's Scholarship of Discovery?
   A. Conducting research on the impact of COVID-19 infection on the quality of life of nursing home residents
   B. Using a new virtual simulation program to help students learn how to conduct a patient interview
   C. Dividing the students into groups in the classroom to compete in a medical terminology game
   D. Planning a service-learning experience to promote health education for a vulnerable population

38. The nurse educator publishes findings from a study conducted with a social worker on meeting the health care needs of homeless veterans. Which of the following scholarship areas does this activity represent?
   A. Scholarship of Teaching
   B. Scholarship of Application
   C. Scholarship of Discovery
   D. Scholarship of Integration

39. Which of the following activities by the nurse educator is an example of Boyer's Scholarship of Application?
   A. Conducting a pilot study for publication
   B. Sharing a new teaching-learning strategy with peers
   C. Planning a service-learning experience
   D. Developing an interprofessional simulation experience

40. Which activity by the nurse educator demonstrates successful socialization as a leader in the academic role?
   A. Joining a professional nursing organization
   B. Reading nursing education journals each month
   C. Advising learners about readiness for graduation
   D. Accepting the chair position for an institutional committee

41. Which action by the nurse educator demonstrates fairness for learners?
   A. Adding points to a test that most learners passed
   B. Notifying learners of academic changes in a clear and timely manner
   C. Allowing learners to leave the clinical site early after care is completed
   D. Developing policies for an acceptable code of conduct

42. Which activity would be the most important for the nurse educator to perform when considering possible curriculum revision?
   A. Conduct a needs assessment.
   B. Identify external frame factors.
   C. Assess population demographics.
   D. Seek input from community stakeholders.

43. The nurse educator assisting with curriculum design for a new nursing program would initially consider which of the following as part of the needs assessment?
   A. Predictions for future nursing workforce needs
   B. Mission, vision, philosophy, and goals of the school
   C. Resources within the nursing program and institution
   D. Organizational structure of the parent academic institution

44. Which statement describes a philosophy statement as a component of the curriculum?
   A. Broad vision for the program
   B. Faculty beliefs and values
   C. Overarching goals for the work being done
   D. Guiding framework for program development

45. In developing the curriculum for a new nursing program, which approach should the nurse educator use for developing course learning outcomes?
   A. Create weekly lesson outcomes that are tied to course outcomes.
   B. Align course assignments and grading criteria with course outcomes.
   C. Crosswalk course outcomes with guiding bodies in nursing education.
   D. Level course outcomes sequentially to align with program learning outcomes.

46. What purpose does curriculum mapping serve in revising a nursing curriculum?
   A. Projects future needs of health care and educational consumers
   B. Determines needed resources for implementation of planned activities
   C. Examines relationships between curricular concepts and stakeholder needs
   D. Ensures essential knowledge and skills are integrated into the curriculum

47. Which domain of learning is addressed in the following course objective: "The learner accurately measures vital signs"?
   A. Affective
   B. Cognitive
   C. Behavioral
   D. Psychomotor

48. Which data would the nurse educator use as an indicator of program effectiveness?
   A. Course evaluations
   B. Graduation rates
   C. Learner course surveys
   D. Learner course exam scores

49. The nurse educator reviewing alignment of the curriculum with nursing regulatory requirements uses which guideline as a reference source for scope of practice?
   A. The state nurse practice act
   B. National accreditation standards
   C. National licensure requirements
   D. The institution's mission statement

50. Which of the following statements is true regarding nursing program accreditation?
    A. Nursing accreditation in the United States is mandatory.
    B. Failure to seek nursing accreditation results in ineligibility for federal monies.
    C. Nursing accreditation bodies provide oversight of licensure requirements.
    D. Learner transfer credits from nonaccredited institutions are typically recognized.

51. What should the nurse educator understand about the primary purpose of systematic program evaluation?
    A. To ensure a process for formal learner complaints
    B. To define programmatic policies and procedures
    C. To ensure national accreditation standards are met
    D. To determine the extent to which the program meets expected outcomes

52. Which source of data can be used as an assessment of external program support?
    A. Course evaluation survey results
    B. Standardized examination results
    C. Learner engagement survey reports
    D. Advisory group meeting minutes

53. Which activity best describes the faculty role in curriculum design?
    A. Confirming physical space is available for planned learning activities
    B. Ensuring concepts and content in the curriculum are complete and relevant
    C. Determining instructional resources are adequate to achieve learning outcomes
    D. Obtaining clinical experiences that are varied and appropriately sequenced

54. What is the primary consideration for the nurse educator when evaluating the effectiveness of teaching-learning strategies?
    A. Ascertaining if learners were satisfied with the strategies used
    B. Judging whether content complexity increased with the strategies used
    C. Assessing if strategies used were designed in accordance with best practice
    D. Determining whether strategies effectively facilitated achievement of learning outcomes

55. The nurse educator recognizes that the primary consideration for selecting a clinical site for learner experiences is which of the following?
    A. The ability for learners to meet learning outcomes in the clinical site
    B. The opportunity for learners to perform complex skills in the clinical site
    C. A clinical site where the nurse educator has practice experience
    D. A clinical site where the patient census remains high most of the time

56. Which statement by the nurse educator about barriers to curriculum development requires follow-up by the mentor?
    A. "Many of the faculty have no experience in curriculum development."
    B. "I'm not sure faculty are going to have the time to work on the curriculum."
    C. "It is not part of the nurse educator's academic role to develop curriculum."
    D. "Faculty may need guidance from an external curriculum expert."

57. The nurse educator is serving on the curriculum committee to evaluate the need for curriculum revision starting with interviewing stakeholders. Which of the following groups are external stakeholders?
    A. Current learners
    B. Clinical partners
    C. Nursing faculty
    D. Nursing dean

58. The nurse educator collaborates with the simulation coordinator to plan high-fidelity learner experiences. Which method is an example of a high-fidelity simulation?
    A. Using task trainers for psychomotor skills
    B. Analyzing unfolding case studies
    C. Practicing oral suctioning on static mannequins
    D. Assessing standardized patients

59. Which domain of learning is addressed in the following course objective: "Compare the physical assessment findings of osteoarthritis, gout, and rheumatoid arthritis"?
    A. Psychomotor
    B. Performance
    C. Cognitive
    D. Affective

60. Which cognitive taxonomic level is this course objective: "Identify the most common social determinants of health for older adults that contribute to health inequity"?
    A. Remembering
    B. Understanding
    C. Applying
    D. Analyzing

61. The nursing faculty is planning to revise the nursing department philosophy. What is the most important consideration when working on this task?
    A. Ensure the nursing department philosophy is congruent with the institution's philosophy and values.
    B. Conduct a thorough literature search for evidence to support the nursing department philosophy.
    C. Include each faculty's opinion in the content of the revised nursing department's philosophy.
    D. Survey learners for their opinion about how the nursing department philosophy should be revised.

62. Which cognitive taxonomic level is this course objective: "Develop a teaching plan for a first-time birth parent who is being discharged to home with a newborn"?
    A. Understanding
    B. Applying
    C. Analyzing
    D. Creating

63. A nursing curriculum committee is analyzing current societal and health care trends in preparation for a curricular revision. Which of the following trends would most likely affect this revision process?
    A. Changes in licensure and certification examinations
    B. Decrease in immigration to the United States
    C. Increase in use of social media for communication
    D. Increased focus on diversity and health equity issues

64. What does the nurse educator recognize as the most important characteristic of a well-designed nursing course?
    A. It is provided in a hybrid format and addresses the varied learning styles of students.
    B. It reflects the program's philosophy and allows students to meet course outcomes.
    C. It addresses current trends in nursing and health care and helps to ensure patient safety.
    D. It is developed by the entire nursing faculty to ensure input from both experienced and novice educators.

65. The graduate nursing program assessment committee analyzes pediatric nurse practitioner certification pass rates. The expected outcome is "85% of each cohort will pass the exam"; the pass rate for the last cohort is 79%. What is the most appropriate recommendation by the committee for action by the full nursing faculty?
    A. Change the expected outcome on the program evaluation plan to a 79% pass rate.
    B. Determine whether there were major changes on the certification exam this past year.
    C. Analyze the possible reasons for the pass rate decline to develop an action plan.
    D. Recommend that the pass rates continue to be monitored for another year.

66. The nurse educator shares the course lesson plans with learners. What is the primary purpose of this action?
    A. To demonstrate that the educator is prepared for each class in the course
    B. To make learners aware of how learning activities align with course objectives
    C. To keep the educator on time during the class to meet all course objectives
    D. To meet nursing regulatory and accreditation curriculum requirements

67. In which activity can the nurse educator engage to best promote change in the nursing profession?
    A. Serve as a faculty advisor to a group of learners.
    B. Obtain grant funding to support leadership initiatives.
    C. Attend a leadership academy to improve leadership skills.
    D. Empower learners and graduates to become leaders in nursing.

68. The nurse educator has the responsibility of fostering which of the following attributes in learners to best advance the profession of nursing?
    A. Critical thinking
    B. Leadership skills
    C. Technology fluency
    D. Communication strategies

69. Which factors most influence the direction for professional nursing education?
    A. Social and political forces
    B. Technologic resources
    C. Teaching best practice guidelines
    D. Learner characteristics and preferences

70. Which approach would be best for the nurse educator to teach cultural competence?
    A. Create instructional strategies that support equity.
    B. Encourage learners to participate in professional groups.
    C. Engage in scholarly work focused on culturally competent care.
    D. Integrate cultural competence content throughout the curriculum.

71. In which activity should the nurse educator engage to contribute to the science of nursing education?
    A. Conduct original clinical research.
    B. Obtain certification in a specialty practice area.
    C. Share teaching innovations with other educators.
    D. Seek grant funding to support scholarly work.

72. Which requirement for nurse educators is the most important for developing a successful scholarship program?
    A. Clinical competence in the assigned teaching area
    B. Continuing education focused on nursing leadership
    C. Training on working with diverse learner populations
    D. Time and resources to establish a firm scholarship foundation

73. An institution committed to expanding diversity to support learning should use which strategy to best promote this effort?
    A. Create a diversity, equity, and inclusion committee.
    B. Integrate diversity, equity, and inclusion content in the curriculum.
    C. Obtain affiliation agreements with clinical sites offering diverse experiences.
    D. Engage learners in scholarship focused on diversity, equity, and inclusion.

74. The nurse educator interested in continuing education to develop leadership skills should pursue which most helpful opportunity?
    A. Attending a nursing leadership conference
    B. Becoming a scholar in a leadership academy
    C. Taking a graduate-level nursing leadership course
    D. Reading journal articles about nursing leadership styles

75. The nurse educator understands that the primary responsibility of a nursing scholar is which of the following?
    A. Use active teaching-learning strategies.
    B. Engage in the spirit of inquiry.
    C. Develop clinical practice expertise.
    D. Conduct literature searches.

76. Which activity by the nurse educator demonstrates Boyer's Scholarship of Teaching?
    A. Conducting interprofessional research on innovative teaching methods
    B. Developing an unfolding case study for groups of learners
    C. Publishing the effectiveness of an innovative teaching strategy
    D. Serving on a nursing education committee for a professional organization

77. Which activity by the nurse educator is an example of scholarly teaching?
    A. Using evidence-based approaches to teaching-learning
    B. Respecting diverse ways of learning
    C. Maintaining high learner satisfaction on course evaluations
    D. Implementing active teaching-learning strategies

78. Nurse educators need to understand that their primary role is which of the following?
    A. Research
    B. Service
    C. Teaching
    D. Leadership

79. The nurse educator is planning to submit a research proposal to the institutional review board (IRB). What is the purpose of the IRB?
    A. Approve the research proposal
    B. Provide funding for the proposed research
    C. Disseminate knowledge about academic research
    D. Ensure protection of research participants

80. Which activity by the nurse educator best demonstrates professional leadership?
    A. Obtaining certification in nursing education
    B. Joining a professional organization
    C. Teaching an online nursing course
    D. Submitting a manuscript for potential publication

81. Which of the following is the most important quality of administrative nursing department leaders?
    A. Communicating frequently with faculty
    B. Creating a vision for the department
    C. Preparing an accreditation self-study report
    D. Participating in the curriculum revision process

82. The nurse educator recognizes that the role of a change agent for a faculty group is which of the following?
    A. Planning the change for the faculty
    B. Implementing the change for the faculty
    C. Determining the need for the change
    D. Ensuring the group is ready for the change

83. Which activity by the nurse educator would likely be the most effective in promoting nursing leadership skills for learners?
    A. Include questions on the final course exam to measure leadership knowledge.
    B. Develop a case study on nursing leadership principles and skills.
    C. Integrate nursing leadership competencies throughout the curriculum.
    D. Assign learners to partner with a nursing leader for a day in the clinical setting.

84. Which activity by the nurse educator demonstrates institutional leadership?
    A. Submitting a research proposal to the institutional review board
    B. Assisting in revising the faculty union contract for the next year
    C. Collaborating with interprofessional faculty to develop a new course
    D. Serving as a guest lecturer for a peer faculty's course

85. Which of the following factors is a requirement for making an effective institutional change?
    A. Hiring an external expert consultant
    B. Ensuring cultural sensitivity and inclusivity
    C. Including every faculty and staff member to make the change
    D. Obtaining approval by the student government association

86. A new administrative nursing leader's goal is to promote faculty satisfaction and to retain educators for the department. Which leadership style would best meet this goal?
    A. Transformational
    B. Participative
    C. Transactional
    D. Authoritative

87. The curriculum committee of a nursing program is planning a curricular change and recognizes that some faculty may not support the change. Using Lewin's theory of change, which initial stage will need to be successful to make the desired change?
    A. Unfreezing
    B. Adapting
    C. Processing
    D. Refreezing

88. Which activity by the nurse educator best demonstrates political advocacy?
    A. Have learners complete a case study on political advocacy.
    B. Serve on a professional organization's legislative committee.
    C. Volunteer to send texts to support a local political candidate.
    D. Assign learners to read about legislative and political advocacy.

89. Which outcome best indicates the effectiveness of a nursing program's admission and progression policies?
    A. Learners are self-directed and require minimal guidance.
    B. Learners meet the clinical outcomes without supervision from their instructors.
    C. Learners exceed minimum grade requirements to progress in the program.
    D. Learners meet the program learning outcomes and graduate.

90. Conducting course evaluations to determine learner achievement of outcomes serves which primary purpose?
    A. Produces data needed for program evaluation and accreditation
    B. Ensures necessary resources for teaching and learning are available
    C. Provides information on effectiveness of teaching and learning methods
    D. Uncovers personal opportunities for improvement for the nurse educator

91. The novice nurse educator effectively uses which method to assess learning in the cognitive domain?
    A. Determine learners' ability to demonstrate safe sterile technique in the insertion of an indwelling urinary catheter.
    B. Observe learners gathering needed supplies to correctly change a peripheral intravenous line dressing.
    C. Ask learners to reflect on their own cultural biases when caring for members of vulnerable populations.
    D. Require learners to describe conflict resolution strategies to promote teamwork among staff in an acute care setting.

92. The novice nurse educator effectively uses which method to assess learning in the psychomotor domain?
    A. Observe verbal and nonverbal communication between learners and their assigned patients.
    B. Review learners' assessment findings documented in the medical record for accuracy.
    C. Determine the learners' ability to safely prepare intravenous medications before administration.
    D. Assess the learners' knowledge of their patients' medications before administration.

93. The novice nurse educator effectively uses which method to assess learning in the affective domain?
    A. Evaluate a learner's written reflection on clinical experience with a dying patient.
    B. Review a learner's competency checklist before doing a dressing change.
    C. Critique a learner's clinical assignment submission and offer feedback for improvement.
    D. Ask the learner to describe the significance of laboratory results for a patient with chronic kidney disease.

94. What is the primary purpose of evidence-based assessment and evaluation practices in nursing education?
    A. To ensure learner satisfaction with the program
    B. To promote engagement in various learning environments
    C. To satisfy state regulatory requirements
    D. To determine whether learners met expected outcomes

95. Which statement is the most important for the nurse educator when developing a grading rubric to evaluate a written assignment?
    A. Specify the number of assignment drafts to be submitted with due dates.
    B. Relate the rubric criteria to the learning objectives of the course.
    C. Provide a template for learners to use when developing the assignment.
    D. Review assignment guidelines with learners before they begin working on it.

96. The nurse educator using course exams understands that this evaluation method best serves which purpose?
    A. Gives insight into learner clinical performance ability
    B. Provides a way of evaluating learning outcome achievement
    C. Assists the nurse educator in determining teaching effectiveness
    D. Allows for prediction of learner performance on the final examination

97. The nurse educator understands that which of the following accurately describes norm-referenced test interpretation?
    A. Scores are judged against preestablished criteria and expectations.
    B. Interpretation involves evaluation of competency-based learning models.
    C. The scores of a group of individuals being evaluated form the basis for comparison.
    D. There is an emphasis on mastery and potential for all learners to achieve competence.

98. The nurse educator understands that which of the following accurately describes criterion-referenced test interpretation?
    A. It reflects whether learners have met predetermined learning outcomes.
    B. It allows for interpretation of learner groups against national criteria.
    C. There is the ability to make comparisons within and outside the learner group.
    D. The criteria for the test are determined by the learners' scores.

99. In developing a test blueprint, the nurse educator completes which of the following actions first?
    A. Determine the weight to be assigned to each content area.
    B. Determine the number and type of items to be used.
    C. Determine the course content to be evaluated.
    D. Determine the learning outcomes to be measured.

100. The nurse educator preparing a test understands which of the following statements about test reliability is correct?
    A. Reliability improves by having other educators review the test.
    B. Test reliability depends on adequate content coverage on the test.

C. Reliability can be addressed by having varying item types on the test.
D. The reliability of test scores increases as the length of the test increases.

101. The nurse educator understands that collaborative testing is an assessment method in which pairs or groups work together on which type of activity?
A. Clinical case studies
B. Unit exams
C. Simulation experiences
D. Scholarly papers

102. While using observation to evaluate learner performance in the clinical learning environment, the nurse educator recognizes that which of the following factors can have an impact on the evaluation process?
A. Educator bias
B. Clinical setting
C. Patient diagnosis
D. Learner attitude

103. The nurse educator appropriately implements learner self-assessment as part of clinical performance evaluation by which of the following?
A. Starting self-assessment at the end of the program
B. Including self-assessment as part of the theory grade
C. Beginning self-assessment with the first clinical course
D. Implementing self-assessment after the educator's evaluation

104. The nurse educator conducting test item analysis would interpret a KR-20 of 0.73 as which of the following?
A. The exam is unreliable.
B. The exam measures intended knowledge.
C. Some of the exam items require revision.
D. The exam demonstrates internal consistency.

105. The nurse educator reviews a test item with a p level of 0.68. What is the accurate interpretation of this value?
A. 68% of learners who took the test got this item correct.
B. The test item did not discriminate between high scorers and low scorers.
C. The test item was not reliable and needs to be revised.
D. 68% of learners who took the test got this item incorrect.

106. The nurse educator reviews the responses of 37 learners who answered the following test item for which C is the correct answer:

A	B	C	D
9	16	5*	7

If using this test item in the future, which two choices would the educator consider revising?
A. Choices A and B
B. Choices B and C
C. Choices A and D
D. Choices C and D

107. The nurse educator reviews the point biserial coefficients for the following test item for which B is the correct response:

Choice	p Level	PBS Value
A	0.15	−0.10
B*	0.42	0.39
C	0.30	0.05
D	0.13	−0.10

What is the educator's interpretation of how this test item discriminated?
A. The point biserial coefficient is not the best measure of item discrimination.
B. This test item was fairly difficult for this group of test takers.
C. This test item needs to be nullified for this group of test takers.
D. This test item discriminated well between high and low scorers.

108. The nurse educator reviews the point biserial coefficients for the following test item for which C is the correct response:

Choice	p Level	PBS Value
A	0.15	−0.10
B	0.42	0.39
C*	0.30	0.05
D	0.13	−0.10

Based on these data, what is the most appropriate action, if any, for the nurse educator to take for the learners who took this test?
A. This test question performed as expected and no action is needed at this time.
B. This test question should be thrown out and not counted in the learners' scores.
C. This test question should be nullified because it poorly discriminated.
D. Learners who selected Choice B should also be given credit for this test item.

109. The nurse educator is preparing to calculate the course grade for a learner based on the following evaluation criteria:

Assignment	Possible Points	Learner's Earned Points
Exams (3) =	150 points	122 points
Scholarly paper =	30 points	27 points
Oral presentation =	25 points	25 points
Quizzes =	20 points	16 points

A = 92%–100%
B = 83%–91%
C = 75%–82%
F = 74% or below

Using the grading scale, what letter grade did this learner earn?
A. Course grade of A
B. Course grade of B
C. Course grade of C
D. Course grade of F

110. The nurse educator recognizes that the primary purpose of a test blueprint is which of the following?
    A. To establish content-related evidence of measurement validity
    B. To establish internal consistency
    C. To help the learners study for the test
    D. To establish interrater reliability

111. Which type of reliability does the nurse educator understand is needed when using a clinical evaluation tool in a faculty team-taught course?
    A. Internal consistency
    B. Interrater reliability
    C. Parallel form reliability
    D. Test-retest reliability

112. Which of the following evaluation tools can be used for formative assessment of learners in a classroom or online course?
    A. Portfolio
    B. Final examination
    C. One-minute paper
    D. Capstone paper

113. Which of the following evaluation methods by the nurse educator would best assess a learner's clinical performance?
    A. Concept map
    B. Care plan
    C. Weekly progress notes
    D. Observation of learner's performance

114. Which statement by the nurse educator about the preceptorship model requires follow-up by the mentor?
    A. "I will monitor and mentor the preceptors to whom my learners are assigned."
    B. "All of the preceptors have been well oriented to their role in this course."
    C. "I gave the preceptors our clinical evaluation tool so they can complete it for each learner."
    D. "I will ask the preceptors and learners to evaluate their clinical experience."

115. Which of the following assessment tools is used for summative evaluation of student learning?
    A. Unit examinations
    B. Comprehensive final examination
    C. Quizzes
    D. Muddiest point

116. How would a nurse educator interpret a test item that has a p level of 0.97?
    A. The test item is likely too easy.
    B. The test item is likely too difficult.
    C. The test item discriminates well.
    D. The test item should be nullified.

117. What does the nurse educator understand to be the most important guideline when providing feedback to learners about their performance?
    A. The feedback should be recorded by the learner.
    B. The feedback should be provided at least twice per semester.
    C. The feedback should be provided at the end of the course.
    D. The feedback should be frequent, timely, and constructive.

118. What is the best method for a nurse educator to assess learning style preferences of students?
    A. Determine learning style based on age of students.
    B. Use a validated instrument for assessing learning style.
    C. Assess learning style based on current student study habits.
    D. Develop and administer a survey asking about learning preferences.

119. Which teaching-learning strategy would be most appropriate for a kinesthetic learner?
    A. Practicing listening to heart sounds in the skills laboratory
    B. Listening to a voice-over slide presentation on heart sounds
    C. Watching a video about types of heart sounds
    D. Taking notes on reading about heart sounds

120. Which of the following resources is essential for nurse educators to competently provide online courses for learners?
    A. Online course management software
    B. Information technology support for learners
    C. Faculty development focused on online instruction
    D. Communication platforms for collaboration with learners

121. The nurse educator understands that which of the following statements best describes Generation X learners?
    A. Are accustomed to structure with very little free time
    B. Are often optimistic, team-oriented, and rule following
    C. Tend to be self-directed, flexible, and technology adept
    D. Absorb information instantaneously and lose interest quickly

122. Which technology should the nurse educator use to promote learner engagement during class activities?
    A. Electronic books
    B. Podcasting or live captures
    C. Drug reference manuals
    D. Audience response systems

123. Which activity describes effective implementation of simulation by the nurse educator as a teaching-learning strategy in the classroom?
    A. Using a virtual simulator in a flipped classroom
    B. Employing Socratic questioning in the classroom
    C. Dividing learners into groups to construct a concept map
    D. Assigning a classroom debate on ethics

124. The nurse educator using debriefing in simulation as a teaching and learning strategy understands that this method is most beneficial in promoting which of the following?
    A. Time management
    B. Clinical skills and techniques
    C. Broadened nursing knowledge base
    D. Clinical judgment and critical thinking

125. The nurse educator interested in providing learning opportunities to develop critical thinking and clinical judgment in the classroom should use which of the following strategies?
    A. Lecture
    B. Case studies
    C. Assigned reading
    D. Written assignments

126. The nurse educator using adult learning theory to guide implementation of teaching-learning strategies would use which teaching-learning activity?
    A. Concept mapping
    B. Group projects
    C. Peer-to-peer teaching
    D. Creating drug cards

127. The nurse educator interested in using experiential learning theory understands that which of the following teaching-learning strategies reflects this theory?
    A. Brief lectures
    B. Practice questions
    C. Clinical care plan
    D. Clinical simulation

128. The nurse educator working to improve clinical education understands that which of the following is key to a positive clinical learning experience?
    A. Clinical site availability
    B. Learner confidence and self-efficacy
    C. Adequate number of patient assignments
    D. Understanding the needs of learners

129. The nurse educator interested in considering life experiences and learner needs should begin by considering which of the following factors?
    A. Military status
    B. Generational differences
    C. Previous work experiences
    D. Racial and ethnic background

130. The novice nurse educator recognizes that which approach best increases retention of diverse learners?
    A. Mentorship
    B. Academic support
    C. Leadership development
    D. English-language programs

131. Which of the following skill sets is most important for nurse educators to teach in the clinical learning environment?
    A. Leadership and management skills
    B. Effective communication skills
    C. Clinical competence in nursing practice
    D. Ability to collaborate with others

132. Which teaching-learning strategy is most effective in developing critical thinking in the classroom environment?
    A. Using class time to clarify and illustrate concepts
    B. Coordinating guest lecturers on specialty topic areas
    C. Placing additional resources on the course learning management system
    D. Asking the learners to take detailed notes during lectures

133. Which strategy would the nurse educator use to best promote critical thinking in the clinical learning environment?
    A. Assigning discussion board assignments focusing on clinical reflection
    B. Requiring learners to complete clinical care plans before the clinical day
    C. Using learning activities that incorporate research utilization
    D. Ensuring learners understand pathophysiology concepts encountered in the clinical setting

134. Which of the following principles would the nurse educator use as a guide to promote a culture of caring in the clinical learning environment?
    A. Minimize communication between peers.
    B. Encourage learners to interact with nursing staff.
    C. Ensure opportunities for collaboration.
    D. Present caring theory content in postconference.

135. The nurse educator interested in creating an interactive learning environment should take which initial step in successfully adopting audience response systems?
    A. Using the technology to assess learning
    B. Integrating the technology into all planned lessons
    C. Surveying learners on their perception of the system
    D. Piloting the system technology

136. The nurse educator understands that clinical instruction opportunities should prioritize which of the following learner outcomes?
    A. Developing clinical decision-making abilities
    B. Performing nursing skills
    C. Completing complex clinical assignments
    D. Providing mentoring for socialization into the profession

137. Which of the following characteristics is most important for ensuring the quality of clinical learning?
    A. Qualified clinical nurse educators
    B. Strong clinical practice partnerships
    C. Validated clinical learning evaluation tools
    D. Integration of high-fidelity simulation in clinical learning

138. Which of the following skills is critical to the successful integration of evidence-based teaching-learning strategies?
    A. Public speaking proficiency
    B. Willingness to take on complex tasks
    C. Ability to critically appraise the literature
    D. Understanding of high-level statistical analyses

139. The nurse educator aiming to engage learners in case studies and role playing would be using which of the following educational technologies?
    A. Static mannequins
    B. App-based practice questions
    C. Electronic information resources
    D. Low-fidelity simulation

140. The nurse educator understands that which of the following is an extrinsic motivational factor for student learning?
    A. Personal values
    B. Cultural beliefs
    C. Work ethic
    D. College degree

141. Which teaching-learning activity would be most appropriate for the auditory learner?
    A. Audio recording of breath sounds
    B. Listening to breath sounds
    C. Interpreting breath sounds
    D. Attending a lecture on breath sounds

142. The nurse educator understands that the advantage of active learning is which of the following?
    A. It is easier for the educator to plan and implement.
    B. It fosters student engagement in the learning process.
    C. It requires group work and collaboration by students.
    D. It is a primary principle of adult learning theory.

143. A nurse educator teaching in the clinical setting overhears staff nurses complaining about learner performance. What is the best action by the educator at this time?
    A. Approach the staff nurses to determine what the learners did to cause the complaints.
    B. Ignore the comments at this time because nursing staff are usually stressed.
    C. Select a later time to talk with staff about how they perceive the learners' experiences.
    D. Report what was said to the nurse manager or chief nursing officer.

144. A nurse educator receives notification that the clinical site is short-staffed and cannot have learners for at least a week. What is the most appropriate action by the educator?
    A. Inform the learners that they will not have a clinical experience but the hours will be made up later.
    B. Provide alternative hands-on clinical experiences in the campus simulation laboratory.
    C. Explain to learners that they will have several clinical paper assignments to make up the missed clinical experiences.
    D. Plan additional classroom and online hours to make up the missed time in the clinical setting.

145. A learner asks the nurse educator to supervise starting a peripheral intravenous line. What is the most appropriate response by the educator?
    A. "Please check with the staff nurses to help you with the procedure because they are the clinical experts."
    B. "You will need to ask the staff nurse to do the IV insertion because I don't have time."
    C. "You don't need to start the IV because you had plenty of practice in the skills lab last week."
    D. "When do you need to start the IV so I can be available to help you?"

146. A nurse educator's goal when assigned to a new acute care clinical site is to develop strong collegial relationships with the nursing staff. Which action by the educator would most likely help relationship building?
    A. Ask staff nurses for help with selecting patient assignments for learners.
    B. Tell learners to report any patient changes to the educator first before the staff.
    C. Attend the unit staff meeting to learn about their policies and procedures.
    D. Offer to provide a staff development session on cultural competence.

147. Which of the following attributes of a nurse educator would best facilitate learning and decrease learner anxiety in the clinical setting?
    A. Clinical competence
    B. Patience
    C. Confidence
    D. Respect

148. Which active teaching-learning strategy is the best for acquiring and retaining knowledge?
    A. Unfolding case study
    B. Concept map
    C. Games
    D. Discussion forum

149. Which of the following approaches by the nurse educator would most likely motivate learners in the clinical setting?
    A. Providing feedback to correct learner errors
    B. Presenting patient cases in postconference
    C. Using a just culture approach
    D. Pairing learners with staff nurses

150. What does the nurse educator recognize as the advantage of using a flipped classroom approach to learning?
    A. Learners conduct a literature search before every class.
    B. Learners take a readiness test at the beginning of each class.
    C. Learners provide group presentations on various topics.
    D. Learners prepare for class by completing learning activities.

Answers and Rationales for Practice Questions

Chapter 2

1. **D.** Psychomotor domain
Rationale: Learning in the psychomotor domain requires "hands-on" experiences, such as when learners practice skills in a laboratory environment. Therefore Choice D is the correct response. The cognitive domain focuses on knowledge and intellectual learning, and the affective domain focuses on attitudes, feelings, and emotions (Choices A and B). There is no visual learning domain (Choice C).
Reference: Billings & Halstead (2020), pp. 188–190

2. **C.** Concept map
Rationale: The concept map is a commonly used graphic organizer that helps learners visualize and organize pieces of information such as patient data. Therefore Choice C is the correct response. The case study and discussion forum are more appropriate for the read/write learner (Choices A and D). Lecture is more appropriate for the aural/auditory learner (Choice B).
Reference: Billings & Halstead (2020), pp. 501–502

3. **A.** "I can let students learn on their own for online learning."
Rationale: The answer to this question is the statement that is not correct. Online learning requires that the nurse educator provide presence and guide the learning. Therefore Choice A is the answer because the statement is incorrect and requires that the mentor follow up with the educator. Educators engaging in online learning would want to give learners prompt feedback and participate when warranted in discussion forums (Choices C and D). Having motivated learners is a benefit for any type of instructional method (Choice B).
Reference: Oermann et al. (2022), pp. 115–124

4. **D.** Working on a case study during class
Rationale: Case studies are active teaching strategies that facilitate knowledge, knowledge transfer, and critical thinking, which represents learning in the cognitive domain. Therefore Choice D is the correct response. Practicing listening to breath sounds is an activity in the psychomotor domain (Choice A). Taking a quiz or exam is not a teaching strategy; it is an assessment of learning methods (Choices B and C).
Reference: Oermann et al. (2022), pp. 65–68

5. **B.** *Jeopardy*
Rationale: *Jeopardy* is a game that is a teaching strategy to help learners gain, recall, or retain knowledge. Games are not used to develop thinking skills; therefore Choice B is the correct response. Case studies and reflective journaling require the use of knowledge and critical

thinking (Choices A and C). Simulation experiences provide learners with the opportunity to transfer knowledge into practice (Choice D).
Reference: Billings & Halstead (2020), p. 294

6. D. Developing a concept map
Rationale: In brain-based learning, deep learning results from making connections between and among the most important concepts. It requires thinking and is not forgotten. Concept maps require the learner build upon previous learned information and rearrange it until it makes sense (Choice D). Superficial learning results from memorization and is short-lived. It can lead to fragmentation and does not require thinking. Choices A, B, and C reflect superficial learning.
Reference: Billings & Halstead (2020), p. 264

7. A. "I will be using concept mapping for clinical assignments."
Rationale: Choice A is the correct answer. Based in constructivism, concept mapping supports the theory that learning is constructed by the learner and builds upon previous learning and experience. Assignments that can potentially be cut and pasted do not require connections to be made or relationships to be discovered. Teaching with a cofaculty member does not determine whether an activity requires new learning connected to previous knowledge (Choices B, C, and D).
Reference: Cannon & Boswell (2016), p. 65

8. D. Write a reflective postclinical paper about the assigned client in DKA crisis.
Rationale: Deep learning results from making connections between and among the most important concepts. Reflection is the foundation of growth through experience. A reflection paper requires the learner to consider, weigh, speculate, contemplate, and deliberate to consider a basis for reasoned action or to gain understanding or attach meaning to an experience. It helps achieve deep learning in the affective domain and results in synthesis of learning (Choice D). Superficial learning results from memorization and is short-lived. It can lead to fragmentation and does not require thinking. Choices A, B, and C can be completed without deep learning.
Reference: Billings & Halstead (2020), p. 264

9. B. Avoid "busywork" assignments.
Rationale: The nurse educator designs learning activities that are relevant and meaningful to all learners. Adult learners are self-directed and have self-controlled learning. They do not appreciate "busy work" and are focused on the task at hand, making Choice B the correct response. Learning is facilitated with collaboration and not competition (Choice A). The nurse educator encourages learners to work together, not decrease their interaction (Choice D). Technology is very useful as a learning tool for all learners and should not be minimized. Most nontraditional learners are either members of Generation X or Y and would therefore be able to use technology.
Reference: Cannon & Boswell (2016), pp. 71, 83

10. D. "I'm going to reduce electronic assignments this semester."
Rationale: Choice D is the correct answer because Generation Z (i-Generation) is the Internet generation and digitally native. These learners absorb information quickly and lose interest just as quickly. The use of social media is often their preference for interaction using technology. Nurse educators use active teaching strategies that engage learners regardless of age. Choices A, B, and C are active learning activities that are indicated to engage Generation Z, and these statements would not require any follow-up.
Reference: Billings & Halstead (2020), pp. 19–20

11. D. Locate S_1 and S_2 as a part of cardiac assessment.
Rationale: Choice D is the correct answer. It is the only choice that involves physical care using a "hands-on" approach. Choices A and B are focused on remembering and understanding

knowledge in the cognitive domain. Choice C represents learning in the affective domain, reflecting values and beliefs.
Reference: Oermann et al. (2022), pp. 65–68

12. D. "I include psychosocial data and the family situation to make it realistic."
Rationale: Choice D is the correct answer. Educators should avoid using textbook scenarios to create a case study, but rather mix up the information to include psychosocial data, family situation, and so forth to make it realistic. The nurse educator develops case studies for learners to apply concepts to real or simulated scenarios, facilitating knowledge transfer and increasing learner confidence. Effective case studies are relevant, realistic, promote engagement, and provide a cognitive challenge for learners (Choice A). Choice B is incorrect because case studies do not have to be graded, although that is an option for the educator. Choice C is incorrect because case studies actively engage learners by providing opportunities to apply concepts to real or simulated scenarios, facilitating knowledge transfer and increasing learner confidence. Effective case studies are relevant, are realistic, promote learner engagement, and provide a cognitive challenge for learners.
References: Oermann et al. (2022), pp. 62–63; Ignatavicius (2019), pp. 9–11

13. A. Reflect
Rationale: The affective domain focuses on learning associated with awareness of values and beliefs and internalizing new values. Therefore "Reflect" is an appropriate verb to use for this domain (Choice A). Choices B, C, and D are verbs that would be better for the cognitive domain, which involves knowledge and using knowledge.
Reference: Billings & Halstead (2020), pp. 453–456

14. B. Team-based learning
Rationale: The only approach in the list of options that requires cooperative learning in groups is team-based learning (Choice B). A flipped or scrambled classroom does not necessarily require the use of cooperative learning, although group work may be part of those approaches (Choices A and C). Structured learning is a broad term for planning teaching-learning (Choice D).
Reference: Oermann et al. (2022), p. 81

15. C. Cognitive
Rationale: Learning in the cognitive domain involves acquiring knowledge and developing thinking, which cannot be directly observed. The learning objective references a thinking activity (Choice C). In the affective domain, learning involves attitudes, values, and beliefs, which cannot be directly observed (Choice A). Learning in the psychomotor domain involves hands-on performance of technical skills, which can be directly observed (Choice B). There is no behavioral learning domain (Choice D).
Reference: Oermann et al. (2022), pp. 65–68

16. B. Discussion board
Rationale: Learning can be either synchronous or asynchronous. In a *synchronous learning* environment, all learners are scheduled for the experience at the same time. Choices A, C, and D are typically implemented in groups who meet at the same time to accomplish the activity. *Asynchronous learning* allows learners to learn at different times. For example, online or remote learning provides an opportunity for students to learn asynchronously, such as when responding to a discussion board or forum (Choice B).
Reference: Oermann et al. (2022), p. 114

17. B. "Games help promote critical thinking and clinical reasoning."
Rationale: Games, either live or electronic, are appropriate active teaching-learning strategies for acquiring and recalling knowledge (Choices A and C), but they do not promote thinking.

Therefore Choice B would require follow-up by the mentor and is the correct response to this test item. Most games take a lot of class or online time to complete, but they tend to be fun (Choice D).
Reference: Billings & Halstead (2020), pp. 294–295

18. B. Concept map
Rationale: As the name implies, graphic organizers are the visual presentation or picture of knowledge that is organized to improve learning. Concept maps, algorithms, and Venn diagrams are examples of these learning tools (Choice B). The other activities are not graphic organizers, but virtual reality is very useful for visual learners (Choices A, C, and D).
Reference: Oermann et al. (2022), p. 264

19. C. Become self-aware using exploration of personal mental health practices.
Rationale: Choice C is the only choice that involves feelings and values for learning in the affective domain. Choices A and B are thinking actions for learning in the cognitive domain. Choice D is the actual "doing" of a skill and represents learning in the psychomotor domain.
References: Oermann et al. (2022), pp. 65–68; Billings & Halstead (2020), p. 454

20. B. Role-playing communication techniques
Rationale: Choice B is the correct answer because the divergent role is more abstract and focused on feelings, which can be observed through role-playing. Choices A, C, and D are examples of the stage of more concrete activities in which the learner is doing something or having an experience. Examples include case studies, role-playing, simulation, concept mapping, skill practice, and games.
Reference: Billings & Halstead (2020), pp. 29–30

21. D. Demonstrate how to insert an intravenous catheter.
Rationale: Choice D is the correct answer, as the psychomotor domain of learning addresses development of manual or physical competencies. The academic nurse educator uses this domain most often in developing nursing skills and competencies for clinical practice. Choice A represents learning in the cognitive domain, which focuses on knowledge and the use of knowledge. Choice B reflects learning in the cognitive and affective domains. Choice C represents learning in the affective domain, which focuses on values, beliefs, and other feelings.
Reference: Billings & Halstead (2020), pp. 29–30

22. C. Watch a film clip and discuss in a think-pair-share activity.
Rationale: Choice C is the correct answer for the visual learner because it involves graphics. Choice A is more appropriate for the auditory learner. Choice B is most appropriate for the read/write learner. Choice D is a kinesthetic activity in the psychomotor domain.
Reference: Billings & Halstead (2020), pp. 453–456

23. D. Find commonalities among the groups and connect with technology.
Rationale: The academic nurse educator finds commonalities and uses a broad range of active learning strategies to help create an engaging and meaningful learning environment. In addition, developing active learning strategies supports success for all learners, regardless of age. Learners today are techno-savvy, and emerging technology educational tools can be used to promote learning and bridge generational differences (Choice D). Although any cooperative learning activity is an active learning strategy, Choice A may not be as preferred by Generation Z learners. Choice B is incorrect because the time of day for study groups does not relate to age. Choice C is an example of technology, but the educator should not assume that online learning would bridge diverse generational learning preferences.
Reference: Billings & Halstead (2020), pp. 17–20

24. B. Deep learning

Rationale: Choice B is the correct answer. Concept maps are an active learning tool that helps learners make connections (relationships) between components of care, which promotes deep learning, not surface or superficial learning (Choice D). Choice A is incorrect because concept mapping results in more than retaining knowledge and does not lend itself to memorization (Choice C). Instead, it helps the learner connect previously learned information to newly learned information.

Reference: Billings & Halstead (2020), pp. 501–502

25. D. Cultural background

Rationale: Choice D is correct because the academic nurse educator modifies teaching strategies and learning experiences based on consideration of learners' diverse needs, including cultural background, past clinical experiences, past educational and life experiences, and generational groups. Choice A creates a positive learning environment and does not need to be modified. Choice B is an example of collaborative learning abilities, but not all learners prefer group work. Clinical sites are selected based on their ability to help learners meet course objectives and do not affect selection of teaching-learning strategies.

Reference: Billings & Halstead (2020), pp. 20–24

26. C. Assign learners to participate in cultural activities on campus.

Rationale: Choice C is the correct answer. Being immersed in a cultural activity promotes learning and experience in the affective and cognitive domains. Behavior change requires affective engagement. Choice A alone will not improve the focus on and understanding of diversity and inclusion in nursing. Choice B is an assessment method, not a learning strategy. One unit focusing on cultural humility is not the best choice because it would likely not have the same impact on learners (Choice D).

Reference: Billings & Halstead (2020), pp. 23–24

27. C. "We first do a personal inventory of our own feelings and beliefs."

Rationale: Choice C is the correct answer because nurse educators need to recognize their feelings and beliefs to uncover explicit or implicit bias. Only after initial self-examination can faculty consider other factors to create an inclusive learning environment. Choices A and D address only one aspect of understanding diversity (testing). Social activities can promote a sense of belonging to a community and should be encouraged, not discouraged (Choice B).

Reference: Billings & Halstead (2020), pp. 22–24, 27

28. A. Have learners practice neurologic assessment in pairs.

Rationale: Choice A is the correct answer. Having learners work in pairs practicing neurologic assessments provides a kinesthetic activity to develop psychomotor skills. As the learners are practicing, the academic nurse educator reinforces or corrects techniques with each pair. Repeating the entire demonstration (Choice B) is not necessary for the entire group. The instructor can provide guidance to each pair of learners as they practice, questions can be clarified, and techniques can be reinforced or corrected. Viewing a film on the nursing care of the client with neurologic deficits (Choice C) does not address the psychomotor aspect of the neurologic assessment but could be helpful in planning home care for the client who has had a stroke. Listening to an audio recording about life after a stroke (Choice D) reaches the auditory learner and the affective domain but is not addressing the "hands-on" psychomotor domain of learning.

Reference: Billings & Halstead (2020), pp. 23–24

29. B. Use a discussion board to establish presence.

Rationale: The correct answer is Choice B; a discussion board initiated before class officially starts as a way of promoting learner-to-learner interaction, giving learners the opportunity to ask questions with faculty present, which can help foster a learning community. Choice A is part

of the evaluation process during and at the end of the course. Having a face-to-face encounter initially is not always possible or even necessary. Some faculty schedule occasional face-to-face meetings to promote a sense of community (Choice C). A learning community can be successfully built online without the participants ever meeting each other. Developing a culture of academic integrity and ensuring test security is a primary responsibility in all settings (Choice D).
Reference: Billings & Halstead (2020), pp. 428–429, 432

30. **A.** Kolb's learning theory
Rationale: Based on experiential learning, Kolb's learning theory is a process that occurs through a transformation of experience, such as clinical simulation learning, and is therefore the correct answer. After an experience, the learner reflects, thinks, and acts for learning to occur (Choice A). Choice B, constructivism, allows learners to discover and build new knowledge using previous knowledge and life experience. Boyer's Model of Scholarship is not a learning or educational theory (Choice C). While not a theory and part of brain-based learning, deep learning occurs as the learner has an intrinsic motivation to understand the material and be able to use that information in practice. Deep learning includes understanding the concept, making decisions, and making connections (Choice D).
References: Bradshaw et al. (2021), pp. 6–7, 26; Billings & Halstead (2020), pp. 264–265

31. **C.** "Special debriefing training is necessary."
Rationale: The formal debriefing process used after a clinical simulation experience requires the facilitator to attend training; therefore Choice C is the correct answer. Several debriefing models can be used in simulation (Choice A). Debriefing is a learner-centered approach (rather than a teacher-centered approach) in which the educator facilitates the learner's reflection immediately after the simulation experience (Choice B). The academic nurse educator guides the learner in a reflective-based conversation, but there is no cognitive retraining involved in debriefing (Choice D).
Reference: Billings & Halstead (2020), pp. 364–367

32. **C.** Concept maps
Rationale: Concept maps are visual representations of the essential elements of client care shown using shapes, colors, lines, arrows, and words on the lines connecting the concepts; therefore Choice C is the correct answer. A case study is a valid method to measure clinical judgment, but it is not a visual strategy (Choice A). Both journaling and debriefing are excellent reflective activities but do not provide graphics, which are preferred by visual learners (Choices B and D).
Reference: Bradshaw et al. (2021), pp. 390–391

33. **C.** "Case studies are not a form of experiential learning."
Rationale: Choice C is the correct answer. Case studies are grounded in experiential learning, which includes reflective observation about the experience; therefore this statement would require follow-up by the mentor. Integrating unfolding case studies in simulation or other learning environments can transform a teacher-centered classroom into a learner-centered active learning environment (Choice A). Faculty development is important to be able to write an effective case study and clinical judgment questions (Choice B). Case studies are more effective when used for complex clinical situations, which require critical thinking to make appropriate clinical judgments (Choice D).
Reference: Billings & Halstead (2020), pp. 220, 297

34. **C.** Guest speakers and debates
Rationale: Choice C is the correct answer. Students who prefer auditory (aural) learning strategies prefer listening to a guest speaker, having a debate, using storytelling, discussions, and chats. Choice A would be preferred by the read/write learner, who prefers diagrams and graphs, designs, concept maps, and charts. Kinesthetic learners prefer cases, trial and error, and experiential

activities (Choice B). Visual learners prefer using colors, shapes, maps and charts, diagrams, and graphs (Choice D).
Reference: Billings & Halstead (2020), pp. 29–30

35. C. What focused assessment will be performed?
Rationale: Choice C is the correct answer. This requires the learner to pull the information together from the data provided. All of the other choices measure knowledge.
References: Billings & Halstead (2020), p. 299; Ignatavicius (2019), pp. 5–6

36. D. Practicing test questions until scoring is consistently above 80%
Rationale: Choice D is the correct answer. Behavioral learning strategies offer a reward for a behavior, such as meeting an 80% score. Drills such as using questions/answers can help learners develop thinking skills using repetition and reinforcement. The other choices have not built in a reward or outcome to achieve.
Reference: Oermann et al. (2022), pp. 32–34

37. B. "Does the learner interact well with the patients and health care team?"
Rationale: The correct answer is Choice B because interacting with others reflects one's values and beliefs, which is an example of learning in the affective domain. Choice A is assessing the psychomotor domain. Choices C and D are examples of questions about activities in the cognitive learning domain.
Reference: Billings & Halstead (2020), pp. 453–456

38. A. Developing an unfolding case study
Rationale: Choice A is correct. Developing a case study is an excellent way for learners to construct new knowledge and meaning. A dosage calculation test is an assessment method, not a teaching-learning activity (Choice B). Choice C involves memorizing facts or steps, which is behavioral learning theory. Practicing in the lab is an example of experiential learning (Choice D).
Reference: Oermann et al. (2022), pp. 79–80

39. A. Psychomotor and cognitive
Rationale: Choice A is the correct answer. The richness of the clinical experience is that it can meld all three domains of learning when providing patient care. Choices B, C, and D include terms that are not learning domains (communicative and behavioral).
Reference: Billings & Halstead (2020), pp. 453–456

40. C. "When do you need me to help you?"
Rationale: Choice C is the correct answer. The educator offers oneself to learners. Every opportunity for practicing a skill in the clinical learning environment is important for professional growth. Choice B does not show an extension of self as a learning facilitator. Choices A and D are not appropriate responses to this item. The clinical educator works to meet learning needs, and the best way to do that is to partner in the learning process in the clinical environment. Being too busy is not a therapeutic answer, nor does it reach out to provide assistance.
Reference: Billings & Halstead (2020), pp. 297–299

41. D. Journaling after a clinical experience
Rationale: Choice D is the correct answer because journaling fosters critical thinking by detailing the learner's personal experiences and connecting those feelings to the learning outcomes. Developing a slide show may or may not foster critical thinking, depending on the assignment (Choice A). Watching a film clip can be a starting point for a discussion that could create a critical thinking discussion, but is not the best answer (Choice B). Reading an article does not help develop critical thinking skills unless additional learning activities are planned (Choice C).
Reference: Oermann et al. (2022), p. 263

42. D. "The staff nurses are accountable for patient care, but I will be available if you need me."
Rationale: The nurse educator is responsible for providing a safe learning environment; Choice D provides reassurance that the patients will be safe and that learners will be monitored. Choice A provides false reassurance, and Choice B is an unrealistic statement. The clinical nurse educator would be available for helping learners with any type of skill, concern, or question and not limit that assistance to invasive skills (Choice C).
Reference: Oermann et al. (2022), pp. 231–238

43. C. Face-to-face
Rationale: Discussing a learner's progress or lack of success is a very emotional topic. Therefore using a face-to-face approach allows the opportunity for both verbal and nonverbal communication (Choice C). The other methods do not allow an in-person or face-to-face approach. These methods are best to communicate short factual information (Choices A, B, and D).
Reference: Oermann et al. (2022), p. 313

44. D. Structured controversy
Rationale: Ethics topics are part of affective learning, especially dilemmas, which can be very controversial. Debates and structured controversy are appropriate teaching-learning activities that are best for affective learning (Choice D). The other activities represent learning in the cognitive domain (Choices A, B, and C).
Reference: Billings & Halstead (2020), pp. 290–291

45. C. Virtual simulation
Rationale: Generation Z learners prefer hands-on experience combined with technology, which can be achieved through virtual simulation (Choice C). This group of learners does not prefer lecture, reading assignments, or slide presentations for learning (Choices A, B, and D).
Reference: Oermann et al. (2022), pp. 97–98

46. A. Concept map
Rationale: A concept map is a visual learning tool that shows connections to promote critical thinking and therefore is appropriate for visual learners. The process of developing the map requires a "hands-on" experience and is appropriate for kinesthetic and read/write learners. If the concept map is explained verbally, auditory learners can benefit. Therefore Choice A is the best answer. A lecture is preferred by auditory learners, and slides are preferred by visual learners (Choices B and C). A final examination is not a teaching-learning strategy, but rather an assessment method (Choice D).
Reference: Oermann et al. (2022), p. 264

47. A. Social media
Rationale: Generation Z learners were born from 1995 to the present, when social media presence markedly increased. Therefore this group prefers communication using social media (Choice A). Generations X and Y prefer email or texting (Choices B and C), and Baby Boomers prefer face-to-face communication (Choice D).
Reference: Billings & Halstead (2020), pp. 47–49

48. C. Psychomotor domain
Rationale: Learning in the psychomotor domain requires hands-on, kinesthetic experiences such as clinical skills performance. Demonstrating wound care is a clinical skill that is learned in a clinical learning environment (Choice C). Affective learning focuses on value, beliefs, and feelings (Choice A); cognitive learning focuses on acquiring and using knowledge and thinking (Choice B). Choice D is not a learning domain.
Reference: Oermann et al. (2022), pp. 65–68

49. D. Identify
Rationale: The remembering cognitive level allows learners to memorize and recall knowledge. The ability to identify knowledge is at the remembering taxonomic level (Choice D) and is therefore the correct answer. *Differentiate* is also a cognitive verb but at a higher thinking level of analyzing (Choice A). *Perform* is an action verb and is most often used for the psychomotor learning domain (Choice B). *Reflect* is a commonly used verb for learning in the affective domain (Choice C).
Reference: Oermann et al. (2022), p. 260

50. A. Case study
Rationale: A good case study requires learners to use critical thinking skills to make appropriate clinical or policy decisions; thinking is part of the cognitive learning domain (Choice A). Journaling and role-playing are commonly used activities for learning in the affective domain (Choices B and D). Skills practice is an activity associated with the psychomotor domain for hands-on learning (Choice C).
Reference: Oermann et al. (2022), pp. 79–80

51. C. Plan a role-play demonstration on communication.
Rationale: Therapeutic communication requires knowledge and the ability to express one's thoughts and feelings using appropriate techniques. Role-playing combines those two requirements (Choice C). Reviewing handouts or reading about communication does not build learner competence or confidence in communication techniques (Choices A and B). Developing a reverse case study on communication requires critical thinking but does not ensure that the learner would then be able to use those skills (Choice D).
Reference: Billings & Halstead (2020), pp. 467–468

52. A. "It can include a large amount of content for a large group of learners."
Rationale: Lecture is a teaching-learning activity that is teacher-centered rather than learner-centered, meaning that most of the communication is one-way from the educator. It is a teaching strategy in which the educator can "cover" a large amount of content for any number of learners. Therefore Choice A shows understanding of the purpose of lecture. Lecture does not allow time for in-depth discussions or critical thinking activities (Choices B and C). As a teacher-centered activity, lecture does not take the needs of diverse learners into account, which is not best practice for effective learning (Choice D).
Reference: Oermann et al. (2022), p. 84

53. A. Unfolding case study
Rationale: An unfolding case study typically presents an initial clinical situation and tells a story in which the situation changes in phases. Each phase is accompanied by multiple thinking questions and is therefore the best teaching-learning activity to help learners with clinical judgment skills (Choice A). All of the other choices are learning activities that stimulate and help develop critical thinking, but they do not allow the learner to make clinical judgments about patient care or other issues (Choices B, C, and D).
Reference: Billings & Halstead (2020), pp. 355–356

54. B. Cognitive domain
Rationale: Most of the classroom and online learning experiences focus on didactic learning, which is when knowledge is shared and learners practice how to use the knowledge through active thinking activities. The cognitive domain focuses on knowledge acquisition and thinking skills; therefore Choice B is the correct answer. Affective learning can also occur in didactic settings, but that is not the primary domain (Choice A). Learning in the psychomotor domain occurs most often in clinical environments (Choice C); there is no behavioral domain (Choice D).
Reference: Oermann et al. (2022), pp. 65–68

55. C. Psychomotor domain

Rationale: Learning in the psychomotor domain occurs most often in clinical environments (Choice C), such as the skills laboratory, clinical simulation, and clinical agencies in the community. Although learners need knowledge to practice skills and could be influenced by feelings associated with affective learning, this learning is not the primary focus (Choices A and B). There is no behavioral domain (Choice D).

Reference: Oermann et al. (2022), pp. 65–68

56. D. Place two to three points of information as summary or key points for each slide.

Rationale: Nurse educators often use a large number of slides for each class, which is unnecessary. Best practice for creating slides includes minimizing the number of slides and the amount of information on each slide (Choice D). A large-size font is preferred over a small-size font (Choice A), and graphic images are preferred over a large amount of text (Choice B). There is no evidence that supports using slides for every class (Choice C).

Reference: Billings & Halstead (2020), p. 400

Chapter 3

1. D. Collaborate with the learner on academic, personal, and professional goals during the meeting.
Rationale: Developmental advising is a collaborative effort that focuses on holistic personal and professional development with the learner. Therefore D is the correct response. Prescriptive advising focuses on information-sharing about courses and places the responsibility for decision making on the advisor (Choices A and C). Advisors may refer learners for tutoring services rather than provide the tutoring (Choice B).
Reference: He & Hutson (2016), pp. 213–240

2. B. Consider each learner's individual needs.
Rationale: Different advisement approaches should be used based on identified learner needs. Therefore Choice B is the correct response and Choice A is incorrect. The developmental, not prescriptive, approach helps learners identify career goals (Choice D). Both developmental and prescriptive forms of advising may be necessary, so one single method may not always be the most effective (Choice C).
Reference: Weir et al. (2005), pp. 74–75

3. A. Diagrams and concept mapping
Rationale: Visual learners learn best by seeing things. Use of diagrams, pictures, concept maps, and demonstrations are preferred methods of learning; therefore Choice A is correct. Small-group discussions are preferred by aural/auditory learners (Choice B). Slide presentations are the preferred learning method of read/write learners (Choice C). Kinesthetic learners enjoy simulation experiences (Choice D).
Reference: Billings & Halstead (2020), pp. 29–30

4. D. Use a variety of interactive teaching-learning strategies, including use of technology, to appeal to multiple generations of learners.
Rationale: Interactive and technology-based teaching strategies will appeal to both tech-savvy and self-directed learners. Therefore Choice D is correct. Focusing on a single teaching-learning strategy will not meet the learning needs of all generational learners (Choices A and B). Technology and multitasking with group work are characteristics of Generation Z (Choice C).
Reference: Billings & Halstead (2020), p. 19

5. B. Use complex vocabulary to help increase their English capacity.
Rationale: To accommodate EAL learners, the educator should use common vocabulary and short, simple sentences. Therefore Choice B is the correct response because it is not appropriate. Allowing audiotaping, role-playing communication techniques, and placing EAL learners in groups with native English speakers are all methods for facilitating learning in EAL learners (Choices A, C, and D).
Reference: Billings & Halstead (2020), pp. 23–32

6. A. Making excessive spelling errors on written assignments like papers
Rationale: Students with learning disabilities often display adequate knowledge and competence in the clinical setting but struggle when taking examinations or writing papers; therefore Choice A is correct. All other options are examples of uncivil behaviors displayed by learners (Choices B, C, and D).
Reference: Billings & Halstead (2020), pp. 67–68

7. A. Providing frequent feedback with clear goals and expectations
Rationale: Millennial learners "want frequent feedback that is tied to their focus on goals and expectations. Communication, feedback, and interactions should concentrate on management and attainment of the goals and expectations established." Millennials prefer to learn with peer

interaction. Therefore Choice A is correct and Choice C is incorrect. It is people from Generation X who do not want public recognition but prefer independence and informality with interactions (Choices B and D).
Reference: Cannon & Boswell (2016), pp. 38–43

8. A. "I should avoid using reflective journaling with adult students as it may bring up past traumas."
Rationale: Adult learners enter education with life experiences and draw on those past experiences when learning new material. Learning activities that allow for reflection on past and current experiences, such as reflective journaling, are effective for adult learners; therefore Choice A is correct and Choice D is incorrect. Adult learners prefer group learning and use of learning contracts that clearly state how they will achieve objectives and be evaluated (Choices B and C).
Reference: Billings & Halstead (2020), pp. 256–257

9. B. To maintain frequent contact with learners at regular intervals
Rationale: According to Chickering and Gamson's (1987) seven principles for good education, encouraging frequent learner–faculty contact is the most important factor in engaging learners with the material to be studied and for facilitating their learning. Therefore Choice B is correct. Additional principles of good education include setting high expectations and helping learners achieve them (Choice C) and creating a collaborative learning environment that is social and cooperative (Choice A). Educators should use a variety of teaching methods to facilitate learners with diverse ways of learning (Choice D).
References: Cannon & Boswell (2016), pp. 71–72

10. D. Complexity of the skill and measure of students' abilities
Rationale: Measure of ability, complexity of task, environmental effects, health status, and gender are all attributes to assess for physical readiness using the PEEK approach; therefore Choice D is correct. Knowledge base, learning disabilities, cognitive ability, and learning styles are all attributes of *knowledge readiness* (Choice A). Level of aspiration, past coping mechanisms, cultural background, locus of control, and orientation are all components of *experiential readiness* (Choice B). Anxiety levels, support systems, motivation, risk-taking behavior, and developmental age are all components of *emotional readiness* (Choice C).
Reference: Bastable (2016), p. 88

11. C. By practicing technical tasks during simulation
Rationale: Convergers prefer technical tasks and finding practical solutions to problems. Problem-solving activities, simulation, and experimentation are teaching strategies preferred by convergers; therefore Choice C is correct. Assimilators prefer learning through readings and lectures (Choice D). Kinesthetic learners prefer videos and demonstrations (Choice A). Read/write learners prefer PowerPoint presentations, whereas visual learners prefer pictures and diagrams (Choice B).
Reference: Oermann et al. (2022), pp. 163–164

12. C. Through email using blunt and direct language
Rationale: Members of Generation X prefer to communicate through email, and the communication is often direct and to the point; therefore Choice C is correct. Millennials use email and voice mail as primary tools of communication, but are usually more polite, positive, and respectful in their communication (Choice D). Baby Boomers tend to prefer face-to-face communication (Choice B). Generation Z members use social media for communication (Choice A).
Reference: Cannon & Boswell (2016), p. 40

13. B. Lack of time to complete academic advising
Rationale: Multiple demands on an educator's schedule can affect the amount of time that can be devoted to academic advisement; therefore Choice B is correct. Technology can be used to aid scheduling of advisement appointments and for quick communication with learners (Choice D).

Although difficulty locating policies and resources may be a barrier, time is the most significant barrier for effective advising (Choices A and C).
Reference: Halstead (2019), p. 50

14. D. Consult with the disability services office and provide the recommended accommodation.
Rationale: According to the American with Disabilities Act (ADA), students with documented learning disabilities must be provided reasonable accommodations in the educational setting upon request while ensuring learning outcomes are met. The disability services department will determine which accommodations are needed; therefore Choice D is correct. Although it is appropriate to provide the accommodations, faculty must maintain confidentiality of the disability and are not permitted to notify other faculty without the learner's permission (Choice B). Learners with disabilities are protected under the ADA and must be provided reasonable accommodations (Choice A). Educators must facilitate learning in all three learning domains; therefore Choice C is incorrect.
Reference: Billings & Halstead (2020), pp. 62–66

15. A. Using simulation equipment to practice urinary catheter insertion
Rationale: Individuals with bodily/kinesthetic intelligence prefer moving their bodies and manipulating tools and items; therefore Choice A is correct. Individuals with spatial intelligence prefer pictures, diagrams, and models (Choice B). Learners with interpersonal intelligence prefer working in groups and sharing information with others (Choice C). Individuals with linguistic intelligence prefer to read, write, and talk (Choice D).
Reference: Cannon & Boswell (2016), pp. 69–70

16. D. "I will group together learners from similar cultural backgrounds so that they may speak their native language."
Rationale: Best practice indicates that the educator should place EAL learners in groups with those who speak the *program's* native language, not the learner's native language; therefore Choice D is the correct response. Highlighting key words, using simple vocabulary, and allowing extra time for completion of assignments and examinations are all methods for facilitating learning in EAL learners (Choices A, B, and C).
Reference: Billings & Halstead (2020), pp. 23–32

17. B. "Learners who need a test reader may choose a friend to sit with them and read the exam questions."
Rationale: Some learners with a documented learning disability may need a reader for examinations, but that reader must be designated by the disabilities office and cannot be a classmate or friend; therefore Choice B is correct. Taking examinations in separate, secure locations; providing extra time for completion of exams; and having a note-taker are all appropriate reasonable accommodations to provide for students with documented learning disabilities (Choices A, C, and D).
Reference: Billings & Halstead (2020), pp. 68–69

18. B. Refer the learner to the campus writing center for support.
Rationale: Campus writing centers can provide assistance to learners with writing strategies and written papers; therefore Choice B is correct. Weekly tutoring by the faculty may be very time-intensive (Choice C). Assigning an additional paper without remediation may not be the most helpful strategy (Choice A). The learner does not appear to demonstrate a learning disability because the learner performs well on both examinations and in the clinical setting (Choice D).
Reference: Billings & Halstead (2020), p. 53

19. D. The learner is a first-generation college student.
Rationale: First-generation college students do not have family members to help provide college mentoring, are typically socioeconomically disadvantaged, and tend to have lower grade

point averages; therefore Choice D is correct. Learners with previous degrees tend to be self-motivated and have developed effective study habits (Choice A). Adult learners tend to be more self-directed and take an active role in the learning process (Choice B). Learning styles help identify how learners perceive and process information but do not necessarily affect academic performance (Choice C).
Reference: Billings & Halstead (2020), p. 22

20. A. Plan to incorporate both prescriptive and developmental advising during the first meeting.
Rationale: The learner has indicated the need for help with both the technical aspects of registering for classes and potential challenges and study strategies; therefore Choice A is correct. Being nervous about starting something new does not warrant a referral to mental health services (Choice B). The learner did not indicate financial difficulties at this time (Choice C). Although the learner would benefit from a list of course sequencing, the learner indicated being nervous about nursing school. The faculty advisor should provide some guidance and strategies about being successful in the nursing program (Choice D).
Reference: He & Hutson (2016), pp. 213–240

21. C. Learners from the Millennial generation
Rationale: Millennial learners typically work well in teams, and interprofessional simulation involves working alongside nursing students and other members of the health care team; therefore Choice C is correct. Generation X learners prefer to work independently and typically do not enjoy group work (Choice A). Individuals with intrapersonal intelligence prefer to work alone (Choice B). Learners with visual/spatial intelligence prefer to learn using pictures, models, and reading (Choice D).
Reference: Cannon & Boswell (2016), pp. 69–70

22. D. Reflective observation and abstract conceptualization
Rationale: Assimilative learners understand best through a combination of watching (reflective observation) and thinking (abstract conceptualization); therefore Choice D is correct. Choice A describes accommodative learners. Choice B describes converging learners. Choice C describes diverging learners.
Reference: Halstead (2019), pp. 50–51

23. D. Use inclusive language on exams and case studies.
Rationale: Reflective journaling, avoiding group work, and meeting with each individual learner are solitary strategies that do not help foster a sense of belonging (Choices A, B, and C). Learning students' names, creating diverse clinical and study groups, and using inclusive language are some of the best methods for fostering a sense of belonging and inclusivity. Therefore Choice D is the correct response.
Reference: Metzger et al. (2020), pp. 12–13

24. D. Ask learners to complete a learning style inventory and a short quiz to determine concept knowledge.
Rationale: Attributes of knowledge readiness include present knowledge base, cognitive ability, learning disabilities, and learning styles; therefore Choice D is correct. Assessment of anxiety and motivation is included in emotional readiness (Choice A). The ARCS model describes factors that educators can use to motivate learners (Choice B). Assessment of cultural background can be used to determine experiential readiness (Choice C).
Reference: Lichtenthal, as cited in Bastable (2016), p. 88

25. A. "Increase the number of high-stakes examinations throughout the semester."
Rationale: High-stakes testing is not considered to be a high-impact educational practice that would help with learner engagement and retention; therefore Choice A is the correct response. Service learning, study abroad programs, and collaborative assignments and projects are all

high-impact educational practices that contribute to deep learning and positive learning outcomes (Choices B, C, and D).

References: American Association of Colleges and Universities (AACU) (2008); Billings & Halstead (2020), p. 32

26. A. "I should expect my learners to be experts upon graduation."
Rationale: This question is looking for the statement that is not correct. The transition to the role of professional nurse is often complicated by reality shock. Benner's novice to expert theory supports that new graduates often start in the early stages (novice, advanced beginner) and that they progress as they gain real-life experience. Therefore Choice A is the correct response. Learners do enter practice at the novice to advanced beginner level and grow over time in their role (Choices B and C). Reality shock does cause learners to often struggle as they transition from academia to the real world (Choice D).
Reference: Billings & Halstead (2020), pp. 257–259

27. B. Role-playing
Rationale: Role-play allows the learner to discover the content in a new way while delving into values and feelings. Socialization to the role of nursing requires an understanding of the values, emotions, and norms, which can all be explored through well-structured role-play. Therefore Choice B is the correct response. The case study is more appropriate for applying concepts to scenarios (Choice A). Lecture and debate are more appropriate to discuss and explore feelings and emotions; however, they are limited in providing active practice at the role of nurse (Choices C and D).
Reference: Billings & Halstead (2020), pp. 467–468

28. D. "Primary responsibility is placed on the learner in online education."
Rationale: Online learning places the responsibility primarily on the learner. Learners have the choice to move at their own speed, focus on the areas they need the most development in, and work following a structured plan. Therefore Choice D is the correct response. Teaching in the classroom versus online has vast differences in the role of the educator (Choice A). Learners will require a detailed, organized plan from the educator. There is a great demand of time from both the educator and the learner (Choices B and C).
Reference: Cannon & Boswell (2016), p. 189

29. B. Internalization of the norms, values, and beliefs is necessary to socialize to the role.
Rationale: Socialization to the role of professional nurse means that an individual embodies the norms, values, and beliefs of the profession. It is necessary to move from learning about the role to internalizing the role to act in accordance with the values and beliefs that are embodied. Therefore Choice B is the correct answer. Learners start socializing to the role during their formal education and continue to develop as they enter professional practice (Choices A and D). Socialization can be developed as the nurse gains knowledge and hands-on experience in the role (Choice C).
Reference: Halstead (2019), pp. 56–57

30. C. "I should model the behaviors that are expected of students in the clinical setting."
Rationale: Setting a positive example by modeling the behaviors of a professional nurse can assist learners in mimicking how to behave in the clinical setting. Learners are continually observing faculty for social cues, and the actions of the educator toward learners model what behavior is appropriate. Therefore Choice C is the correct answer. Teaching learners the policies of a facility does not provide socialization on professional behaviors such as values and therapeutic communication (Choice A). Learners need preparation for the different learning settings they encounter and need to learn about inappropriate behaviors that they may encounter and strategies to identify and deal with such behaviors (Choices B and D).
Reference: Cannon & Boswell (2016), pp. 117–120

31. C. "The clinical setting is the only place for the student to develop the values and norms of nursing."
Rationale: This question is looking for the statement that is not correct. The clinical setting (including laboratory and simulation) is an appropriate setting for the learners to grow in their professional roles. Learners are exposed to their instructors in addition to health care professionals in the practice environment who can help them understand better what it is to be a nurse. Therefore Choice C is the correct answer. Socializing to the role of nursing can take place across all learning environments the learner encounters (Choices A and D). The nurse educator has a responsibility to model the professional values and behaviors of a nurse (Choice B).
Reference: Billings & Halstead (2020), pp. 328–329

32. A. Discuss the concerns with the student privately and stress the values of nursing.
Rationale: Discussing the concerns noted with the learner in private is necessary to facilitate trust between the educator and learner. It is important to offer the opportunity for the learner to talk rather than jump to conclusions. Educators have a responsibility to tailor their response to the unique needs of the learner. Therefore Choice A is the correct answer. It is not accurate to tell learners they will be removed from nursing school or to report the learner to administration before first having a conversation (Choices B and D). Discussing the concerns with other learners is unprofessional and does not model appropriate behavior or engage the learner in a safe environment (Choice C).
Reference: Billings & Halstead (2020), pp. 38–39

33. B. Conceptualizing
Rationale: This question is looking for the incorrect answer. Values are important standards that nurses live and act on as professionals. Conceptualizing is part of the psychomotor domain of learning and is not a value. Therefore Choice B is the correct answer. Caring, diversity, and integrity are all considered values of nursing (Choices A, C, and D).
Reference: Billings & Halstead (2020), p. 38

34. A. Motivation
Rationale: Online learners need motivation to be self-directed for success in this mode of instructional delivery. Therefore Choice A is correct. Caring, inclusivity, and organization (Choices B, C, and D) are important traits for an individual to have, but they are not specific to success in the online learning environment.
Reference: Cadet (2021), pp. 209–215

35. D. Learners should set personal goals based on their own self-reflection and needs.
Rationale: Personal goal setting is tied to achievement in the academic setting. Goal setting can be taught and engages learners as active participants in their education. Therefore Choice D is the correct answer. Course outcomes can aid in guiding goal development; however, goals should be developed by each individual learner (Choices A and B). Setting goals is important to move the learner toward achieving more complex outcomes and is a skill that is necessary in professional practice.
Reference: Billings & Halstead (2020), pp. 27–28

36. B. Regularly leaving class early without explanation
Rationale: This question is looking for which behavior is appropriate. Uncivil learner behaviors can vary widely in severity. Raising the hand to ask questions during class is not disruptive and is an expected behavior (Choice C). Requesting that the faculty consider changing an assignment due date is not uncivil unless the learners start demanding this change (Choice D). Although turning off the camera when online may be considered by some as disrespectful, this behavior is a learner's right (Choice A). Leaving class early on a regular basis is very disrespectful and is considered to be uncivil. Therefore Choice B is the correct answer.
Reference: Cannon & Boswell (2016), p. 115

37. B. Immediately take the two learners involved to a private setting to discuss the matter, and follow the incivility policy of the program.

Rationale: Incivility can be noted in many different learning environments. Speaking inappropriately about another learner is uncivil behavior. Adding that the learners were discussing such a matter in front of a patient adds another element to the incivility. Patient safety is directly affected by uncivil acts; therefore this action needs to be addressed immediately and privately. The institution policy regarding incivility should be followed. Therefore Choice B is the correct answer. Holding a conference that includes the learner who was being disrespected or simply notifying the learner of the matter is not the appropriate way to address the learners directly engaged in uncivil behavior (Choices A and C). Reprimanding both learners in the middle of the clinical setting is inappropriate and demonstrates uncivil behavior on the part of the faculty (Choice D).
Reference: Billings & Halstead (2020), p. 279

38. A. Preventive action can be an early intervention to avoid uncivil behavior.

Rationale: Being proactive about what professional behavior looks like is an important tool to prevent incivility. Although the learners are adults, it should not be assumed that they automatically know what is appropriate for the course and to the educator. Therefore Choice A is the correct answer. Listing out inappropriate behaviors does not model what the expectations are for the learner (Choice B). Learners may understand some norms regarding higher education; however, it should not be assumed that all learners inherently understand what the educator expects as professional behavior (Choice C). Not including language regarding professional behaviors does not model what is appropriate for the learner and opens the door to confusion on the part of both the learner and educator (Choice D).
Reference: Billings & Halstead (2020), pp. 274–275

39. C. Cognitive

Rationale: The cognitive domain of learning refers to intellectual development and thinking. The use of lecture, group discussions, and case studies are all teaching strategies in the cognitive domain. Therefore Choice C is the correct answer. Diverging comes from Kolb's learning styles and includes those who observe and gather information and those who are open minded to view multiple perspectives (Choice A). The psychomotor domain involves performing hands-on skills to gain competency, and the affective domain is learning about feelings, attitudes, and beliefs (Choices B and D).
Reference: Billings & Halstead (2020), pp. 188–189

40. A. Applying

Rationale: The cognitive domain of the learning hierarchy includes six levels, from knowledge to create. *Interpreting, applying, assessing,* and *examining* are all verbs that can be used to describe the application level of the cognitive domain. Therefore Choice A is the correct answer. Remembering includes verbs such as *define, describe,* and *identify* (Choice B). Evaluating includes verbs like *support, appraise,* and *justify* (Choice C). Analyzing includes *explain, compare,* and *relate* as examples of action verbs (Choice D).
Reference: Billings & Halstead (2020), pp. 188–189

41. D. Skill demonstration

Rationale: Teaching a hands-on skill is part of the psychomotor domain of learning. Practicing skills in a laboratory setting after demonstration is appropriate for learning a new skill. Performing skills in the clinical setting and at simulations are all ways to learn and grow in the psychomotor domain once hands-on experience has been mastered. Therefore Choice D is the correct answer. High-fidelity simulation is part of the psychomotor domain, but a skills demonstration is more appropriate for first being introduced to a skill (Choice A). Lecture is a teaching strategy that is best used for the cognitive domain (Choice B). Reflective journaling can best be used to grow the affective domain (Choice C).
Reference: Billings & Halstead (2020), pp. 190–191

42. A. Demonstrate safe technique in the insertion of an intravenous catheter in the assigned patient.

Rationale: The precision level of the psychomotor domain of learning involves a learner who can perform a skill independently. Demonstrating a hands-on skill is part of the precision level. Therefore Choice A is the correct answer. Following steps falls under the imitation level of the psychomotor domain when a learner is just developing the process of how to perform a certain skill (Choice B). Analyzing and describing steps both fall under the cognitive domain of learning (Choices C and D).

Reference: Billings & Halstead (2020), pp. 190–191

43. D. Affective

Rationale: The learning outcome presented in the question is related to attitude and values. The learner promoting autonomy is a skill that involves feelings and emotions and particularly for the hospice patient. This learning outcome represents the affective domain. Therefore Choice D is the correct answer. The cognitive domain refers to intellectual development and thinking (Choice A). Kinesthetic is a learning style, and it is associated with psychomotor skills (Choice B). The psychomotor domain involves performing hands-on skills to gain competency (Choice C).

Reference: Billings & Halstead (2020), pp. 189–190

44. B. Discuss the values of the role of practical/vocational nursing.

Rationale: The affective domain of learning includes values, feelings, beliefs, and attitudes. Discussing the values of the role of nursing encompasses the affective domain. Therefore Choice B is the correct answer. Demonstrating a hands-on skill is learning in the psychomotor domain (Choice A). Apply a pathophysiologic process and describe risk factors both fall under the cognitive domain of learning (Choices C and D).

Reference: Billings & Halstead (2020), pp. 189–190

45. D. "Feedback is meant to punish the learner."

Rationale: Providing feedback to learners is an important skill for the nurse educator. This question is looking for which statement is incorrect. Feedback is intended to help the learner grow. Punitive feedback is not appropriate, as feedback is not meant to be a form of punishment. Therefore Choice D is the correct answer. Feedback should enhance the success of learners by providing communication that is timely, relevant, and includes concrete examples and ways to improve (Choices A, B, and C).

References: Billings & Halstead (2020), pp. 50–51; Cannon & Boswell (2016), pp. 69–72; Christensen & Simmons (2020), p. 12

46. A. Allow learners to reflect on their clinical performance.

Rationale: Self-evaluation is important for learners to develop as they prepare to enter professional practice. Reflection is a critical element of self-evaluation that can help learners identify strengths and weaknesses and begin goal setting. Self-evaluation should encourage reflecting on what has been learned in addition to the feelings about that. Therefore Choice A is the correct answer. Allowing learners to grade their own examinations or quizzes does not allow the learner to reflect and use feedback (Choices B and C). Allowing the learner to evaluate peers is not self-evaluation (Choice D).

Reference: Billings & Halstead (2020), pp. 258–259, 495–496, 504–505

47. C. Learners should be provided with clear guidance and a rubric to use for evaluation.

Rationale: Learners should be taught to engage in peer evaluation, as it is an important skill for developing the role of professional nurse. Educators should guide the learner in how to engage in peer evaluation and provide the tools to guide the feedback. Peer evaluation can assist in preparing learners for interprofessional practice. Therefore Choice C is the correct answer. Learners should receive guidance in what to evaluate and how to do so along with concrete examples. It is

not appropriate to use negative language (Choices A and B). It is important to learn how to work in a team, and peer evaluation can assist in developing those skills (Choice D).
Reference: Billings & Halstead (2020), pp. 496, 504–505

48. A. Learners do not need to engage in professional development; they are already in school.
Rationale: This question is looking for which statement is incorrect. Professional development is part of lifelong learning that nurses must engage in. Educators should begin fostering professional development for learners. Therefore Choice A is the correct answer. Professional development is one element of the role of the nurse (Choice B). Service learning presents the opportunity for learners to begin to engage in professional development (Choice C). Educators and learners working side by side in professional development allows the educator to model appropriate practices (Choice D).
Reference: Billings & Halstead (2020), pp. 220–221, 318

49. C. Educators should model participation in professional organizations.
Rationale: Membership in professional nursing organizations encourages lifelong learning. Educators should model participating in professional organizations for the learner. Explaining the benefits to learners can encourage them to engage in nursing organizations that are of interest to them professionally. Therefore Choice C is the correct answer. Professional organizations do not teach learners how to be a nurse, and the educator should not require the learner to join a particular organization (Choices A and B). Learners should begin engaging in professional organizations while still in school (Choice D).
Reference: Christensen & Simmons (2020), p. 12

50. B. Lifelong learning
Rationale: Engaging in professional development activities is imperative for faculty. Educators should also model this behavior for learners. Learning about inclusivity and diversity is an important concept for nurses and represents engaging in lifelong learning. Therefore Choice B is the correct answer. Caring and autonomy are both values of the nursing profession (Choices A and C). Dissemination of information can be facilitated through membership in professional organizations (Choice C).
References: Billings & Halstead (2020), pp. 104, 139–140; Christensen & Simmons (2020), p. 12

Chapter 4

1. D. Identifying the purpose of the evaluation

Rationale: The first step in the evaluation process is identifying the purpose of an evaluation; therefore Choice D is correct. Selecting an evaluator is the third step in the evaluation process (Choice A). Selection of a framework is the fourth step in the evaluation process (Choice B). Selection of an instrument occurs after choosing a framework for evaluation (Choice C).

Reference: Billings & Halstead (2020), pp. 439–440

2. B. Formative evaluation

Rationale: Formative evaluation occurs while learning is taking place and provides opportunity for feedback and improvement; therefore Choice B is correct. Norm-referenced evaluations are tests designed to rank learners (Choice A). Summative evaluations occur at the end of an activity or course and are used to make judgments about the learner's performance (Choice C). High-stakes tests are rigorous examinations used to determine admission or progression in a program (Choice D).

Reference: Billings & Halstead (2020), pp. 451, 475–476

3. A. Interrater reliability

Rationale: Interrater reliability refers to the consistency and consensus of multiple raters to score the evaluation of learner performance; therefore Choice A is correct. Validity of an instrument refers to the ability of that instrument to accurately assess what the evaluator intends (Choice B). Formative evaluation refers to an evaluation while learning is still taking place (Choice C). Learner evaluations can be useful for making improvements to teaching practices or classroom environments, but do not help eliminate bias in grading among multiple raters (Choice D).

Reference: Oermann & Gaberson (2021), p. 37

4. C. Patient simulation

Rationale: Patient simulation requires learners to role-play, make clinical decisions, and demonstrate clinical skills and therefore can be used to evaluate all three domains of learning (Choice C). Reflections and essays can be used to evaluate only the cognitive and affective domains (Choices A and B). Concept mapping typically is used to evaluate learning in the cognitive domain (Choice C).

Reference: Billings & Halstead (2020), pp. 457–458

5. D. "I will use formative assessments to determine final course grades for my students."

Rationale: This test item is asking to determine which statement is incorrect and, therefore, needs follow-up. Formative assessments are ongoing and are performed throughout a course while learning is taking place; therefore Choice D is the statement that needs follow-up and is the correct answer. Choices B and C are true statements. Summative evaluation involves making a judgment about student achievement; therefore Choice A is also a true statement.

Reference: Cannon & Boswell (2016), pp. 164–165

6. B. Reflection papers can be used to evaluate high-level cognitive and affective domains of learning.

Rationale: Reflection requires learners to contemplate an experience or question and to self-reflect, which can be used to evaluate both the cognitive and affective domains; therefore Choice B is correct. Reflection does not require performance of technical skills and does not adequately evaluate learning in the psychomotor domain (Choice A). Reflection is a solitary activity and does not foster collaboration or learner interaction (Choice C). Reflection does allow for assessment of critical thinking skills (Choice D).

Reference: Billings & Halstead (2020), pp. 457–460

7. C. Formative evaluation

Rationale: Classroom assessment techniques allow the nurse educator to gain evaluation data while learning is occurring. Formative evaluation aligns with using classroom assessment techniques that gather data in real time to help learners improve. Therefore Choice C is the correct response. Summative evaluation occurs at the end of a course and evaluates what the student has learned overall (Choice A). Norm referencing and criterion referencing are methods to measure learner achievement on an assessment (Choices B and D).
Reference: Cannon & Boswell (2016), p. 164

8. A. The assessment tools measure the course learning outcomes.

Rationale: The assessment tool used by the nurse educator should be guided by the course learning outcomes. The course outcomes can guide which domain is most appropriate for assessment. Therefore Choice A is the correct response. Program learning outcomes should be an overall factor that is considered, but is not the most important, as course outcomes should be guided by overall program outcomes (Choice B). What the nurse educator finds as important is not relevant in choosing an assessment tool, and accrediting bodies do not specify outcomes for the individual course (Choices C and D).
Reference: Billings & Halstead (2020), p. 451

9. D. Explanation of each level of performance

Rationale: A rubric should include a description of the assignment, scale, the necessary elements of the assignment, and an explanation of each level of performance. A rubric is used to grade or score an assessment. Therefore Choice D is the correct response. Multiple-choice items would not be included on a rubric (Choice C). Measurement of affective behaviors and evidence of observation would be items that could be included in a clinical evaluation tool (Choices A and B).
Reference: Oermann & Gaberson (2022), pp. 165–172

10. C. "Keep detailed notes in a secure location regarding each learner."

Rationale: Keeping detailed notes on learners can be an effective method to track observational data that are collected from the clinical experience. Data should be kept in a secure location. Therefore Choice C is the correct response. Concerns about learners should be addressed immediately; however, observational data should be tracked because there are often multiple learners, and this can be challenging to remember from week to week (Choices A and B). Having a phone available in the clinical setting is not always appropriate (Choice D).
Reference: Billings & Halstead (2020), p. 495

11. B. To establish interrater reliability

Rationale: Rubrics are often used by multiple faculty, and it is very important that a rubric is used by multiple faculty in the same way. Interrater reliability refers to the percentage of agreements in scores when multiple faculty are using the rubric. Therefore Choice B is the correct response. It is necessary to use the same rubric when it is a shared assessment, and each faculty member should not create individual rubrics (Choices A and C). Statistics are most often used with testing and do not apply to this scenario (Choice D).
Reference: Billings & Halstead (2020), pp. 452–453

12. B. Final clinical evaluation tool

Rationale: Summative evaluation occurs at the end of a learning experience to assess the learner overall. Clinical experiences can best be evaluated using a formal clinical evaluation tool that measures the outcomes defined by that clinical course. Therefore Choice B is the correct response. A portfolio showcasing multiple courses is more appropriate for the end of a program (Choice A). A self-evaluation tool can be part of a final clinical evaluation; however, it should not be the only criteria for assessment (Choice C). A rubric alone is not an appropriate tool to use for a clinical experience (Choice D).
Reference: Billings & Halstead (2020), pp. 507–508

13. A. Demonstrate skill in using patient care technologies.
Rationale: Clinical learning outcomes should align with course outcomes. Outcomes should be specific and measurable. Therefore Choice A is the correct response. Developing further knowledge and skills is vague and does not relate to a specific outcome (Choice B). It is not appropriate to include patient diagnoses in outcomes (Choice C). Administering medications independently is not appropriate for the learner in the clinical setting (Choice D).
Reference: Billings & Halstead (2020), pp. 499–500

14. D. Ensure privacy for the learner to provide feedback.
Rationale: Safety is paramount in the clinical setting. Feedback should be done in private, particularly when addressing a concern. Therefore Choice D is the correct response. Documenting the instance should be done, but feedback should also be given immediately to the learner (Choice A). Waiting to address the issue is a safety concern. Giving feedback in front of peers or the patient is inappropriate (Choices B and D).
Reference: Billings & Halstead (2020), pp. 50–51

15. C. "The clinical setting only evaluates learners in the psychomotor domain."
Rationale: Evaluation in the clinical setting involves input from multiple types of experiences and interactions. Learners should be evaluated based on behaviors, patient care, and safety, just to name a few. These areas represent learning in the cognitive, psychomotor, and affective domains. Therefore Choice C is the correct response. The nurse educator should keep detailed notes in order to provide detailed feedback on an ongoing basis and during final evaluation (Choices A and B). Clinical objectives should be readily available and discussed with learners (Choice D).
Reference: Cannon & Boswell (2016), pp. 230–231

16. A. This exam is reliable.
Rationale: The KR-20 is used to assess reliability of exam scores. An ideal KR-20 is above 0.80; however, above 0.70 is considered acceptable. Therefore Choice A is the correct response. In order to determine if revision is necessary, a further item analysis must be conducted (Choices B and C). The KR-20 is an indicator of reliability, not validity (Choice D).
Reference: Billings & Halstead (2020), pp. 486–487

17. B. 15 learners taking the exam
Rationale: An inadequate test length of fewer than 40 questions and inadequate sample size of fewer than 25 learners can lower the reliability of an exam. The strength of questions can also affect exam reliability. Therefore Choice B is the correct response. Forty questions on the exam are adequate and the minimum to ensure good reliability (Choice A). Time to take the exam and the average score are adequate for the exam (Choices C and D).
Reference: Billings & Halstead (2020), pp. 486–487

18. C. Poor exam reliability
Rationale: The KR-20 represents the reliability of an exam. In order to be adequate exam reliability, the KR-20 should be at least 0.70. Therefore Choice C is the correct response and not Choice A. KR-20 does not indicate exam validity (Choice B). Discrimination is determined for each item after further analyzing an exam (Choice D).
Reference: Billings & Halstead (2020), pp. 486–487

19. D. "An exam blueprint can help ensure content-related validity."
Rationale: An exam blueprint can assist in ensuring an exam is including the content intended and connects each question to the intended student learning outcomes (SLOs). Content-related validity ensures that an exam is measuring the SLOs. Therefore Choice D is the correct response. An exam blueprint is not for nursing administration (Choice A). Statistics such as those used to determine item discrimination and reliability are not in an exam blueprint (Choices B and C).
Reference: Billings & Halstead (2020), p. 486

20. **A.** Provide clearer directions.
Rationale: Several factors can negatively affect exam validity, such as inadequate sampling, poor items, and uncertain directions. Poor items that are only associated with a specific question type could be related to a lack of direction. Therefore Choice A is the correct response. The items do not need to be removed or rewritten if directions can be provided (Choices B and C). Poor scores on items can affect overall validity (Choice D).
Reference: Billings & Halstead (2020), p. 486

21. **C.** "I should ensure that all learners pass the exam."
Rationale: Exam analysis includes an overall assessment and a closer assessment of each item and item response. Exam analysis is for the purpose of editing and improving items as supported by the data. Therefore Choice C is the answer to this item because it is an incorrect statement. Exam analysis does not ensure that all learners pass the exam. Making needed adjustments to item scoring and improving the exam for future use based on an analysis of each item is the purpose behind exam analysis (Choices A, B, and D).
Reference: Billings & Halstead (2020), pp. 486–491

22. **B.** Choice B
Rationale: Point biserial is an indication of how well an item discriminates. The correct response in the test-item analysis (Choice C) should have a positive point biserial, which it does, whereas the distractors should ideally have a very low or negative point biserial. In this scenario, Choice B is a distractor but has a high positive point biserial. This indicates that Choice B needs revision before reusing the question. A negative point biserial is ideal for distractors; therefore Choices A and D do not need revision.
Reference: Billings & Halstead (2020), pp. 489–490

23. **A.** This item requires no revision.
Rationale: The p values for this item are within appropriate range. Fifty-six percent of learners answered correctly, and the item is highly discriminating. The distractors were all chosen and show they also discriminate. Therefore Choice A is the correct response. The responses for this item do not need to be revised based on the statistics (Choices B and D). This item should not be nullified (Choice C).
Reference: Billings & Halstead (2020), pp. 489–490

24. **C.** 35% of learners answered the item correctly.
Rationale: A p level indicates the percentage of learners that answered the item correctly. A p level of 0.35 indicates that 35% of learners answered the item correctly. Therefore Choice C is the correct response. The p value does not indicate the item must be nullified (Choice A). Sixty-five percent of learners answered the item incorrectly, not correctly (Choice B). This p value is below the acceptable range and indicates the item may be too difficult (Choice D).
Reference: Billings & Halstead (2020), pp. 489–490

25. **C.** This indicates the exam was too easy.
Rationale: The mean score is the average score of all learners in the sample. A score of 90% is a high score, indicating the exam may have been too easy. Therefore Choice C is the correct response. Consider whether any outliers could have altered the mean. This finding is not appropriate for a distribution of scores (Choice A). A score of 90% is a high passing score, indicating the exam was not difficult (Choice B). An exam should not be nullified, but rather individual questions should be nullified as necessary (Choice D).
Reference: Billings & Halstead (2020), p. 488

26. **A.** Revise the distractors.
Rationale: This item shows that 100% of learners answered correctly. None of the distractors were chosen by any learners. This is an easy item, and the point biserial remains 0.00 because

there is no ability to discriminate. Therefore Choice A is the correct response. This item shows it is easy and that it does not discriminate, so action should be taken before using it again (Choice B). The correct response likely does not need revision (Choice C). It is not necessary to nullify this item because learners were able to score well (Choice D).
Reference: Billings & Halstead (2020), pp. 489–490

27. B. "The KR-20 will help me predict exam validity."
Rationale: This test item is asking which statement is incorrect and, therefore, requires intervention. A KR-20 relates to the reliability of an exam. Validity assesses whether an exam has measured what was intended. Therefore Choice B is the answer to this item because it is an incorrect statement. The KR-20 can range from 0 to 1.00, but the acceptable level is 0.70 or above (Choices A and C). Reliability refers to measuring the internal consistency of an exam (Choice D).
Reference: Billings & Halstead (2020), pp. 486–487

28. D. This is a highly discriminating test item.
Rationale: This test item shows that 57% of learners answered correctly with a high point biserial. The high point biserial indicates that this item discriminates learners from nonlearners. Therefore Choice D is the correct response. The p value indicates how many learners got the item correct (Choice A). Validity is not measured in item statistics (Choice B). The high level of discrimination shown means that high-scoring learners answered correctly (Choice C).
Reference: Billings & Halstead (2020), pp. 489–490

29. B. Choice B
Rationale: All choices have an appropriate p level. The point biserial for Choice C indicates this is a discriminating item. However, Choice B shows that high-scoring learners chose that option. Therefore Choice B is the correct response to this question. Choices A, C, and D do not need revision, as they demonstrate discrimination between the learners and nonlearners. Only Choice B requires revision in the item.
Reference: Billings & Halstead (2020), pp. 489–490

30. D. Outcomes approach
Rationale: Evaluators who use the outcomes approach rely on goals, objectives, and outcomes to evaluate courses, lessons, and programs; therefore Choice D is correct. One who applies a service approach uses a values-based holistic perspective to identify strengths, weaknesses, and progress towards a goal when evaluating learner performance (Choice A). A constructivist focuses heavily on the value of stakeholders who will be affected by program graduates (Choice B). Evaluation from a judgment perspective reflects a focus on assigning a numeric or letter grade when evaluating learner performance (Choice C).
Reference: Billings & Halstead (2020), p. 439

31. C. Paper
Rationale: A written paper can evaluate learners' organizational skills, critical thinking, and learning in the affective domain; therefore Choice C is the correct answer. A checklist is used to evaluate learner performance of a clinical procedure (Choice A). A test question only evaluates learning in the cognitive level (Choice B). A questionnaire can be used to measure feelings and attitudes, but will not provide the opportunity for learners to articulate the differences in personal and professional values and responsibilities.
Reference: Billings & Halstead (2020), pp. 443, 462

32. A. Criterion-referenced test
Rationale: Criterion-referenced tests are used to evaluate mastery of content and are constructed according to specific learning outcomes; therefore Choice A is correct. A reflection journal is mostly used for formative assessment and would not be appropriate for summative mastery of

content (Choice B). Formative assessment evaluates learning as it is occurring, not mastery of content (Choice C). A norm-referenced test provides a ranking of each learner's performance among other learners, not mastery of content (Choice D).
Reference: Billings & Halstead (2020), pp. 475–476

33. D. Analyzing
Rationale: The question requires that the learner analyze the client's situation and decide which action to take first; therefore Choice D is correct. The action required by the learner requires more than remembering, understanding, and applying (Choices A, B, and C).
Reference: McDonald (2018), pp. 134–147

34. B. Formative assessment
Rationale: The educator wants to assess student learning as it is taking place in order to provide feedback or improvement; therefore Choice B is correct. Summative assessment is used to determine evaluation of learner performance and outcomes (Choice A). Criterion-referenced tests are used to determine mastery of subject matter (Choice C). Norm-referenced tests are used to provide a relative ranking of learners (Choice D).
Reference: Billings & Halstead (2020), pp. 450, 475–476

35. C. Summarize how to conduct a health history.
Rationale: Behavioral objectives written at the understanding level require learners to explain, interpret, or summarize understanding of a concept; therefore Choice C is correct. Choices A and D are written at the remembering (knowledge) level. Formulating a plan of care requires learners to create or develop something, which is a behavior at the creating level of the cognitive domain (Choice B).
Reference: Billings & Halstead (2020), pp. 188–189

36. D. It helps establish content-related validity.
Rationale: The test blueprint can provide evidence of content-related validity; therefore Choice D is correct. Interrater reliability refers to the ability of two different raters to obtain the same evaluation results (Choice A). Test blueprints do not assess readiness to learn (Choice B). The test statistics, not the blueprint, provide item discrimination information (Choice C).
Reference: Billings & Halstead (2020), pp. 486–487

37. D. "I will have learners develop a concept map so that I can evaluate the psychomotor domain."
Rationale: Concept mapping can be used to evaluate the cognitive and affective domains, but cannot be used to evaluate psychomotor learning; therefore Choice D is the answer to this item because it is an incorrect statement. Reflection journals are used for the affective domain (Choice A). Test questions in the high-level cognitive domain can be used to assess critical thinking (Choice B). Checklists can be used to evaluate learners' performance of clinical procedures, which are part of the psychomotor domain (Choice C).
Reference: Billings & Halstead (2020), pp. 457–458

38. C. Ask learners to perform insertion on a simulation mannequin.
Rationale: The objective requires learners to "demonstrate" a technique. Having learners perform the psychomotor skill of insertion on a mannequin would be most appropriate; therefore Choice C is correct. Giving a quiz would evaluate the cognitive domain (Choice A). Group discussions would not allow the instructor to evaluate proper technique (Choice B). An essay can be used to evaluate cognitive and affective domains, but not psychomotor (Choice D).
Reference: Billings & Halstead (2020), pp. 457–458

39. A. Grading rubric
Rationale: Grading rubrics help facilitate interrater reliability of evaluations among multiple raters; therefore Choice A is correct. A Likert scale would not be appropriate for grading a paper

(Choice B). Test blueprints are used for exams, not scholarly papers (Choice C). Peer evaluations would not be appropriate for assigning grades to scholarly papers (Choice D).
Reference: Billings & Halstead (2020), p. 500

40. B. Achievement of learning outcomes at the end of the semester
Rationale: Evaluation of all the learning at the conclusion of the semester would be an example of summative evaluation; therefore Choice B is correct. Evaluation at midterm would not include all the learning objectives for the semester (Choice A). Learner evaluations of the clinical site are important, but are not an example of summative evaluation (C). Evaluation of learning after a lesson is an example of formative assessment (Choice D).
Reference: Billings & Halstead (2020), p. 438

41. C. Provide a quiz that includes factors that can alter mobility.
Rationale: The objective is written at the knowledge (remembering) level of the cognitive domain; therefore a quiz would be appropriate for assessing this objective (Choice C). Having learners demonstrate the use of canes and walkers does not effectively assess their understanding of factors that affect mobility (Choice A). Creation of a care plan assesses learning at a much higher cognitive level and would not be appropriate for this objective (Choice B). Learner performance of range of motion would be a psychomotor assessment, not cognitive (Choice D).
Reference: Billings & Halstead (2020), pp. 456–460

42. A. Calculate the proper dose of acetaminophen for a pediatric patient.
Rationale: Having a learner perform a dosage calculation requires applying previous knowledge to solve a problem; therefore Choice A is correct. Matching, identifying, and listing information are all at the knowledge (remembering) level of the cognitive domain (Choices B, C, and D).
Reference: Billings & Halstead (2020), pp. 456–460

43. D. "I will develop a test blueprint after writing the test questions and provide it to the students."
Rationale: The test blueprint should be used to guide the development of test questions, not be created after the test is written; therefore Choice D is the correct response for this question because it is an incorrect statement. Blueprints are used to make sure the content objectives are being tested (Choice A). Having plausible distractors and using action verbs consistent with the cognitive process are both hallmarks of writing effective test questions (Choices B and C).
Reference: Billings & Halstead (2020), pp. 478–479

44. B. Have learners maintain a comprehensive portfolio of assignments throughout the program.
Rationale: Because portfolios are a collection of learners' works, they can be used to evaluate all three domains of learning, achievement in individual courses, or as an outcome measure of a program; therefore Choice B is correct. A comprehensive final exam and a high-stakes exam will only measure cognitive learning and are not appropriate for evaluation of program outcomes (Choices A and C). A self-reflection paper will not adequately demonstrate achievement of all program outcomes (Choice D).
Reference: Billings & Halstead (2020), pp. 456–460

45. C. Policies must be ethically sound and based on current evidence.
Rationale: Admission policies should be fair, ethical, and evidence-based; therefore Choice C is correct. Learners are allowed a pathway for filing grade grievances, so Choice A is incorrect. Changes in health care delivery may influence policy decisions, but they are not the only reason for modifications (Choice B). Formative assessments are used to provide feedback to learners about their performance (Choice D).
Reference: Billings & Halstead (2020), pp. 532–535

46. A. To ensure that students receive an education that prepares them to be competent in practice

Rationale: Knowledge of current clinical and educational research is necessary for educators when preparing students to meet the needs of clients in practice; therefore Choice A is correct. All educators are expected to incorporate evidence-based practices and teaching regardless of promotion and tenure requirements (Choice B). Evidence-based teaching practices are necessary for both the classroom and clinical (Choice C). The faculty, not individual educators, are expected to collectively maintain expertise in all methods of assessment and evaluation; therefore Choice D is incorrect.

Reference: Halstead (2019), pp. 68–69

47. C. Student learning outcomes

Rationale: Evaluation techniques should be chosen based on the learning outcomes they are intended to evaluate; therefore Choice C is correct. Certification examination pass rates should not influence the evaluation strategies chosen for an individual course; therefore Choice A is incorrect. Trends in health care would not be an influential factor in the type of evaluation strategy chosen for a course (Choice B). The learning outcomes, not individual learning styles, will primarily influence the evaluation method chosen by the educator (Choice D).

Reference: Billings & Halstead (2020), pp. 450–451

48. D. As a formative assessment of student learning

Rationale: Classroom assessment techniques (CATs) are quick, formative evaluations used to assess student learning; therefore Choice D is correct. CATs are not used as a form of summative assessment (Choice A). They cannot be used to determine final course grades (Choice B). Because they are formative in nature, they cannot be used as an alternative to a comprehensive final examination (Choice C).

Reference: Cannon & Boswell (2016), pp. 164–165

49. C. Focus on evaluation of learners using a pass/fail approach.

Rationale: Evaluation from a judgment perspective focuses on assigning grades or a pass/fail approach; therefore Choice C is correct. An outcomes approach to evaluation involves relying on goals and objectives (Choice A). Those who use the service approach to evaluation emphasize the student learning process and identification of strengths and weaknesses (Choice B). Using peer evaluations is not an element of the judgment perspective of evaluation (Choice D).

Reference: Billings & Halstead (2020), p. 439

50. B. The learners were able to guess the correct answer.

Rationale: In this sample item, two of the distractors were not picked by any learners. When a distractor does not function, it increases the odds that a learner could guess to get the correct answer. Therefore Choice B is the correct response. This item is unacceptable because not all distractors were chosen (Choice A). Choices A and B in the sample item need revision to be more plausible as distractors (Choice C). Although this item does show an acceptable level of discrimination, Choice C is also positive, indicating that learners who scored well also chose that item. Overall, the item requires revision (Choice D).

Reference: Billings & Halstead (2020), pp. 489–490

51. A. Learners who scored lower on the exam got this test item correct.

Rationale: This item shows an appropriate p level above 0.50. The point biserial for this item is negative, indicating that lower-scoring learners got this item correct. Therefore Choice A is the correct response. All distractors were chosen, meaning that it is not likely that learners were guessing (Choice B). This item does not show a high level of discrimination because nonlearners were able to answer correctly (Choice C). Validity cannot be inferred from these statistics (Choice D).

Reference: Billings & Halstead (2020), pp. 489–490

52. C. Nullify this test item.

Rationale: The p value for this item is below the acceptable range. The point biserial for this item is negative, indicating that those who scored lower on the exam got this item correct. It is appropriate to nullify this item based on the statistics. Therefore Choice C is the correct response. This item is not appropriate based on the statistics for the correct response and because no learners chose distractor Choice B (Choice A). Accepting multiple choices is not appropriate in this situation because this item shows poor discrimination (Choice B). It is not appropriate to change a correct response after a test has been administered (Choice D).

Reference: Billings & Halstead (2020), pp. 389–490

53. D. "You should keep data to compare over time to enhance the teaching and learning process."

Rationale: Assessment and evaluation data in a course should be tracked over time by the nurse educator. Comparing norms and interpreting data can help the educator make improvements moving forward and better understand the teaching-learning process. Therefore Choice D is the correct response. Keeping data is necessary to make improvements and track trends (Choice A). Data do not necessarily need to be submitted to the university unless specified by a certain type of course in a curriculum (Choice B). Nursing programs should have policies regarding the length of time to keep data; however, the nurse educator should understand the importance of keeping data for improvements is separate from any policies on data retention (Choice C).

Reference: Billings & Halstead (2020), pp. 446–447

54. B. Consult with a clinical expert in the area being tested.

Rationale: It is important to assess validity in multiple ways. Gaining expert help can help validate what is being tested compared with what knowledge is needed in clinical practice. Therefore Choice B is the correct response. Academic affairs is not a unit that is an expert on nursing content, nor are faculty who are outside of nursing (Choices A and C). Consulting with learners after the exam is a poor method to establish validity, as the educator guides the learners through the objectives and the content that is tested (Choice D).

Reference: Billings & Halstead (2020), pp. 486–487

55. D. Testing, administration, and evaluation information must be available for learners.

Rationale: Standardized testing products must have information available for educators regarding the actual tests, how to administer, and evaluation information. Therefore Choice D is the correct response. Policies must be created based on the data available to ensure fair and consistent use among learners. Cost is a consideration but not the most important one (Choice A). Personal preferences should not play a role; choices should be learner-centered to be a supplement and should not replace the teaching-learning expertise of the nurse educator (Choices B and C).

Reference: National League for Nursing (2020), www.nln.org/fairtestingguidelines

56. A. "It is important to provide clear evaluation data early so that learners know how to achieve the objectives."

Rationale: Learners must be aware of what they are being evaluated on in order to meet the objectives of the assessment. Grades are often tied to assessment and rubrics; learners need the opportunity to know in advance what is required of them. Therefore Choice A is the correct response. Learners do need access to rubrics in order to ensure fair, equitable grading (Choice B). A 1-week lead time is often not enough time to grade papers. The length of the assessment and time required to complete it should be considered when determining the timing of providing a rubric (Choice C). Evaluation data should be provided to all learners at the same time; therefore Choice D is not correct.

Reference: Cannon & Boswell (2016), p. 159

Chapter 5

1. **C.** Defines expectations for graduates broadly and in general terms
Rationale: Choice C is the correct response because program learning outcomes (PLOs), also known as *end-of-program learning outcomes,* are broad statements that stand the test of time, reflect the organizing framework for the program, and define expectations for graduates. Choice A describes a course outcome, Choice B describes a course objective, and Choice D is a false statement unrelated to curricular outcomes.
Reference: Billings &Halstead (2020), pp. 122–130

2. **B.** Formulate safe and effective clinical judgements guided by the nursing process, clinical reasoning, and evidence-based practice.
Rationale: Choice B is the correct response because program learning outcomes are broad statements that stand the test of time, reflect the conceptual framework for the program, and define specific expectations for graduates. Choices A and D could be course outcomes, and Choice C is a course objective because it is the most specific outcome among all of the options.
Reference: Billings & Halstead (2020), pp. 122–130

3. **C.** 80% of graduates will pass the family nurse practitioner certification examination on their first attempt.
Rationale: Program outcomes are measured *after* graduation to determine program effectiveness. Choice C is the correct answer because family nurse practitioner students have to pass the national certification examination after graduation to practice. Choice A is not measurable and would not be a reasonable outcome. Following graduates for 6 to 12 months after graduation to determine whether they are employed is a nursing accreditation requirement—not within 3 months after graduation (Choice B). Choice D is an outcome to be measured *before* graduation and would not be appropriate as a program outcome.
Reference: Ignatavicius (2019), pp. 10–12

4. **A.** Formulate a plan of care that promotes health and safety of the pediatric patient.
Rationale: Choice A is the correct answer because the word *formulate* is a high-level revised Bloom's taxonomy verb at the creating cognitive level, which would be appropriate for a senior-level student. Choice B is at the level of understanding. Choice C is at the applying level, and Choice D asks the learner to use a plan to determine effectiveness, which is at the analyzing level.
Reference: Billings & Halstead (2020), pp. 188–189

5. **C.** "The curriculum committee selects and assigns all course outcomes for the curriculum."
Rationale: Choice C is the correct answer and would require further intervention because nursing faculty own the curriculum, and all faculty should be involved in the selection of course outcomes. Choices A, B, and D are all correct regarding course outcomes and would not require follow-up by the mentor.
Reference: Billings & Halstead (2020), p. 110

6. **D.** Foundations' skills laboratory
Rationale: Choice D is the correct answer because, to meet this objective, the learning environment needs to allow students the opportunity to demonstrate the skill at the desired level. Therefore the foundations' skills laboratory is the best learning environment to introduce and meet this objective. Choice B does not provide an adequate setting for demonstrating a skill. Choices A and C are inappropriate settings for introducing this skill because learners should be competent in this skill before entering these clinical settings.
Reference: Billings & Halstead (2020), p. 126

7. **C.** Summarize an example of two quality initiatives that influenced nursing practice.
Rationale: All of the options in this item are examples of SMART course objectives because they are specific, measurable, achievable, relevant, and timely. However, Choices A, B, and D are performance objectives and not within the cognitive learning domain. Therefore Choice C is the correct response. *Summarize* is a verb commonly used for the understanding level of the revised Bloom's cognitive taxonomy.
Reference: University of Buffalo (n.d.), http://www.buffalo.edu/ubcei/enhance/designing/learning-outcomes/high-quality-learning-outcomes.html

8. **A.** "I will need to adjust these course objectives to align with my learning activities."
Rationale: Choice A would likely require follow-up by the nurse educator mentor because a change in course objectives (and likely content) could leave a curricular gap. When choosing learning activities, faculty need to consider how these activities align with learning outcomes. Learning activities should support outcomes—outcomes should not be changed to support learning activities. Choices B, C, and D are appropriate interventions for selecting learning activities. Learning activities should be appropriately leveled, active, help learners achieve course objectives, and fit within the context of the course.
Reference: Billings & Halstead (2020), pp. 184–185

9. **D.** Advance knowledge in health assessment and communication skills.
Rationale: Choice D is the correct answer and would require follow-up by the mentor because this objective is not measurable or specific. Choices A, B, and C are all specific, measurable, achievable, relevant, and timely.
Reference: University of Buffalo (n.d.), http://www.buffalo.edu/ubcei/enhance/designing/learning-outcomes/high-quality-learning-outcomes.html

10. **B.** Journal assignment
Rationale: Choice B is the correct response because journaling is an effective method for helping learners detail personal experiences in the clinical setting and connect them to learning outcomes. The learners' experiences related to ethical considerations represent learning in the affective domain. Choice A is for demonstrating kinesthetic skills, Choice C is a passive activity and does not lend itself to discussion, and Choice D is an evaluative method, not a learning activity.
Reference: Billings & Halstead (2020), p. 299

11. **D.** Technology activity supports course objective
Rationale: Choice D is the most important consideration for selecting any learning activity; faculty must consider how learning activities and technology align with course objectives. Choices A, B, and C are also relevant logistical factors, but they are not as essential as Choice D when planning technological learning activities.
Reference: Billings & Halstead (2020), p. 184

12. **C.** Experience supports course outcome
Rationale: Choice C is the most important and the correct response because the purpose of clinical experiences is to provide learners with an opportunity to meet course outcomes and objectives. Choices A, B, and D include considerations that the educator keeps in mind while selecting clinical experiences, but they are not as important as Choice C.
Reference: Billings & Halstead (2020), p. 333

13. **D.** Medical/surgical unit
Rationale: Choice D is the correct response because this setting is most appropriate for learners to care for older adult patients with chronic health problems. Faculty must consider how clinical experiences align with course outcomes and objectives. Choices A and C are

critical care areas for patients with emergent and acute complex health problems. Choice B does not provide experiences for learners to work with older adults.
Reference: Billings & Halstead (2020), p. 333

14. A. Alignment of clinical experience with course outcomes
Rationale: Choice A is the correct answer because it is the most important information for learners to understand regarding clinical experiences. Faculty must communicate to learners the relationship between clinical experiences and course outcomes. Choices B, C, and D are also important logistics related to ensuring that learners are prepared for their clinical experience, but these factors are not as important as Choice A to communicate.
Reference: Billings & Halstead (2020), p. 334

15. B. Scholarly paper
Rationale: Choice B is correct because the objective represents learning in the cognitive domain. Cognitive learning can be measured through a written assignment. Choice A is not an appropriate evaluative method for cognitive learning. Choices C and D are cognitive evaluative methods but do not allow the learner the opportunity to examine or explore content.
Reference: Oermann & Gaberson (2021), p. 162

16. A. Cognitive
Rationale: Choice A is correct. Written assignments evaluate learning in the cognitive domain, and concept maps are objective written assignments. Choice B is not a learning domain. Learning in the psychomotor domain (Choice C) is measured by direct observation. Learning in the affective domain (Choice D) can be measured by journaling or another reflective evaluative method.
Reference: Billings & Halstead (2020), p. 453

17. B. Describes the purpose of the program in preparing nursing graduates
Rationale: Choice B is the correct answer; the mission statement describes the purpose for the program. Choice A is the definition for a philosophy statement, Choice C defines a vision statement, and Choice D focuses on values for the program.
Reference: Ignatavicius (2019), p. 9

18. A. "I need to review the nursing program's philosophy statements so that I am familiar with the definition of scholarship for this university."
Rationale: Choice A is the correct response because it is the *institutional philosophy statement* that would provide the definition of scholarship for faculty. Therefore this statement would require follow-up by the mentor. Choices B, C, and D are all correct statements about program philosophy statements.
Reference: DeBoor (2023), pp. 93–94

19. D. Faculty beliefs regarding adult learning theory
Rationale: Choice D is the correct response because the nursing program philosophy statement should include faculty beliefs regarding adult learning supported by educational theory. Choices A, B, and C are not components of or sources of evidence for a program philosophy.
Reference: Ignatavicius (2019), p. 9

20. B. It helps to prepare graduates for what they may face as new nurses.
Rationale: Choice B is the correct answer because review of nursing trends helps programs be accountable to adequately prepare graduates for today's practice settings. Choice A is incorrect because these topics need to be included into nursing curricula. Although the curriculum may inform the nursing handbook, it is not the purpose for including content on incivility and violence; therefore Choice C is incorrect. Including incivility and violence in nursing does not promote empathy and understanding for nursing colleagues (Choice D).
Reference: Billings & Halstead (2020), p. 84

21. **D.** "Our faculty will need to develop curriculum that has a local focus because learners are not likely to practice outside our area."

Rationale: Choice D would require follow-up by the faculty mentor because national and global health issues should be incorporated into nursing curriculum. Choices A, B, and C are all important to incorporate into a nursing curriculum (technology for health care, interprofessional collaboration, and community health priorities).

Reference: Billings & Halstead (2020), p. 89

22. **C.** "We should examine QSEN Safety Standards to make sure our curriculum incorporates them."

Rationale: Choice C would require follow-up by the faculty mentor because QSEN is not a community priority, which is what this test item is assessing. Choices A, B, and C are all community health-related issues that would be relevant to research (infant mortality, chronic health conditions, crime rates, and violence) for designing a new curriculum.

Reference: DeBoor (2023), p. 97

23. **D.** Write a research paper discussing access to health care in the United States.

Rationale: Choice D is the correct answer because access to health care is a social determinant that examines the issue from a national perspective. Choice A is a health care–related trend; Choices B and C are both community health–related issues.

Reference: U.S. Department of Health and Human Services (USDHHS). (n.d.), https://www.healthypeople.gov/2020/topics- objectives/topic/social-determinants-of-health

24. **A.** Concept-based curriculum

Rationale: Choice A is the correct answer. A curriculum based on key concepts and exemplars is a concept-based model, and students engage in conceptual learning. Choices B and C are other curricular models; Choice D is an educational learning theory.

Reference: Ignatavicius (2019), p. 26

25. **A.** "Concept-based curricular models often overload learners with content."

Rationale: Choice A would require intervention by the faculty mentor because concept-based curricula are designed to prevent content overload. The other three options are all correct statements (Choices B, C, and D).

Reference: Ignatavicius (2019), p. 28

26. **B.** Scope of practice for the state

Rationale: Choice B is the correct answer. State boards of nursing in the United States provide regulations for nursing programs and the scope of nursing practice at varying levels, which can help guide nursing curricular design. Choices A, B, and C are all important nursing standards but do not provide regulatory guidance.

Reference: Ignatavicius (2019), p. 5

27. **C.** Experiential learning theory

Rationale: Choice C is the correct response because simulation with debriefing is an example of experiential learning theory in which students have hands-on learning experiences with reflection on their learning. Simulation is valued by learners and can help them translate knowledge into realistic practice. Choices A, B, and D are appropriate educational theories applied by faculty in curriculum and instruction but are not the main theories used in simulated learning experiences.

Reference: Billings & Halstead (2020), p. 253

28. **B.** Narrative pedagogy

Rationale: Choice B is the correct answer. Journaling is an example of narrative pedagogy in which learning experiences are focused on using dialogue to help students process and gain

knowledge from experiences. This written assignment is not consistent with experiential learning ("hands-on" learning) and constructivism (building on previous knowledge or experience) (Choices C and D). Adult learning theory is a broad-based theory that focuses on adult motivation to learn and goal orientation (Choice A).
Reference: Billings & Halstead (2020), p. 253

29. **C.** Segments of lecture are interspersed with application activities.
Rationale: Choice C is the correct answer; a scrambled classroom is an active learning environment in which small segments of lecture are interspersed with active learning application activities. Therefore Choice A that refers to passive learning is not the correct definition. Although group activities may be used in a scrambled classroom, group learning is not required (Choices B and D).
Reference: Ignatavicius (2019), p. 80

30. **D.** Documentation assignment in a simulated electronic health record (EHR)
Rationale: Choice D is the correct response. Simulating actual documentation with an EHR provides learners an authentic care situation. Nursing education must incorporate health care technology to stay current with practice demands. Choices A, B, and C all focus on allowing learners to practice or reflect on nursing care, but Choice D actually simulates a realistic technology that represents actual nursing and health care practice.
Reference: Billings & Halstead (2020), p. 253

31. **B.** "I would like to customize my course LMS so that it stands out from other program courses."
Rationale: Choice B is the correct answer and would require follow-up by the faculty mentor. The LMS provides organization for the course, and a consistent look across courses helps students' familiarity with the program learning environment. All other options are correct statements about an LMS (Choices A, C, and D).
Reference: Iwasiw et al. (2020), p. 497

32. **C.** Participating in care of a simulated, laboring patient using a high-fidelity obstetric mannequin
Rationale: Choice C is the correct answer. High-fidelity simulated clinical care experiences are an evidence-based method for providing students with "hands-on" clinical learning experiences that are more realistic than additional didactic content (Choice A), skills lab practice with a mid-fidelity mannequin (Choice B), or a concept map (Choice D).
Reference: Billings & Halstead (2020), p. 353

33. **B.** Task trainer for IV insertion
Rationale: Choice B is the correct answer. Task trainers for IV insertion are low-fidelity simulation technology. Choice A is mid-fidelity, and Choices C and D are high-fidelity learning experiences.
Reference: Billings & Halstead (2020), p. 354

34. **A.** National nursing education consultant
Rationale: Choice A is the correct answer. Although consultants should not develop a nursing curriculum because that is the faculty's role, a national consultant in nursing education can be an appropriate leader to facilitate curricular design. Newly hired educators do not have enough knowledge or experience to lead curriculum redesign (Choice B). The entire faculty cannot lead the curricular change but should participate in the process (Choice D). The vice president of academic affairs, who is typically not a nurse, is not qualified to lead a curriculum redesign (Choice C).
Reference: Billings & Halstead (2020), p. 130

35. B. Faculty who do not have experience or educational background in curriculum development
Rationale: Choice B is the correct answer. The major barrier in planning curricular design that must be considered by the leader is that many faculty do not have experience or educational background in curricular development. Faculty may have preferences for what they want to teach, but that is more easily resolved (Choice A). A reduction in the number of faculty needed for a new or revised curriculum is not likely (Choice C). Learners are often excited that the curriculum is changing or being redesigned and are therefore not resistant to the process or result of the change (Choice D).
Reference: Billings & Halstead (2020), p. 131

36. B. Assign them an experienced mentor during the design process
Rationale: Choice B is the correct response. The curriculum design leader should assign a novice nurse educator to a mentor to develop knowledge and understanding of curriculum design. Mentorship is more effective than a conference or curriculum textbook, although these resources can be very valuable to provide knowledge about curriculum design (Choices C and D). Assigning the new educator to develop a course without the needed knowledge and experience is not a reasonable choice (Choice A).
Reference: Billings & Halsted (2020), pp. 7–8

37. C. Lesson plans
Rationale: Choice C is the correct answer. Course design begins with program learning outcomes (PLOs) that should be aligned with course outcomes. The lesson plans consist of course objectives, learning activities, and assessment of learning methods. The development of calendars, course outcomes, and course objectives happens before development of lesson plans (Choices A, B, and D).
Reference: Billings & Halstead (2020), p. 182

38. A. Learning activities must align with course objectives.
Rationale: Choice A is the correct answer because it is essential that learning activities align with course objectives and outcomes. All of the other statements are true, but if the activity does not align with course objectives, it is an irrelevant activity for the course (Choices B, C, and D).
Reference: Billings & Halstead (2020), p. 185

39. D. "When designing a new course, I will need to examine my own educational philosophy."
Rationale: Choice D, the correct response, would require follow-up by the faculty mentor. One's personal educational philosophy is not a consideration when designing a curriculum. All other statements are true regarding curricular design (Choices A, B, and C).
Reference: Billings & Halstead (2020), p. 182

40. A. Selecting a change model for the revision process
Rationale: Choice A is the correct response because selecting a change theory would be the *most* important intervention before making curricular changes so that the process of change can be successfully facilitated. Choice B is important to identify champions that can support the change during the curriculum process, but it is not the most important factor. The other two, Choices C and D, occur after curricular revisions have been made.
Reference: Iwasiw et al. (2020), p. 48

41. C. Many faculty members are inexperienced with curriculum design.
Rationale: Choice C is the correct answer because inexperienced faculty is a major common barrier that the nurse leader must expect and mitigate. Choices A, B, and D are not barriers *to* curricular revision, but they may occur *as a result of* curricular revision.
Reference: Billings & Halstead (2020), p. 156

42. **D.** "While teaching out the old curriculum, we will need to make sure that all current learners are able to join the new curriculum if desired."

Rationale: Choice D is the correct answer. Learners would remain in the current "old" curriculum that is being phased out as per the school's student handbook and catalog with which they were admitted. They would not transfer to the new curriculum if they desired to do so. Choices A, B, and C are all correct statements.

Reference: Billings & Halstead (2020), p. 158

43. **A.** Graduates will complete the nursing program within 150% of the degree plan time frame.

Rationale: Choice A is the correct response because monitoring program completion rates helps demonstrate the program's effectiveness. Tracking program completion rate is an example of a program outcome (PO) that is measured after graduation. The other three options are examples of expected results to measure whether learners have met program learning outcomes (PLOs) before graduation (Choices B, C, and D).

Reference: Ignatavicius (2019), p. 10

44. **B.** Review program learning outcomes to determine whether updates are needed.

Rationale: Choice B is the correct answer. Any major changes to the AACN's *Essentials* document should prompt a review of program learning outcomes to determine whether a revision is needed to maintain alignment. The other three options (Choices A, C, and D) are not affected by changes in the AACN's *Essentials* document.

Reference: DeBoor (2023), pp. 145–146

45. **A.** Course outcomes

Rationale: Choice A is the correct answer. Any revision of the program learning outcomes will likely result in changes needed in competency statements, including course outcomes and objectives. The other three options (Choices B, C, and D) would occur after curricular revisions have been developed.

Reference: Billings & Halstead (2020), p. 125

46. **D.** Inviting student representatives to attend faculty meetings

Rationale: Option D is the correct response because it is the best way to actively involve learners in the process of curriculum revision. Inviting learner representatives to attend faculty meetings provides an avenue to keep learners informed such that they feel supported and aware of the changes being implemented. The other three options (Choices A, B, and C) may provide some supportive information, but they are passive and do not actively engage learners.

Reference: Iwasiw et al. (2020), p. 394

47. **B.** Direct observation

Rationale: Choice B is the correct response. The objective is assessing learning in the psychomotor domain because the action verb in the statement is *perform*. Skill performance is a kinesthetic activity, which is best measured through direct observation. Choices A, C, and D are evaluative methods to assess learning in the cognitive domain.

Reference: Billings & Halstead (2020), p. 333

48. **A.** "We are so excited for you to begin our new curriculum; you will be our test group for determining how successful the program will be."

Rationale: Choice A is the correct answer and requires follow-up by the faculty mentor. Learners in the new curriculum should not be referred to as "a test group" because this negative statement does not instill confidence or provide reassurance regarding the new curriculum. Choices B, C, and D are all statements that are positive and encouraging to learners regarding the new curriculum and should be followed through during curriculum implementation.

Reference: Iwasiw et al. (2020), p. 394

49. A. Use of simulated electronic health record
Rationale: Choice A is the correct answer. Nursing education must incorporate skills and competencies related to health care technology into the curriculum to meet the needs of current practice. Faculty beliefs, social media topics, and learner demographics/culture preferences are not evidence-based sources for ensuring currency of curriculum (Choices B, C, and D).
Reference: Billings & Halstead (2020), p. 88

50. B. Global health
Rationale: Choice B is the correct answer. Global health focuses on protecting the world population against health threats and delivery of health care services worldwide. The COVID-19 pandemic is not an example of demographics, environmental challenge, or natural disaster (Choices A, C, and D).
Reference: Billings & Halstead (2020), p. 89

51. A. Personal devices can be used in class to simulate what will be expected in practice.
Rationale: Choice A is the best answer. Use of personal devices can provide learners the opportunity to apply course content in a real-world setting. Depending on what app is used, personal devices may also help with knowledge acquisition or retention, but they do not promote better understanding of the knowledge (Choice D). Choice C is not a true statement. Choice B would indicate that learners have access to assignments and exams, which would not be appropriate.
Reference: Billings & Halstead (2020), p. 381

52. D. Area clinical preceptors
Rationale: Choice D is the correct answer because clinical preceptors are the only external stakeholders among the choices. All the other choices are internal stakeholders (Choices A, B, and C). External stakeholders' knowledge and experience can contribute greatly to a creation or revision of a curriculum.
Reference: Iwasiw et al. (2020), p. 133

53. A. Education specialist with the state board of nursing
Rationale: Option A is the correct answer. Nursing board representatives are external stakeholders who advise on the legal scope of nursing practice in a state and determine whether nursing education programs meet established criteria. Choices B and D are internal stakeholders. Nursing accrediting bodies review programs to determine compliance with national standards, not state standards or scope of practice (Choice C).
Reference: Billings & Halstead (2020), p. 148

54. C. Reviewing the current state of the curriculum
Rationale: Choice C is the correct answer. The process of curricular revision may include a consultant employed to lead the revision process, which usually begins with a review of the current curriculum. Faculty are responsible for the design of the curriculum and would be responsible for Choices A, B, and D.
Reference: Billings & Halstead (2020), p. 130

55. A. Some faculty may have a lack of confidence in the new curriculum.
Rationale: Choice A is the correct answer. Faculty may not have confidence or buy-in with the new curriculum. It is very important to be prepared for this issue so it can be addressed early. Clinical sites are not typically resistant to curricular changes (Choice B). Faculty will need assistance with buy-in because some educators may be resistant to curricular change (Choices C and D).
Reference: Iwasiw et al. (2020), p. 17

56. D. The entire faculty must be fully informed of all key curricular elements.

Rationale: Option D is the correct answer because faculty need to be fully informed and supportive of all key elements of the new curriculum and how each part fits together. Although the other three statements are true, it is more important for the faculty to be fully familiar with all components of the curriculum (Choices A, B, and C).

Reference: DeBoor (2023), p. 38

57. C. Part-time faculty should be aware of how their course fits with the curriculum.

Rationale: Choice C is the correct answer; part-time faculty should be aware of how their course fits with the curriculum and program learning outcomes (PLOs). However, it is not necessary or as important for part-time faculty to understand all the details of the curriculum (Choices A, B, and D).

Reference: DeBoor (2023), pp. 104–105

58. D. Students learn expectations of the practice environment.

Rationale: Choice D is the correct answer because learning in the clinical area orients learners to the norms of current nursing and health care practice. The classroom is not a clinical learning environment (Choice B). The laboratory is an ideal setting to learn skills, but skill performance is only a small part of clinical learning. Therefore Choices A and C are not correct.

Reference: Billings & Halstead (2020), p. 328

59. B. Interprofessional collaboration

Rationale: Students need to learn all of these skills and the knowledge needed to become a professional nurse. However, Choice B is the correct answer because participating in interprofessional collaboration in a clinical agency is a *priority* for today's practice arena. The other options (Choices A, C, and D) can be practiced in a skills lab setting.

Reference: Billings & Halstead (2020), p. 335

60. A. "Students need to be in the hospital setting for clinical experiences to learn how to provide patient care."

Rationale: Choice A is the correct response that requires follow-up by the mentor. Students can learn how to provide patient care in a variety of clinical settings, not just hospital settings. Clinical experiences in the community setting are highly valuable for learners in addition to the acute care setting (Choices B, C, and D).

Reference: Billings & Halstead (2020), p. 329

61. B. Mid-program standardized exam scores

Rationale: Choice B is the correct answer because formative evaluations occur during a course to provide learners with feedback on their progress. Formative evaluation allows learners to improve on any areas that are identified by the tool, such as a mid-program exam. Choices A, C, and D all are summative evaluation methods used at the end of the course or program.

Reference: Billings & Halstead (2020), pp. 191–192

62. A. Progress toward tenure

Rationale: Choice A is the correct answer. In most universities and colleges, faculty progress toward tenure is prescribed by the institution and can be used as a faculty outcome for program assessment. Choice B is determined by state boards of nursing and nursing accrediting bodies, although institutions may also require specific credentials for employment. Choice C is not a program assessment measurement, and Choice D is a measurement for learners.

Reference: Billings & Halstead (2020), p. 335

63. A. Scores on standardized exit exam

Rationale: Choice A is the correct answer. Standardized exit exam scores are a direct measure of performance for assessing the ability of students to meet program learning outcomes. Choices B,

C, and D are all indirect methods of measurement because they are opinions rather than actual learner performance methods.
Reference: Ignatavicius (2019), p. 238

64. D. Ensure quality improvement and adherence to accreditation standards

Rationale: Choice D is the correct answer. The purpose of program assessment is to ensure a quality improvement process while demonstrating adherence to accreditation outcome standards. The program assessment plan guides the faculty in ongoing systematic evaluation. Part of program assessment may include determining learner satisfaction, but that is not the purpose of a program assessment plan (Choice A). Regulations for faculty workload are determined by the state board of nursing and are not the purpose of program assessment (Choice B). Although the assessment plan must be consistent with state guidelines and documents assessment activities for accrediting bodies, that is not the purpose for the program assessment plan (Choice C).
Reference: Ignatavicius (2019), p. 238

65. A. Review of program historical data

Rationale: Choice A is the correct answer because it is important to set benchmarks for the nursing program that are reasonable and based on factors such as past performance and data. Textbooks, similar programs, and faculty recommendations are not sound evidence for developing expected outcomes as part of program assessment (Choices B, C, and D).
Reference: Oermann (2017), p. 49

66. B. Advisory committee members

Rationale: Option B is the correct answer. Advisory committees are external stakeholders who provide input about the changing needs of the marketplace for incorporation into the program assessment plan, also known as the systematic plan for evaluation of the program. Institutional administration and nursing program faculty are internal stakeholders (Choices A and C). Although area program directors are external stakeholders, they would not be able to provide data that are directly relevant for the program (Choice D).
Reference: Billings & Halstead (2020), p. 552

67. D. "Accreditors are only concerned with the data collected."

Rationale: Choice D is the correct answer because this statement needs follow-up by the faculty mentor. Accreditors are not only concerned with data that are collected but also are concerned with the plan of action and progress toward completion of those actions. All of the other statements are true because all faculty participate in program assessment, program assessment can identify problems with the curriculum, and the process is often led by a program assessment committee (Choices A, B, and C).
Reference: Billings & Halstead (2020), p. 557

68. A. The SPE may need to be adjusted to measure IPC or provide an action plan for improvement.

Rationale: Choice A is the correct answer. As faculty and other stakeholders use the plan, they should identify areas in which the benchmarks or criteria need to be changed. Feedback from an advisory committee on performance of graduates provides important data that may require an adjustment in a plan of action for improvement. It should affect the SPE and be addressed when concerns arise rather than at the next meeting (Choices B and C). Data collected from both internal and external stakeholders are essential, and data are shared, not confidential (Choice D).
Reference: Oermann (2017), p. 56

69. C. Accreditation standard for program completion

Rationale: Option C is the correct answer. As accreditation standards change, the program assessment plan may need revision. Nursing accreditation standards currently specify program

completion rate calculations. Learner demographics, admission requirements, and faculty load are not typically part of the program assessment plan (Choices A, B, and D).
Reference: Oermann (2017), p. 56

70. **A.** Clinical partners
Rationale: Choice A is the correct answer because clinical partners can offer valuable information about current nursing and health care practice that would help guide curriculum design. Although area nursing program directors would be able to share information about relevant nursing practice, they may not be current and do not work in the program where the curriculum is being designed (Choice B). Institutional administration and general education faculty are typically not nurses and would not be able to provide useful information about nursing and health care practice (Choices C and D).
Reference: Billings & Halstead (2020), p. 123

71. **D.** Incidence of coronary artery disease in the county
Rationale: Choice D is the correct answer and is an example of a local health care trend. Health issues related to the communities where people live and work must be addressed to prepare nurses for providing care. Choices A, B, and C do not provide local health information.
Reference: Billings & Halstead (2020), p. 84

72. **A.** Participation in clinical learning
Rationale: Choice A is the correct answer. Adult learning theory espouses that students are able to apply learning to real-world problem-solving and where learning is relevant. Choices B and D involve active learner discussion but do not have "real-world" experience opportunity. For Choice C, the learners observe a skill demonstration by the instructor rather than practice the skill themselves.
Reference: Billings & Halstead (2020), p. 253

73. **B.** "I will include extra content on cardiac heart rhythms due to my extensive clinical experience in this area."
Rationale: Curriculum development requires faculty to design curriculum that extends beyond their preferences and experience. Therefore wanting to include content that matches the novice educator's expertise and does not match course outcomes requires follow-up by the mentor, which makes Choice B correct. Choices A, C, and D are all correct statements about course outcomes and designing learning activities.
Reference: Iwasiw et al. (2020), p. 28

74. **B.** Program learning outcomes
Rationale: Option B is the correct answer because program learning outcomes reflect the knowledge, skills, and behaviors a graduate is expected to achieve upon program completion. Course outcomes (Choice A) and course competencies (Choice C) are outcomes that are met during the program. There are no curricular outcomes in nursing curriculum (Choice D).
Reference: Billings & Halstead (2020), p. 122

75. **C.** The flipped/scrambled classroom requires advanced preparation by students with class time for application of learning.
Rationale: Choice C is the correct answer. The flipped or scrambled classroom requires advanced work assignments so that learners come to class prepared to engage in active learning activities. The traditional class tends to focus primarily on lecture with PowerPoint slides. This teaching method is not necessarily concept-based or the preferred evidence-based method for promoting student learning and knowledge retention (Choices A and D). Choice B is incorrect because a flipped or scrambled classroom does not include extensive lecture and note-taking.
Reference: Ignatavicius (2019), p. 80

Chapter 6

1. A. Empowerment of graduates to be leaders
Rationale: Choice A is the correct answer. Empowering learners to be leaders provides for continual advancement of the nursing profession. Changing a national health care policy (Choice B), creating nursing research (Choice C), and providing community leadership (Choice D) do advance change in nursing, but empowering graduates to be leaders can effect change on an exponential level.
Reference: Halstead (2019), p. 107

2. D. Authoritarian
Rationale: Choice D is the correct answer; the nurse administrator is demonstrating an authoritarian leadership style, which defines outcomes without group input. Choice A would involve all faculty in the decision making for the policy, Choice B involves providing rewards and punishments. In Choice C, the administrator would delegate the policy development to faculty.
Reference: International Institute for Management Development (2021), https://www.imd.org/imd-reflections/reflection-page/leadership-styles/

3. B. Transactional
Rationale: Choice B is the correct answer; the nurse administrator is demonstrating a transactional leadership style by providing a reward for meeting an administrator-designed outcome. Choice A would involve all faculty in the decision making for the policy. For Choice C, the administrator would delegate the policy development to faculty, and for Choice D, the administrator would simply require mandatory attendance at faculty committee meetings.
Reference: International Institute for Management Development (2021), https://www.imd.org/imd-reflections/reflection-page/leadership-styles/

4. C. Transformational
Rationale: Choice C is the correct answer because a transformational leader inspires a team with a vision and then empowers the team to achieve the vision. Choice A would require the team to develop the vision, Choice B is more focused on achieving specific goals and tasks rather than a shared vision, and Choice D would impose the expectation for the vision rather than empowering the team to achieve the vision.
Reference: International Institute for Management Development (2021), https://www.imd.org/imd-reflections/reflection-page/leadership-styles/

5. C. Shared beliefs of the organization
Rationale: Choice C is the correct answer. Organizational culture is the shared patterns of behavior, meanings, values, beliefs, norms, and assumptions. Organizational culture is not shared work (Choice A), demographics (Choice B), or abilities of the organization (Choice C).
Reference: Iwasiw et al. (2020), p. 36

6. D. Ensuring openness and respect for all opinions to be shared
Rationale: Choice D is the correct answer. Successful implementation of change will be enhanced by a culturally sensitive environment that ensures openness and respect for all opinions to be shared. Allowing unlimited discussion is not a feasible choice (Choice A). Allowing leaders extra time for feedback does not allow for all opinions to be shared equally (Choice B). Setting limits on the discussion (Choice C) does not allow for openness and limits discussion to only what the leader wants.
Reference: Billings & Halstead (2020), p. 131

7. B. Involve key faculty and faculty leaders in presenting the change to the group.
Rationale: Choice B is the correct answer because involving key faculty and key faculty leaders will enhance successful implementation of the change. Providing reassurance to faculty regarding the release time is out of the scope for the educator (Choice A). Limiting discussion to only experienced faculty is uncivil (Choice C). Timelines should be set as a group and not by the leader (Choice D).
Reference: Billings & Halstead (2020), p. 131

8. B. Accreditation is not required but is voluntary.
Rationale: Choice A is the correct answer because accreditation *is* a voluntary process, but learners in nonaccredited programs are not eligible for financial aid. Program approval by the state is required, not voluntary (Choice A). Program approval's purpose is to protect the welfare of the state. Accreditation is not primarily focused on the welfare of the state (Choice C). Program assessment is required both by accreditors and program approval regulators (Choice D).
Reference: Oermann & Gaberson (2021), p. 352

9. A. Provide frequent communication of the proposed change using a variety of methods.
Rationale: Choice A is the correct answer. Providing frequent communication regarding the proposed change using a variety of communication methods so that all faculty are clearly informed of the change is the best method for managing any barriers. It is helpful to identify potential threats to the change but not for the purpose of reporting them (Choice B). Choice C, curricular change at this level, is not typically required by accreditors. And telling other faculty how easy this is to implement is not always helpful (Choice D). Although it may seem easy or obvious to you, this might not be perceived the same by others.
Reference: Oermann (2017), p. 352

10. D. Site visit by accrediting agency
Rationale: Choice D is the correct answer. The site visit by the accrediting agency peer evaluators provides an *external* method for evaluation. Faculty review of mission (Choice A), drafting of the self-study (Choice B), and documenting program outcome achievement (Choice C) are all *internal* evaluative activities.
Reference: Oermann & Gaberson (2021), p. 351

11. A. Modeling of professional behaviors in the clinical setting
Rationale: Choice A is the correct answer. Modeling is an effective leadership tool for directly affecting learner understanding of civility. Serving on a university committee (Choice B) provides leadership to learners in an indirect manner by developing policies for them. Participating in a faculty discussion (Choice C) may or may not affect learners. Developing a measurement tool for research (Choice D) does not provide leadership to learners.
Reference: Iwasiw et al. (2020), p. 108

12. C. Developing an interactive presentation on asthma for active learning
Rationale: Choice C is the correct answer. This activity provides leadership within the program for learners to acquire knowledge. Choices A and B provide leadership at the institutional level, and Choice D provides leadership at the national level.
Reference: Billings & Halstead (2020), p. 9

13. A. Serving on a committee to develop faculty policies for the institution
Rationale: Choice A is the correct answer. This activity provides leadership within the institution by collaborating with other disciplines to develop a larger context of knowledge. Serving on a nursing program committee (Choice B) provides leadership at the program level, participating in a community health clinic with learners (Choice C) is an example of the Scholarship of

Application, and mentoring a faculty member (Choice D) provides leadership at the institutional level and is an example of the Scholarship of Teaching and Discovery.
Reference: Billings & Halstead (2020), p. 9

14. C. Scholarship of Application

Rationale: Choice C is the correct answer because developing a service-learning project is an example of the Scholarship of Application in which professional service is demonstrated. The Scholarship of Discovery (Choice A) is related to research activities. The Scholarship of Teaching (Choice B) is related to the ability to effectively teach learners. Choice D, the Scholarship of Integration, is related to working with members of the interprofessional or interdisciplinary team to discover or incorporate knowledge.
Reference: Billings & Halstead (2020), p. 9

15. A. Participating in an interdisciplinary research project with the college of pharmacy to promote safety for patients on a ventilator

Rationale: Choice A is the correct answer; research projects that involve collaboration with other college disciplines are institutional discovery activities. Creating a dimensional analysis activity (Choice B) is a teaching activity. Collaborating with departments outside the program and participating in interdisciplinary committees (Choices C and D) are both interdisciplinary service activities that provide institutional leadership to help the community and are related to the Scholarship of Application.
Reference: Billings & Halstead (2020), p. 9

16. B. "I need a nurse faculty mentor in order for me to learn more about conducting research at this institution."

Rationale: Choice B would require further intervention; experienced interdisciplinary faculty can also serve as excellent mentors for research for novice faculty. Serving on an institutional committee to revise a mission statement (Choice A) is an example of integration. Taking learners to a community health event on behalf of the institution (Choice C) is an example of institutional leadership. Serving on institutional committees for faculty affairs involves oversight of tenure policies (Choice D).
Reference: Billings & Halstead (2020), p. 9

17. B. Providing continuing education to area clinical partners

Rationale: Choice B is the correct answer; serving as a content expert providing continuing education to area clinical partners is leadership on a community level. Coordinating clinics abroad (Choice A) is related to global leadership. Presenting research at a national conference provides national leadership (Choice C). Participating in statewide collaborations provides regional/state leadership (Choice D).
Reference: Billings & Halstead (2020), p. 94

18. D. Having learners work with a case manager who coordinates care

Rationale: Choice D is the correct answer; learning about case management for community-based care is essential for developing student leadership skills at the community level. Providing care in an acute care setting (Choice A) does not provide community-level leadership. Clinical postconference discussions provide the opportunity for a leadership discussion but do not necessarily develop leadership behaviors (Choice B). Creating a care plan (Choice C) does not develop leadership abilities at the community level.
Reference: Billings & Halstead (2020), p. 9

19. A. Participating with the local health department to provide an immunization clinic

Rationale: Choice A is the correct answer. Participating in community partnership activities such as an immunization clinic is an important method for developing learners' understanding of

leadership through interdisciplinary collaboration. Participating in international studies (Choice B) promotes leadership at a global level. Speaking at a state conference (Choice C) promotes leadership at the state level. Observing collaboration by others (Choice D) is an observational activity and may or may not develop understanding of leadership at the community level.
Reference: Billings & Halstead (2020), p. 235

20. **C.** Serving as a representative on the board of a nursing education committee
Rationale: Choice C is the correct answer; serving as a member on the board of nursing education committee provides leadership on a state level. Serving on a professional conference committee (Choice A) provides national leadership. Serving on a university outreach committee (Choice B) provides leadership within the institution. Serving on a professional nursing organizational committee (Choice D) provides national leadership.
Reference: Billings & Halstead (2020), p. 108

21. **A.** "Joining a professional organization is optional and is focused on networking."
Rationale: Choice A is the correct answer and would require intervention. Participating in professional organizations provides opportunities for networking, but this is not the primary focus of the organization. Choices B, C, and D are all correct statements; professional organizations give nursing a larger voice, provide an opportunity to participate in state or regional leadership, and enhance the visibility of nursing.
Reference: Billings & Halstead (2020), p. 117

22. **C.** "Obtaining a professional certification in nursing education demonstrates standards of excellence have been met."
Rationale: Choice C is the correct answer; certification in nursing education demonstrates high standards of excellence in facilitating nursing education have been met. Certification in nursing education (Choice A) is as important as clinical professional certification and demonstrates excellence in teaching and learning. Certification in nursing education demonstrates leadership (Choice B). Certification in nursing education does not measure or ensure clinical knowledge (Choice D).
Reference: National League for Nursing (2019), http://www.nln.org/Certification-for-Nurse-Educators

23. **D.** Providing a service-learning experience to discourage negative mental health stigma on campus
Rationale: Choice D is the correct answer. A campus-wide service-learning experience addresses health care needs within the institution. A county immunization coalition (Choice A) addresses needs at the local level but not at the institutional level. A service-learning experience at a food pantry (Choice B) is also at the local level. A legislative event (Choice C) could be at the local, state, or national level.
Reference: Halstead (2019), pp. 107–109

24. **A.** Conducting an environmental scan to determine and prioritize institutional health-related needs
Rationale: Choice A is the correct answer. An environmental scan to determine and prioritize health-related needs would be an important first step. Developing appropriate level materials (Choice B), aligning projects to course objectives (Choice C), and evaluating projects (Choice D) are all important, but they are not first steps.
Reference: Billings & Halstead (2020), p. 97

25. **B.** Institutional level
Rationale: Choice B is the correct answer; this is an example of addressing health-related needs at an institutional level. It is beyond the level of the program (Choice A). But the teaching activity does not extend to the community (Choice C) or region (Choice D) beyond the institution.
Reference: Billings & Halstead (2020), p. 84

26. B. Clinical education experience providing client care at a practice partnership clinic
Rationale: Choice B is the correct answer. Practice partnerships between faculty and health care agencies serve the needs of the community but also help prepare learners for future practice as nurse leaders within their community. Providing care at a county hospital does not necessarily provide leadership opportunities (Choice A). Providing education at a day care center or senior health fair does not necessarily provide leadership development (Choices C and D).
Reference: Billings & Halstead (2020), p. 95

27. C. Environmental scanning of the community is used to identify health needs to guide the curriculum.
Rationale: Choice C is the correct answer. Environmental scanning is used to identify the health needs of the community to guide the curriculum. Environmental scanning is not an accreditation requirement (Choice A). It does not generally inform selection of clinical sites (Choice B). Environmental scanning for health-related needs is done by the nursing faculty (Choice D).
Reference: Billings & Halstead (2020), p. 97

28. A. Analysis and review of county health statistics
Rationale: Choice A is the correct answer. Analysis and review of county health statistics will result in data that can inform faculty on the priority health care needs for the local community and are based on sound evidence. Focus group discussions of health care concerns with area interest groups (Choice B) provide anecdotal evidence and do not necessarily represent the community. Review of the local news reports for the area on health care needs (Choice C) is also anecdotal. Review of nursing textbooks on community health (Choice D) provides evidence-based information, but it is not necessarily targeted to the local community.
Reference: Billings & Halstead (2020), p. 98

29. D. Working with international populations within the community
Rationale: Choice D is the correct answer. Working with international populations within the community can aid students' learning of global health issues and is easily implemented. Participating in a study-abroad women's health clinic (Choice A) or providing care at an international medical mission (Choice B) promotes understanding of global health concerns, but neither is easy to implement. Completing a concept map diagramming a major global health issue (Choice C) will only introduce learners to one issue, whereas working with diverse populations will introduce them to many.
Reference: Billings & Halstead (2020), p. 238

30. A. An enlarged worldview
Rationale: Choice A is the correct answer. The greatest benefit learners gain from involvement in international partnerships is an enlarged worldview (Choice A). Learners may have the opportunity to experience other languages (Choice B), network with other providers (Choice C), or have hands-on experiences, but these are not as great a benefit as the enlarged worldview gained from the experience.
Reference: Billings & Halstead (2020), p. 240

31. C. Social determinants of health
Rationale: Choice C is the correct answer. The social determinants of health found in Healthy People 2020 and 2030 outline key health priorities for the United States (Choice C). The QSEN competencies are more related to safety guidelines (Choice A). The essentials (Choice B) provide guidelines for nursing programs but do not necessarily cover specific health care priorities for the region. A scope of practice statement does not address health care priorities for populations (Choice D).
Reference: U.S. Department of Health and Human Services (n.d.), https://health.gov/healthypeople/objectives-and-data/social-determinants-health

32. A. Lewin's model

Rationale: Choice A is the correct answer. Lewin's three-step model describes the process for change as unfreezing, moving to a new level, and freezing the new change to sustain the change. Lippitt's change theory is a seven-step theory and includes the role of the change agent (Choice B). Roger's theory describes the rate of adoption of change by group members (Choice C). Social cognitive theory emphasizes the interaction between person, environment, and behavior, and a focus is on achieving self-efficacy, which will aid in sustaining/maintaining the desired change (Choice D).

Reference: Iwasiw et al. (2020), p. 35

33. B. SWOT analysis

Rationale: Choice B is the correct answer. The SWOT analysis examines the strengths, weaknesses, opportunities, and threats related to a potential change. Lewin's model (Choice A) is a three-step model of unfreezing the current level, moving to a new level, and freezing the new change. Roger's theory describes the rate of adoption of change by group members (Choice C). Social cognitive theory emphasizes the interaction between person, environment, and behavior and has a focus on achieving self-efficacy, which will aid in sustaining/maintaining the desired change (Choice D).

Reference: Iwasiw et al. (2020), p. 35

34. C. Roger's diffusion of innovations

Rationale: Choice C is the correct answer. Roger's theory describes the rate of adoption of change by group members. Lewin's model (Choice A) is a three-step model of unfreezing the current level, moving to a new level, and freezing the new change. The SWOT analysis (Choice B) examines the strengths, weaknesses, opportunities, and threats related to a potential change. Social cognitive theory emphasizes the interaction between person, environment, and behavior, and a focus is on achieving self-efficacy, which will aid in sustaining/maintaining the desired change (Choice D).

Reference: Iwasiw et al. (2020), p. 35

35. B. Lippitt's change theory

Rationale: Choice B is the correct answer. Lippitt's change theory is a seven-step theory and includes the role of the change agent. Lewin's model (Choice A) is a three-step model of unfreezing the current level, moving to a new level, and freezing the new change. Roger's theory describes the rate of adoption of change by group members (Choice C). Social cognitive theory emphasizes the interaction between person, environment, and behavior, and a focus is on achieving self-efficacy, which will aid in sustaining/maintaining the desired change (Choice D).

Reference: Iwasiw et al. (2020), p. 35

36. D. Selection of a change theory to guide the intended change

Rationale: Choice D is the correct answer. Selection of a change model for implementation of a change would be the most important first step. Analysis of faculty rate of acceptance for change (Choice A), review of leadership strategies for the change agent (Choice B), and creation of a timeline (Choice C) are important parts of the process, but selection of a change model is an important first step.

Reference: Iwasiw et al. (2020), p. 34

37. A. "Some faculty may have differing views on whether this change should be implemented."

Rationale: Choice A is the correct answer. Whenever a change is proposed, faculty may have differing views on accepting the change. Change is often not easily accepted (Choice B) or embraced, even if described as forward thinking (Choice C). And elimination of a favorite course can create feelings of fear, which can inhibit acceptance of change and creation of a timeline (Choice D).

Reference: DeBoor (2023), p. 32–34

38. B. "The nurse administrator needs to create a timeline for implementation of the change."
Rationale: Choice B is the correct answer and would require intervention. A shared timeline will need to be created by the group rather than a timeline created by the nurse administrator. Key faculty will need to be involved in the change (Choice A), and agreed-upon goals will need to be set by the group (Choice C). Data to support the change will be a powerful motivator for acceptance (Choice D).
Reference: Billings & Halstead (2020), p. 131

39. A. "Serving on the institutional faculty committee will ensure that nursing has a voice in policy development."
Rationale: Choice A is the correct answer. Nursing faculty serving on an institutional-level committee ensures nursing has a voice in institutional policies. Serving on an institutional committee is a service activity, not discovery (Choice B), and the decisions of the committees will greatly affect the nursing program (Choice C). All faculty members should consider participating in an institutional committee—this is not limited to experienced faculty members (Choice D).
Reference: Halstead (2019), p. 49

40. C. "Nursing does not need a representative for the institutional assessment committee, as we have our own program assessment plan."
Rationale: Choice C is the correct answer and would require intervention. An institutional assessment committee would be an excellent committee for nurse faculty members because of their extensive experience with program assessment. Providing a nursing perspective on institutional committees is paramount (Choice A) and is a service activity (Choice B). It is important to review the committee duties to see which would be a good fit for faculty interests (Choice D).
Reference: Halstead (2019), p. 49

41. D. Developing a curriculum that includes evidence-based leadership competencies
Rationale: Choice D is the correct answer. Developing a curriculum that incorporates evidence-based leadership competencies is the best method for promoting leadership in learners. Serving as a role model (Choice A), self-reflective leadership assignments (Choice B), and providing peer mentors (Choice C) do promote leadership abilities among learners, but designing a comprehensive curricular experience that incorporates evidence-based leadership competencies is the best way to develop leadership abilities.
Reference: Halstead (2019), p. 108

42. D. Working with an experienced faculty member to develop a course
Rationale: Choice D is the correct answer. Assigning the new faculty member to work with an experienced faculty member would best promote leadership abilities. Serving as the curriculum committee chair (Choice A) would not be appropriate for an inexperienced faculty member. Teaching a course on leadership does not necessarily promote leadership abilities for the faculty member (Choice B). Assigning them to create a research team for a new project would be too overwhelming for a new faculty member without a mentor (Choice C).
Reference: Billings & Halstead (2020), pp. 122–123

43. A. "I will need to try to obtain resources for the new faculty to attend the leadership conference this fall."
Rationale: Choice A is the correct answer. Providing resources for opportunities to develop leadership best promotes the growth of faculty members. Teaching an upper-level course (Choice B) would not necessarily promote the development of leadership abilities. Meeting only once at the end of the year will not promote leadership abilities (Choice B). Ongoing meetings and providing feedback better promote leadership abilities. New faculty should be included in curricular development (Choice D) but should be mentored by an experienced faculty member.
Reference: Iwasiw et al. (2020), p. 123

44. **B.** "I will need to attend the advisory committee meeting for this fall so we can ask clinical partners for their input on this curricular decision."

Rationale: Choice B is the correct answer. Gathering information about current practices from clinical partners is an effective method for gaining relevant information for curricular change. Curriculums need continual evaluation for change, and keeping them the same (Choice A) would not necessarily promote a current curriculum. All faculty need to participate in environmental scanning for trends, not just experienced faculty (Choice C). It is also important to involve external stakeholders such as clinical partners in curricular decisions, not just nursing faculty (Choice D).

Reference: Billings & Halstead (2020), p. 109

45. **D.** "Global health care trends are not as relevant for nursing curriculum, as they may not affect our community."

Rationale: Choice D is the correct answer. Global trends should be monitored for inclusion in the nursing curriculum. Ongoing review of accreditation standards (Choice A), attending a nursing conference to obtain updated information on clinical care (Choice B), and participating in professional organizations (Choice C) are the responsibility of all nursing faculty and result in gaining up-to-date information that can inform curriculum.

Reference: Iwasiw et al. (2020), p. 169

46. **A.** Flexibility

Rationale: Choice A is the correct answer. Faculty who are flexible and responsive to change best promote adaptability. Curricular knowledge (Choice B), clinical expertise (Choice C), and advanced degrees (Choice D) are all important characteristics, but flexibility is critical for successfully adapting to change.

Reference: Billings & Halstead (2020), p. 99

47. **B.** Failure to achieve a desired outcome

Rationale: Choice B is the correct answer. Failure to achieve a desired outcome often creates a sense of urgency among the team to make a change. Incivility (Choice A), selection of a new leader (Choice C), or disagreement on values and beliefs (Choice D) do not result in a sense of urgency for change.

Reference: University of Minnesota Libraries (2010), https://open.lib.umn.edu/organizational behavior/chapter/15-5-creating-culture-change/

48. **A.** Creating shared values and beliefs for the organization

Rationale: Choice A is the correct answer. Creating shared values and beliefs for the organization will result in commonality among group members. Promoting civility (Choice B), providing leadership development/support (Choice C), and providing a reward system do not necessarily result in commonality.

Reference: Iwasiw et al. (2020), p. 134

49. **A.** Incivility among team members

Rationale: Choice A is the correct answer. Incivility is a major barrier to a successful culture of change. It is the responsibility of all faculty to maintain an environment of civility. Failure to achieve a desired outcome often creates a sense of urgency among the team to make a change. Failure to achieve desired outcomes (Choice B), inexperienced leaders (Choice C), or external stakeholder views (Choice D) are not usually barriers to change.

Reference: Halstead (2019), p. 160

50. **A.** "This curricular discussion should be limited to faculty who are experienced."

Rationale: Choice A is the correct answer and would require intervention. The discussion should not be limited to experienced faculty—novice faculty bring a fresh perspective to discussions that

can move the group forward. Learner input should be obtained when considering program decisions (Choice B). Faculty should consult external stakeholders when considering change (Choice C), and organizations require collaboration to create a culture of change (Choice D).
Reference: Iwasiw et al. (2020), p. 136

51. B. Inability to participate in or influence decisions that affect nursing
Rationale: Choice B is the correct answer. Failure by nursing faculty to participate in institutional governance results in the inability to influence institutional decisions that affect nursing. It does not necessarily affect tenure or promotion (Choice A). It does not always result in a loss of budgetary resources (Choice C). In addition, although it does limit opportunities to network, this is not as major of an impact as the inability to participate in decisions that affect nursing (Choice D).
References: Halstead (2019), p. 156

52. D. "I will teach my learners health care policy and political processes."
Rationale: Choice D is the correct answer. The best method for advocating for nursing in the political arena is to educate learners to become familiar with health care policy and political processes to advocate for change. In this way, the nurse educator has created exponential advocacy for nursing in the political arena. Joining a state board of nursing committee (Choice A), a national nursing organization (Choice B), or developing nursing research (Choice C) are all important methods for advocating for nursing but do not have as great an impact as all the learners the faculty will affect with their teaching.
Reference: Halstead (2019), p. 111

Chapter 7

1. B. Asks to be a nursing committee member
Rationale: A nurse educator would be determined to be socialized to the academic role if asking to be part of a committee, so Choice B is the correct response. Choices A and C are part of usual faculty–learner interactions and are not specific to socialization into the role. Choice D is a nurse educator scholarship activity.
Reference: Halstead (2019), pp. 124–125

2. A. The individual nurse educator's experience and needs
Rationale: The orientation process should be customized based on the individual nurse educator's experience and needs. Experienced educators usually do not need the same basic information that a novice educator does. Therefore Choice A is the correct response. Choices B, C, and D are factors related to orientation, but the nurse educator's orientation does not depend on these factors.
Reference: Billings & Halstead (2020), pp. 12–13, 538

3. C. Developing a new curriculum
Rationale: Developing a curriculum is considered a midcareer role and is therefore not part of the orientation process (Choice C). In order for new nurse educators to navigate and function within their new environment, they must attend departmental meetings, meet and socialize with other faculty, and become familiar with the policies and procedures with their department and their college or university as part of their orientation (Choices A, B, and D).
Reference: Billings & Halstead (2020), pp. 12–13

4. D. Lecturer
Rationale: The lecturer, sometimes called the instructor, is not part of an institution's ranking system and is considered a prerank position for educators who do not meet the credentialing requirements for tenure, which makes Choice D correct. Table 7.1 defines each of the other non-tenure academic roles (Choices A, B, and C).
Reference: Billings & Halstead (2020), p. 6

5. A. Identifying active teaching strategies
Rationale: According to the National League for Nursing, mentorship in the early-career time of the nurse educator includes guidance about teaching and evaluation practices (see Table 7.4). Therefore Choice A is the correct response. Choices B, C, and D are mentorship activities needed in the educator's midcareer.
Reference: National League for Nursing (NLN) (2006), pp. 110–113

6. B. One
Rationale: New nurse educators should volunteer for one committee during their first year as they socialize into their role. Committee membership is considered during the evaluation process, and being part of a committee will help the new nurse educator meet other faculty.
References: Billings & Halstead (2020), pp. 4–6; Cannon & Boswell (2016), pp. 48–49

7. B. Engaging in lifelong learning experiences
Rationale: Choice B would be the *most* important commitment for the nurse educator. The dynamic nature of nursing education requires that nurse educators commit to a variety of lifelong learning, which may include taking continuing education classes (not a certain number required) and meeting certifications (usually not yearly). Increasing knowledge in clinical expertise is an expectation associated with the educator's role in teaching.
Reference: Halstead (2019), pp. 149–150

8. D. Serving as a member of a board of national nursing organization
Rationale: Nurse educators are evaluated on three elements: teaching, scholarship, and professional service. Examples of professional service would include serving on a committee within the organization and serving on a board of a national nursing organization. Facilitating an online nursing course would be an example of teaching. Giving a presentation and publishing an article in a peer-reviewed journal would be examples of scholarship.
References: Billings & Halstead (2020), pp. 4–10; Cannon & Boswell (2016), pp. 47–48

9. B. Conducts research about the characteristics of a mentor
Rationale: Boyer's Scholarship of Discovery can include primary empirical research, analysis of large data sets, theory development, and methodologic studies. Therefore Choice B is the correct response. Choices A, C, and D demonstrate Boyer's Scholarship of Application.
Reference: Billings & Halstead (2020), pp. 8–9

10. B. Advise the novice nurse educator to take additional training classes on simulation.
Rationale: The novice nurse educator may lack confidence or feel intimidated by questions from a more experienced peer. Choice B is therefore the correct option. Advising the novice nurse educator to take additional training classes will help fill any gaps in knowledge and demonstrate scholarship and initiative for lifelong learning. Training classes would also help the novice nurse educator to become more confident with simulation. The other options do not help the novice nurse educator to feel welcomed to the department and are not professional actions to foster a positive work environment.
Reference: Billings & Halstead (2020), pp. 8–10

11. B. Discovery and Integration
Rationale: When the educator is appointed to the rank of associate professor, the educator should have already mastered the Scholarship of Teaching and Application. Choices A, C, and D include these scholarship areas. Rather, the associate professor focuses more on research (Scholarship of Discovery), especially in collaboration with other health professions' faculty (Scholarship of Integration). Therefore Choice B is the correct response. Table 7.1 summarizes this information.
Reference: Billings & Halstead (2020), pp. 8–9

12. C. Reviewing literature about service learning and developing a multidisciplinary service-learning project in a course
Rationale: Choice C is correct. The Scholarship of Integration involves integrating knowledge from various disciplines or professions. Choice A is an example of the Scholarship of Discovery. Choice B is an example of the Scholarship of Application. Choice D is an example of the Scholarship of Teaching.
Reference: Billings & Halstead (2020), pp. 8–9

13. A. "I am going to apply for the department chair position next week."
Rationale: The novice nurse educator is in an early academic career period and should be focusing on Boyer's Scholarship of Teaching and Application. Helping with curriculum review and using faculty policies to guide practice demonstrate a focus on the Scholarship of Teaching (Choices B and C). Attending a professional development workshop shows the educator's commitment to lifelong learning, which demonstrates the Scholarship of Application. Novice educators may not comprehend that they are not qualified to seek a leadership position, which therefore needs follow-up by the faculty mentor. Therefore Choice A is the correct response.
Reference: Billings & Halstead (2020), pp. 8–9

14. B. Provide guidance in transitioning the faculty member into an academic leadership position.
Rationale: According to the National League for Nursing as delineated in Table 7.4, one of the midcareer mentorship activities should be helping the nurse educator transition into an academic

leadership position and learn about the responsibilities of that position. Therefore Choice B is the correct response. Choices A, C, and D are mentorship activities that occur in a nurse educator's early career.
Reference: National League for Nursing (NLN) (2006), pp. 110–113

15. A. Prioritize activities and then complete them in that order.
Rationale: Choice A is the correct answer. Teaching responsibilities have the highest priority per the contractual agreement. The other choices are not going to help refocus energy and accomplish what is needed to develop in the role as the nurse educator.
Reference: Billings & Halstead (2020), pp. 4–7

16. C. "Professional organization involvement will help me grow professionally and personally."
Rationale: Being an active member of a professional organization is an example of the Scholarship of Application. The primary purpose for being actively involved in an organization is the growth that educators can gain. Therefore Choice C is the correct response. Choices A, B, and D are all true statements, but they are not the best response for why educators should join professional organizations.
Reference: Billings & Halstead (2020), p. 9

17. D. Completing a doctoral degree to be eligible for promotion and tenure
Rationale: Seeking an advanced degree is formal education that shows the nurse educator is committed to lifelong learning. Therefore Choice D is the correct response. All of the other choices are examples of the educator's commitment to service.
Reference: Halstead (2019), pp. 127–128

18. C. Presenting the results of collaborative interprofessional research at a national conference
Rationale: Boyer's Scholarship of Integration requires the nurse educator to collaborate with interprofessional health care team members to interpret and synthesize knowledge to create new models of care or teaching. Choice C is an example of that activity and is the correct response. Choices A and D are examples of the Scholarship of Teaching. Choice B is an example of the Scholarship of Application.
Reference: Billings & Halstead (2020), pp. 8–9

19. A. Obtaining and maintaining the Certified Nurse Educator® credential
Rationale: Choice C represents the Scholarship of Discovery. Choice D is an example of service, and Choice B is an educator responsibility in preparation for applying for promotion and tenure. Therefore Choice A is the correct response because it demonstrates the expertise of the nurse educator within the nursing profession.
Reference: Billings & Halstead (2020), pp. 8–9

20. A. FERPA
Rationale: Choice A is the correct answer. The Federal Educational Rights and Privacy Act (FERPA) protects the privacy of student educational records and reports for all institutions that receive funding through the U.S. Department of Education. Parents or guardians wanting information must have written permission from the 18-year-old or older student. Choice B is the Individuals with Disabilities Education Act (IDEA), which ensures learner with disabilities have equitable education. Choice C is the Health Insurance Portability and Accountability Act (HIPAA), which protects individuals' medical records and other personal health information. Choice D stands for Public, Educational, and Governmental Access (PEG), which prohibits obscene or sexually explicit content on cable channels.
Reference: Cannon & Boswell (2016), pp. 89–90

21. A. Providing prenatal care for women in Appalachia

Rationale: Service learning involves a hands-on collaborative effort between the service community (in this case Appalachia) and the institution and is designed to help students learn social responsibility and civic engagement. It is an active learning experience designed to meet student learning outcomes and the health care needs of a selected community. Choice A meets these requirements and is therefore the correct response. Choices B, C, and D do not meet the requirements to qualify as service learning.

Reference: Billings & Halstead (2020), pp. 218–219

22. D. Conducting health and blood pressure screenings for senior citizens

Rationale: Choice D is the correct response because performing screenings is an excellent opportunity to provide an actual direct care or screening service. Health education classes, either face-to-face or via podcasts (Choices A and B), and a booth at a job fair (Choice C) do not provide actual direct care or screening services.

Reference: Billings & Halstead (2020), pp. 218–220

23. B. Develops cultural awareness

Rationale: Service-learning experiences are often graded as pass/fail rather than letter graded. Therefore participating in service learning does not necessarily affect a learner's grade point average (Choice A). Choice C is incorrect because this experience enhances collaborative learning. Not all service-learning projects require travel, because the experience might occur in a nearby community (Choice D). Service learning should always increase cultural awareness of various populations and groups. Therefore Choice B is the correct response.

Reference: Billings & Halstead (2020), pp. 218–219

24. A. Portfolio

Rationale: The portfolio is a collection of documents used to display one's work when applying for appointments, promotions, and tenure. Therefore Choice A is the correct response. A resume is a short summary of one's education, work history, credentials, and skills (Choice B). Choice C, the concept map, is a graphic organizer used as a teaching-learning strategy by students. The curriculum vitae may be part of the portfolio and is an extensive document that delineates the nurse educator's educational history, employment history, scholarship activities such as publications, and awards and honors (Choice D).

Reference: Billings & Halstead (2020), pp. 456–460

25. B. Publishing an article in a peer-reviewed journal

Rationale: A publication in a peer-reviewed journal is preferred over publication in a journal that does not have the same rigorous process. Professional publications are considered part of the nurse educator's scholarship activities. Therefore Choice B is the correct response. Choices A, C, and D are examples of service activities.

Reference: Billings & Halstead (2020), pp. 5–7, 539–540

26. C. "I need to pay close attention to the summary of learner evaluations of my course to decide how to improve."

Rationale: Feedback from a variety of sources can be helpful for nurse educators to pursue quality improvement (QI). Learner course evaluations are the most important source of this feedback and should be carefully considered by the educator. Therefore Choice C is the correct response. Self-reflection is important but is not the best source of feedback (Choice A). The process for peer evaluation is not a choice for the educator to accept or not; some institutions do not support peer evaluation (Choice B). Choice D is incorrect because it is essential that the nurse educator receive feedback as part of continuous QI.

Reference: Billings & Halstead (2020), pp. 528–531

27. A. Have access to own education records

Rationale: Postsecondary students have rights outlined by federal law (FERPA). The only student right that is included in this law is Choice A, which makes it the correct answer. Choice B, C, and D are not student rights.

Reference: Billings & Halstead (2020), p. 43

28. C. "Students are expected to make errors because they are learners."

Rationale: A just culture avoids blame and uses errors as learning opportunities for quality improvement. This environment accepts that students are going to make mistakes and learn from them. Therefore Choice C is the correct response. Choices A, B, and D are punitive in approach.

Reference: Walker et al. (2020), pp. 133–138

29. A. Notify current and future learners 6 to 12 months before the change.

Rationale: Learners have the right to be informed of program changes in a timely and effective manner. Implementation of a revised or new curriculum can affect current and future learners. Therefore the learners need adequate notice of this major change, usually 6 to 12 months before implementation, as specified in the correct response (Choice A). Choices B, C, and D may be part of the process but are not required.

Reference: Billings & Halstead (2020), p. 156

30. D. Hobbies and special interests

Rationale: The curriculum vitae (CV) is a detailed and extensive document that reflects the nurse educator's educational and employment history, professional organization memberships, scholarship activities, and professional awards and honors. It is a professional reflection of the nurse educator's career and would *not* include the educator's hobbies or interests. Therefore Choice D is the correct response.

Reference: Christenbery (2014), pp. 267–268

31. A. Student incivility

Rationale: All of the choices are legal/ethical issues that nursing faculty may encounter. However, students learn appropriate professional behavior from faculty. If faculty are uncivil, learners may think incivility is acceptable in the nursing profession. Therefore faculty need to act professionally such that students can learn from their role modeling, which makes Choice A the correct response. Role modeling would likely not influence the other legal/ethical issues (Choices B, C, and D).

Reference: Billings & Halstead (2020), pp. 270–274

32. C. LinkedIn

Rationale: Choice C is the correct answer because this social media tool is designed for professionals and professional communications. Members can access employment information, current trends, professional news, and information about marketing. The other social media platforms listed are for personal communication and special interests.

Reference: Billings & Halstead (2020), pp. 57–58, 387

33. C. Standardized tests should be used for assessment purposes only.

Rationale: Choice C is the correct answer because standardized exams should be used for assessment of learning rather than as high-stakes testing (Choices B and D). These tests are not predictive of which learners will definitely pass or fail licensure or certification exams (Choice A). The National League for Nursing's Fair Testing Guidelines for Nursing Education support appropriate testing and evaluation methods that provide feedback for student learning and curriculum effectiveness.

Reference: Billings & Halstead (2020), pp. 58–59

Chapter 8

1. A. Awarding promotion and tenure to faculty
Rationale: Boyer's Model of Scholarship is used as a guide to make decisions about promotion and tenure for faculty; therefore Choice A is correct. Assigning courses to teach is usually based on the faculty member's expertise and the current teaching needs (Choice B). Boyer's model is not used to make decisions about grant awards or for identifying specific learner needs (Choices C and D).
Reference: Billings & Halstead (2020), p. 8

2. C. Obtain institutional review board approval for the study.
Rationale: When participating in research with human subjects, it is necessary to obtain institutional review board (IRB) approval to confirm that research protocols are ethical and ensure the rights and welfare of the learners participating in the research activities are protected; therefore Choice C is correct. A pretest to determine the current level of knowledge of online learning does not measure learners' perceptions (Choice A). Before applying for a grant to fund the study or consulting with a statistician, the researcher will want to obtain IRB approval for the study (Choices B and D).
Reference: Marzinsky & Smith-Miller (2019), p. 1

3. B. Publish findings of use of an innovative classroom learning activity.
Rationale: Using and publishing findings of innovative teaching methods is an example of the scholarship of teaching; therefore Choice B is correct. Serving on a faculty governance committee is an example of service to the institution (Choice A). Conducting a study on pet therapy is generation of new knowledge and would be an example of the scholarship of discovery (Choice C). Interdisciplinary grants for service learning would be an example of achievement in the scholarship of integration (Choice D).
Reference: Billings & Halstead (2020), pp. 8–9

4. B. Formulate a PSCOT question and begin a literature review.
Rationale: Evidence-based teaching involves using educational techniques supported by evidence. The first step in the process of evidence-based teaching is to develop a question and search the literature; therefore Choice B is correct. Choices A and C are incorrect because the other instructors may not necessarily be using evidence-based teaching practices. Choice D is incorrect because the search involves finding information about the correct procedure, not on the most effective teaching/learning strategy.
Reference: Cannon & Boswell (2016), pp. 11–16

5. D. Use the PSCOT to identify keywords and concepts when searching the literature.
Rationale: PSCOT is a format for developing an education-focused question that identifies keywords for use in a literature search; therefore Choice D is correct. The next step after developing the PSCOT question is to use it to search the literature; therefore Choices A and B are incorrect. A PSCOT does not help identify current gaps in learner knowledge (Choice C).
Reference: Cannon & Boswell (2016), pp. 14–17

6. D. Publishing two peer-reviewed articles on implementation of innovative teaching methods
Rationale: Publishing articles on innovative teaching practices is an example of the scholarship of teaching; therefore Choice D is correct. Creation of an interprofessional simulation is an example of the scholarship of integration (Choice A). Academic advisement is a service activity and not an example of scholarship of teaching (Choice B). Maintaining consistently high learner evaluations of teaching is an example of good teaching but does not reflect the scholarship of teaching (Choice C).
Reference: Billings & Halstead (2020), pp. 8–9

not appropriate without review (Choice C). The findings cannot ...

7. D. Scholarship of teaching

Rationale: Educators who apply principles of both good teaching and scholarly teaching, with the distinction of also disseminating scholarship, are exhibiting the scholarship of teaching and learning, which makes Choice D correct. Educators who apply Chickering and Gamson's principles of good practice in education are demonstrating good teaching (Choice A). Educators who apply good teaching principles, reflect on teaching, use evidence-based approaches, and regularly engage in discussion with colleagues and reading the literature are demonstrating scholarly teaching (Choice B). The scholarship of integration involves demonstrating scholarship through the interpretation and synthesis of knowledge across disciplines (Choice C).

Reference: Halstead (2019), pp. 139–140

8. B. Receiving a grant award supporting teaching and learning

Rationale: Receiving a grant or other type of award for teaching is an example of recognition of scholarly work; therefore Choice B is correct. Serving on a department committee and reviewing textbooks are essential practices for educators but do not demonstrate recognition of one's scholarly work (Choices A and C). Volunteering at a food bank is an example of community service and does not demonstrate recognition of scholarship (Choice D).

Reference: National League for Nursing (NLN) (2016), pp. 3–6

9. B. Undergoes the institutional review board process for a research study

Rationale: Integrity as a scholar involves upholding ethical obligations. The use of an institutional review board (IRB) is one way the nurse educator can demonstrate integrity. Therefore Choice B is the correct response. Gaining consent for research on learners by the nurse educator conducting the study and analyzing test scores for research without gaining consent are both unethical practices (Choices A and C). Sharing data that have been collected about learners in order to conduct research is also unethical without consent (Choice D).

Reference: Halstead (2019), pp. 137–138

10. A. Meet with other medical-surgical nursing faculty to discuss the method and findings.

Rationale: Sharing expertise with colleagues regarding teaching practices is an important part of the nurse educator role and can help build a community. Testing a new method in the classroom should first be shared with other faculty to discuss the method and findings. Therefore Choice A is the correct response. Publishing the results in a journal and presenting at a national conference are not appropriate at this point, as the nurse educator has not conducted any formal studies (Choices B and D). Although academic freedom is important, it does not mean that faculty should not share practices (Choice C).

Reference: Halstead (2019), p. 142

11. D. Write a proposal to be reviewed by the institutional review board (IRB).

Rationale: After establishing a PSCOT and determining a plan of action for research, the nurse educator should prepare a proposal to be reviewed by the IRB. Approval by the IRB must take place before any further steps can be taken. Therefore Choice D is the correct response. Any process that begins collecting data and selecting specific learners is unethical (Choices A and B). Investigating journals for publication can be an early step; however, initiating the IRB process is the most important (Choice C).

Reference: Grady (2015), pp. 1148–1155

12. A. Develop a proposal for review to retroactively study the data collected.

Rationale: Nurse educators can retroactively look at data collected to provide evidence for novel teaching practices. To present such data, it is important to undergo the ethical review process before moving further. Therefore Choice A is the correct response. Removing all identifying data will be necessary; however, it is not the first step (Choice B). Going back to ask for consent is

not appropriate without review (Choice C). The findings cannot ethically be presented without a review (Choice D).
Reference: Lafayette (2021), https://irb.lafayette.edu/the-three-types-of-irb-review/

13. **D.** Apply for a grant to obtain funding.
Rationale: Gaining new knowledge to implement best teaching practices and studying the impact of those practices are excellent ways to engage as a nurse scholar. Obtaining grant funding is an appropriate option to consider. Therefore Choice D is the correct response. Dropping the idea because of a shortage of funds is not appropriate. Many national organizations have prioritized nursing education research (Choice A). Asking the simulation director or dean are not appropriate sources of funding (Choices B and C).
Reference: Vajoczki et al. (2011), article 2

14. **B.** Require the students to complete the CITI Program training.
Rationale: Learning about integrity as a nurse scholar is critical to uphold ethical practices in research. This work is often engaged in as a graduate student, and it would be most appropriate to have them complete the CITI Program. Therefore Choice B is the correct response. Developing a PowerPoint presentation is not appropriate to provide thorough context surrounding ethical training, and neither is an assignment (Choices A and C). Reminding learners to simply use their judgment does not role-model integrity as a nurse scholar (Choice D).
Reference: CITI Program (n.d.), https://about.citiprogram.org/get-to-know-citi-program/

15. **C.** Developing a collaborative assignment to be used based on a review of current nursing education literature
Rationale: Demonstration of evidence-based teaching is a necessary part of effective teaching by the nurse scholar. Developing teaching practices based on evidence is an appropriate way to demonstrate evidence-based teaching. Therefore Choice C is the correct response. Teaching the way one was previously taught and using material from a colleague both do not show evidence of growth as an educator (Choices A and B). Engaging learners based on their needs can be helpful; however, learners are not experts in the knowledge they need to gain (Choice D).
Reference: Cannon & Boswell (2016), pp. 7–10

16. **D.** Present at a national conference for nursing education.
Rationale: Disseminating scholarly findings is an important part of promoting the growth of nursing education. Presenting at a national conference will allow results of a study to be widely distributed and reviewed by peers. Therefore Choice D is the correct response. Publishing or presenting findings only to one's department does not widely disseminate new evidence or widely create the opportunity for review and critique (Choices A and B). Informally presenting to colleagues is not the most effective method to share research findings (Choice C).
Reference: Oermann et al. (2022), pp. 381–384.

Chapter 9

1. **C.** "Content on caring for patients with infections should be increased in the curriculum."
Rationale: Social forces that influence program decisions, including curricular revision, include health issues that are prevalent in society or in a local region. The COVID-19 pandemic illustrated the need for nurses to be very knowledgeable in how to take care of patients with infections, especially viral infections for which there was initially no available drug therapy (Choice C). Choice A is an incorrect statement because most nursing programs are experiencing increased enrollments. Choices B and D are institutional forces that influence program decisions.
Reference: Iwasiw et al. (2020), pp. 156–157

2. **A.** Need to address health equity issues and the role of the professional nurse
Rationale: The COVID-19 pandemic affected people of color more than White individuals, with more severe disease, hospitalizations, and deaths. This fact created dialogue about differences in disease outcomes based on race and ethnicity and fueled a movement to address health equity (Choice A). This issue is much more important than learning about infection statistics (Choice B). The initial problem with personal protective equipment (PPE) was lack of adequate PPE, not lack of nursing knowledge (Choice C). There was also no evidence that nurses lacked knowledge regarding how to perform sterile technique (Choice D).
Reference: Iwasiw et al. (2020), p. 154

3. **B.** "We should increase our maternal–infant clinical hours because more babies are being born now."
Rationale: Choices A, C, and D are true statements about clinical experiences in a nursing program based on social forces. However, Choice B is not correct because there has not been a major recent increase in births; this statement therefore requires follow-up by the mentor.
Reference: Billings & Halstead (2020), pp. 87–88

4. **D.** "Some small colleges and universities have closed or merged in recent years."
Rationale: Choices A and B are incorrect statements. Academic faculty are paid less than clinical practice nurses. Most learners graduate from all types of programs with a high student loan debt. Choice C is not correct because college enrollments have been generally lower than usual over the past few years. Nursing enrollments have often increased, however. Choice D is the correct response to this test item because lack of financial resources and financial constraints have resulted in multiple strategies by educational institutions, including merging or closing.
Reference: Halstead (2019), pp. 156–157

5. **B.** For-profit institutions
Rationale: Proprietary schools are private and for-profit, making Choice B correct. As private entities, they do not directly receive local and state funding to operate (Choice A). Therefore tuitions are typically higher for learners when compared with public schools, especially community colleges. Proprietary schools are usually not governed by a board, and they typically have adequate, well-prepared faculty (Choices C and D).
Reference: Billings & Halstead (2020), pp. 545–548

6. **A.** Modeling political advocacy
Rationale: Although any of the choices could be an expectation for a particular nurse educator, Choices B, C, and D are not expectations of any or every educator. All of these expectations depend on where the educator is employed, what educator credentials are required, and what the role description delineates. However, any and all nurse educators should model political advocacy to help learners recognize the need and learn how to be politically active as practicing nurses, making Choice A correct.
Reference: Halstead (2019), pp. 162–163

7. **A.** Adjunct
Rationale: As shown in Table 9.1, the definition of an adjunct faculty member is one who works part-time and may teach either in a didactic or clinical setting. The other faculty positions (Choices B, C, and D) are usually full-time and have different roles and responsibilities.
Reference: Billings & Halstead (2020), pp. 5–8

8. **D.** Serve the workforce of the community
Rationale: Public community colleges were developed to serve the needs of their local community and are funded partially by those communities, which makes Choice D correct. Because of that funding, they can offer low-tuition programs compared with most public universities or private schools, but that is not their primary purpose (Choice A). The mission of community colleges does not include conducting research, although some faculty may engage in research (Choice B). Most community colleges offer programs that award associate degrees of certificates to their graduates (Choice C), but this is not the primary reason these schools were founded.
Reference: Iwasiw et al. (2020), pp. 145–146

9. **D.** Public university
Rationale: Faculty who are employed by public universities typically have the best opportunity for participation in the governance of the institution, making Choice D correct. In many public universities, faculty are unionized or have contracts that outline the process for self-governance. Nurse educators working in a community college or vocational-technical school have fewer opportunities for this experience because of faculty workloads and organizational culture (Choice C). Private institutions are often under pressure to make a profit or are non-profit Choice B). Many of these institutions, especially private career schools, function within a business model rather than an educational model (Choice A), thus limiting faculty and staff input.
References: Billings & Halstead (2020), pp. 544–545; Halstead (2019), pp. 155–156

10. **A.** To demonstrate the ability to meet quality educational standards
Rationale: The primary purpose of regional or national accreditation of schools, colleges, and universities is to show that the institution has achieved excellence in meeting quality educational standards; therefore Choice A is the correct response. Being accredited may allow the institution to apply for grants and be competitive, but these are secondary benefits of accreditation (Choices C and D). The type of program in Choice B is irrelevant.
Reference: Billings & Halstead (2020), p. 560

11. **D.** Access to necessary hardware and Internet for learners
Rationale: Success in education refers to the outcomes for learners. Therefore the years of experience and type of nursing program that the nurse educator teaches in are not relevant to success (Choices B and C). Learners at any point in their program can benefit from online education, so Choice A is not correct. Learners need to have the necessary computer hardware equipment and high-speed Internet to be able to access and participate in the online course. Therefore Choice D is the correct response.
Reference: Iwasiw et al. (2020), pp. 404–414

12. **C.** "Your main responsibility now is to gain expertise in teaching."
Rationale: The priority for a new nurse educator is to acquire expertise in teaching and learning. The other university expectations associated with scholarship, research, and service are not essential until the educator is effective in teaching; therefore Choice C is the correct response. The mentor should not help with the new educator's responsibilities (Choices A and D), and it would be inappropriate to make the comment in Choice B.
Reference: Halstead (2019), pp. 154–155

13. **A.** "The college will be able to give the nursing faculty a raise in their salaries."
Rationale: Some nursing programs are expanding or have recently expanded to offer an optional track or increase enrollments because there is a nursing shortage, causing a high demand for new nurses (Choice C). Increased enrollments can increase revenue for the college or university because learners have to complete general education courses in the arts, sciences, and humanities; therefore Choice B is an accurate statement. Choice D is also an accurate statement because a strong nursing program is well respected by community stakeholders. Choice A is not an accurate statement and therefore would require follow-up by the mentor. Nursing faculty are generally paid on the same pay scale as other college or university faculty.
Reference: Halstead (2019), pp. 156–160

14. **B.** Lack of adequate nursing faculty
Rationale: Many college and university students today are interested in becoming nurses, especially since the COVID-19 pandemic. Therefore Choice A is not the correct response to this test item. Expanding a nursing program would net additional revenue to purchase more learning resources, indicating that Choice C is also not correct. Classroom space may also be a challenge (Choice D), but lack of adequate nursing faculty is a major factor that limits program growth across the country, making Choice B the correct response.
Reference: Billings & Halstead (2020), p. 2

15. **C.** Participating in professional development
Rationale: Advanced practice nurses (APNs) are experts in clinical practice but have little to no formal training in education or nursing education. Therefore the priority activity for these new faculty is professional development in teaching and learning, technology in education, and assessment of learning, making Choice C correct. The other three activities (Choices A, B, and D) may be pursued at a later time to meet the requirements of the academic role and/or requirements for promotion and tenure.
Reference: Billings & Halstead (2020), pp. 536–539

16. **A.** Shared values, expectations, and attitudes
Rationale: Choices B, C, and D are more aligned with the definition of institutional climate and norms rather than institutional culture. Choice A is the definition of organizational culture, making it the correct response.
Reference: Iwasiw et al. (2020), p. 146

17. **C.** Providing timely constructive feedback to learners
Rationale: Organizational climate includes the shared perceptions of and meanings attached to policies and procedures and employee behaviors that are expected, supported, and rewarded. Choice C meets that definition by providing prompt constructive feedback to learners as part of ongoing learning assessment. Although engaging learners in active learning is expected, it is a part of institutional culture if it is shared among all faculty (Choice A). Obtaining the terminal degree is for personal growth and to meet promotion and tenure requirements rather than meeting the definition of organizational climate (Choice D). To respect professional boundaries, a luncheon with learners is not appropriate; therefore Choice B is not correct.
Reference: Iwasiw et al. (2020), p. 146

18. **D.** High productivity and satisfaction
Rationale: Choices A and B are not positive behaviors or outcomes and would therefore not be part of a positive institutional climate. Increasing faculty salaries would not be the result of a positive climate (Choice C). However, a positive institutional climate would result in both faculty and learner satisfaction. Faculty satisfaction usually leads to high productivity, making Choice D correct.
Reference: Iwasiw et al. (2020), p. 146

19. B. Encouraging a learner to transfer to a program in another role

Rationale: Choices A, C, and D are positive, civil behaviors and activities that would be appropriate for formative and summative assessment of learning. Only Choice B is an example of an uncivil behavior by faculty. It is not appropriate to judge learners regarding their career goals.

Reference: Billings & Halstead (2020), p. 271

20. C. Abusing an assigned patient

Rationale: Disrupting class, usually by excessive talking, is an example of learners being annoying, rather than being criminal (Choice D). Cheating on an examination and plagiarizing are examples of administrative violations rather than criminal ones (Choices A and B). However, physical, emotional, or financial abuse of any patient is an example of a criminal act or conduct because the patient is harmed, making Choice C correct.

Reference: Billings & Halstead (2020), pp. 271–274

21. D. "I plan to weed out those learners who should not become nurses."

Rationale: Choices A, B, and C are all appropriate statements about assessing learner performance using formative (Choice C) and summative evaluation methods (Choices A and B). However, Choice D is an example of faculty incivility and requires follow-up by the mentor.

Reference: Billings & Halstead (2020), pp. 271–274

22. B. Role modeling by faculty

Rationale: Learning how to avoid uncivil behaviors represents learning in the affective domain. Learning strategies in the affective domain include reflective journaling and role modeling by faculty; therefore Choice B is the correct response to this test item. Choices A, C, and D are examples of learning strategies in the cognitive domain and would not be appropriate for affective learning.

Reference: Billings & Halstead (2020), pp. 271–274

23. C. Mission and values

Rationale: The mission and values of the educational institution shape the mission, values, and curriculum of the nursing program. Therefore Choice C is the correct response. Choices A, B, and D would be considered when examining the feasibility of implementing the newly revised curriculum, but they are not the most important considerations.

Reference: Iwasiw et al. (2020), pp. 145–146

Answers and Rationales for Comprehensive Practice Exam

1. C. Are technologically proficient

Rationale: Both the latchkey kids (Generation X), born between 1965 and 1979, and Millennials (Generation Y), born between 1980 and 1994, work well in groups rather than individually (Choice D). Baby Boomers, born between 1945 and 1964, prefer face-to-face learning (Choice A). Generation Y learners like quick access to instruction and frequent feedback on their learning performance (Choice B). Although Generation X learners are not digital natives, they are technologically savvy; Generation Y learners are digital natives and typically very proficient in technology from a very young age. Therefore Choice C is the correct answer.

Reference: Cannon & Boswell (2016), pp. 33–43

2. A. Provide positive feedback and reinforcement.

Rationale: As a group, adult learners are very self-directed and motivated to learn. To help foster that motivation, they need positive, constructive feedback and reinforcement (Choice A). Most adults do not prefer lecture or reading because these are passive learning strategies; adults prefer to be engaged in the learning process (Choices B and D). Taking a survey to determine learning preferences can assist the educator to select the most appropriate learning strategies but does not promote motivation for adult learners (Choice C).

Reference: Billings & Halstead (2020), pp. 338–339

3. C. Ask the disruptive learners to share their comments with the class.

Rationale: An important part of managing the classroom is motivating learners to pay attention. Policies regarding attendance and engagement can be helpful. Despite these policies, learners at times will still disrupt class, which requires the nurse educator to directly address the behavior. Although it can be uncomfortable to implement this action, using strategies such as asking the disruptive learners to share their comments with the class can be helpful (Choice C). Telling the learners to leave the classroom (Choice A) is counterproductive and would put these learners at a disadvantage in missing important learning. Randomly assigning seats to break up the group (Choice B) can be a good strategy, but not at the exact time of the disruption. Advising learners that their grades will be affected by their behavior (Choice D) is not a positive way to encourage accepted behavior and can be viewed as threatening.

Reference: Cannon & Boswell (2016), pp. 161–162

4. B. Family and work responsibilities can be stressors.

Rationale: A heavy academic workload in addition to family and work responsibilities are major stressors, making Choice B correct. These learners tend to not identify with and model their peers (Choice A) and are intrinsically rather than extrinsically motivated (Choice C). In addition, nontraditional learners tend to have diverse characteristics in terms of professional and life experiences (Choice D).

Reference: Halstead (2019), p. 49

5. **D.** Employing nurse educators who are technology experts

Rationale: Leveraging technology in the classroom is an expectation in academia. To successfully integrate technology in the classroom to support learning, tech-savvy faculty or educators need to lead the transition and can do so over multiple sections or courses over time (Choice D). The leader in this initiative needs to be a part of the nursing discipline to understand the nuances of the content being learned. Ensuring adequate institutional technology support (Choice A) is helpful and important for sustainability, but it is not the best method to support the nurse educator in incorporating more technology. Additionally, holding a faculty development session focused on technology use in the classroom (Choice B) can provide benefit, but it is not the best method in supporting the nurse educator because of the likely lack of follow-up in the implementation of the change. Obtaining funding to provide mobile devices for learners and faculty for classroom engagement is helpful in relieving financial burden and in providing resources, but it does not specifically support the transition or ensure successful use of the technology (Choice C).
Reference: Oermann et al. (2022), pp. 93–94

6. **B.** Use a skills checklist to observe the learner performing the skill and provide constructive feedback.

Rationale: Competency evaluation involves seeking visible evidence of psychomotor skill learning and can be done either formatively or summatively. When formatively evaluating a learner's ability to safely perform a nursing procedure such as urinary catheter insertion, the nurse educator could use a skills checklist to observe the learner perform the skill and provide feedback at that time (Choice B). Assessing the learner's understanding of how to safely perform the procedure on a written examination and assigning a written case study on urinary catheter insertion and evaluating the responses (Choices A and D) may provide formative evaluation data but are not competency-based methods of evaluation. Observing the learner performing the skill in clinical and documenting in the final clinical evaluation (Choice C) is a competency-based approach but is a summative evaluation method.
Reference: Oermann et al. (2022), pp. 202–204

7. **A.** Emphasize that uncertainty is acceptable in learning.

Rationale: Strategies that promote learner development and foster a productive learning environment include regarding uncertainty as a safe position in which questions and mistakes are expected and encouraged for learning. Emphasizing that uncertainty is acceptable in learning (Choice A) will foster a productive learning environment. The educator would not want to select or call on some learners to answer questions but rather allow any learners to answer the educator's questions (Choice C). The nurse educator should not protect learner identities during class discussions. The nurse educator should not divert attention away from tense or uncomfortable topics (Choice B). Asking individuals to speak on behalf of others in the class (Choice D) does not promote learner development and therefore should be avoided.
Reference: Oermann et al. (2022), pp. 48–49

8. **A.** Learning outcomes

Rationale: The nurse educator should primarily consider the learning outcomes for the course to determine whether the teaching methods used are a good fit for student learning. The outcomes are the criteria used to determine learning, thereby providing evidence of effectiveness of the teaching methods (Choice A). Other considerations include learner preferences (Choice B), available resources (Choice C), and administrative support (Choice D), but these factors do not provide a specific measure of success in learning when compared with outcomes.
Reference: Oermann et al. (2022), p. 65

9. **D.** Communication between learners and faculty

Rationale: The nurse educator teaching an online course should employ good online teaching practices that center on communication between learners and faculty (Choice D). Use of active

rather than passive learning (Choice A) is another essential practice. Completion of tasks *on time* to ensure progression in the course (Choice B), not an emphasis on task completion, is an important practice. *Prompt* faculty feedback (Choice C) is important but is not an essential concept for best practices in online learning. Other best practices include reciprocity and cooperation among learners, communicating high expectations, and respecting diverse ways of learning.
Reference: Oermann et al. (2022), pp. 113–123

10. **C.** Giving prompt constructive feedback on learner work
Rationale: Curricular and co-curricular learner support significantly contributes to improved learner satisfaction and is tied to learner success. Giving prompt feedback on learner work (Choice C) supports learners and helps them to be successful. Engaging in mentored research projects (Choice B), discussing grades and course progression (Choice A), and discussing ideas from class during open office hours (Choice D) are examples of curricular activities, but they are course activities and do not necessarily promote the faculty–learner relationship.
Reference: Oermann et al. (2022), p. 54

11. **D.** Learners with disabilities may perform well in certain areas and may not perform well in other areas.
Rationale: Learning disabilities are the most common type of limitation for learners at the college level. In nursing education these learners may perform well in the clinical area, for example, but may be unable to demonstrate the same ability in other areas such as written examinations (Choice D). Learners often need assistance navigating barriers, and campus resources are available to assist (Choice A). Learners should be referred to the appropriate counselors for assistance with identifying helpful and necessary resources (Choice B). Often, learners with disabilities do not have documented evidence before starting their college careers (Choice C).
Reference: Oermann et al. (2022), pp. 55–56

12. **A.** "Other than talking to me, how have you addressed this concern so far?"
Rationale: Nurse educators often serve in the role of academic advisor for nursing learners, which is meant to assist individual learners or small groups of learners in personal empowerment and success in the program and profession. Desirable attributes of academic advisors include knowledge of advising; knowledge of institutional policies, procedures, resources, and curricula; good interpersonal and communication skills; problem-solving and goal-setting abilities; values learner advocacy; and is organized, timely, welcoming, and authentic. In this scenario the faculty advisor should assist the learner initially by getting a sense of what actions the learner has already taken (Choice A), which allows the advisor to determine the next appropriate steps to address the concern. Telling the learner that the instructor is an expert disregards the learner's concern and does not demonstrate learner advocacy (Choice B). Deferring to the grievance policy at this time may not be necessary; until the advisor knows what has already been done, the advisor cannot determine whether this would be needed (Choice C). Reviewing the assignment with the learner is inappropriate and does not respect the authority of the instructor evaluating the learner; therefore this action should be avoided to prevent crossing boundaries (Choice D).
Reference: Billings & Halstead (2020), p. 549

13. **C.** Affective
Rationale: Domains of learning include cognitive, psychomotor, and affective. The affective domain (Choice C) is about professional identity development and internalizing values of the profession. Performing a self-assessment requires reflection on the learner's strengths and areas needing improvement. Self-evaluation, a critical part of the learning process, is effective in evaluating growth in the affective learning domain. The cognitive domain (Choice B) focuses on knowledge attainment. The psychomotor domain (Choice D) relates to skill acquisition. Social learning (Choice A) is a learning theory but is not a learning domain.
Reference: Billings & Halstead (2020), pp. 505–506

14. C. Analyzing laboratory results for a patient case scenario
Rationale: Domains of learning include cognitive, psychomotor, and affective. The nurse educator should plan learning activities that address all three learning domains. Analyzing laboratory results for a patient case scenario (Choice C) addresses the cognitive domain of learning, as it requires the learner to rely on previously learned knowledge to come to a conclusion using critical thinking. Writing a personal health improvement plan and listening to a patient's lived experience (Choices A and D) are activities that address the affective domain of learning. Transferring a patient from the bed to the chair safely (Choice B) addresses the psychomotor domain of learning.
Reference: Oermann et al. (2022), pp. 65–68

15. D. Graphic images
Rationale: A common way to identify learners is using the VARK learning preferences: visual, auditory, read/write, and kinesthetic learners. Visual learners learn best from pictures, graphic images, and videos (Choice D). Auditory learners would likely prefer hearing traditional lecture (Choice A), and kinesthetic learners would likely prefer the hands-on experience required to practice technical psychomotor skills (Choice B). Reflective journaling requires writing, which would be a preferred learning activity for the read/write learner.
Reference: Billings & Halstead (2020), p. 30

16. A. Adults are not responsible for their own learning.
Rationale: Initially described by Knowles, adult learning theory specifies that adults are responsible for their own learning, are self-directed (Choice B), and are goal-oriented (Choice D). They also have minimal interest in doing "busywork" assignments but rather prefer assignments that help them learn (Choice C). Therefore the incorrect statement is Choice A.
Reference: Oermann et al. (2022), pp. 30–41

17. B. "I asked my learners to volunteer for a diversity committee to manage any problems."
Rationale: Although a diversity and inclusion committee can be helpful to develop policies, this statement does not address learner diversity and requires follow-up and guidance from the mentor (Choice B). Instead, the educator would ask learners what they need and prefer to meet those needs (Choice A) and respect all learners (Choice D). The educator would also solicit information about the diverse characteristics of the learners to better understand their needs (Choice C).
Reference: Billings & Halstead (2020), pp. 32–33

18. B. Veterans work very well in groups or teams to meet the desired outcome.
Rationale: Active military and veteran students have strong shared cultural characteristics, including working very well in groups or teams with loyalty (Choice B); they do not tend to prefer individual work or learning (Choice A). Although many veterans have experienced physical and mental disabilities, there is not a high incidence when considering all veterans as a group (Choice C). There are no data to support that veterans are first-generation college learners (Choice D).
Reference: Billings & Halstead (2020), pp. 21–22

19. C. To socialize learners into the professional role
Rationale: The nursing faculty would want guidelines or policies regarding incivility so that students can learn how to conduct themselves as professional nurses (i.e., socialize into the professional role) (Choice C). Policies would not necessarily help promote learner success or increase affective learning (Choices A and B). Using civil behaviors would be more welcoming than uncivil behaviors (Choice D), but that is not the most important reason that incivility policies are needed.
Reference: Billings & Halstead (2020), pp. 270–284

20. D. Completing a reflective journal
Rationale: Learning in the affective domain is about professional identity development and internalizing values of the profession. One of the best ways for learners to be aware of their values

and identity is through reflective journaling (Choice D). Choices A and C represent learning in the cognitive domain. Taking a history of a standardized patient is part of clinical performance in which cognitive, affective, and psychomotor learning occur (Choice B).
Reference: Oermann et al. (2022), p. 67

21. C. "I don't let learners attend professional development conferences because they will miss class."
Rationale: Nurse educators are obligated to help learners develop professionally. To help them learn how to professionally develop, sharing one's own experience and role modeling desired behavior can be very helpful for learning (Choices A and C). Referring learners to opportunities for professional growth is also an appropriate way to help develop them (Choice D). However, the educator should allow learners to attend professional development opportunities, even if class time would be missed. Attending a professional conference, for example, is just as important as being in a nursing classroom. Therefore the statement in Choice C requires follow-up by the mentor.
Reference: Halstead (2019), pp. 124–126

22. A. Role modeling of civil behaviors by nurse educator
Rationale: Learning about appropriate professional nursing behaviors is within the affective domain. One of the best ways to ensure affective learning is to role model appropriate behaviors for learners (Choice A). Choices B and C are learning activities in the cognitive domain, which help learners gain knowledge about professional behaviors but do not demonstrate those behaviors. Keeping a diary can help provide insight into learner behaviors but does not help learn how to practice or use them (Choice D).
Reference: Billings & Halstead (2020), pp. 270–284

23. B. "I will be sure we have that device for you before you come to lab for practice."
Rationale: According to the Americans with Disabilities Act (ADA), organizations are obligated to make reasonable accommodations for an individual's disability. Providing an amplified stethoscope is a reasonable accommodation for a learner's hearing loss and is a low-cost device (Choices B and C). Choice A indicates that the educator would be willing to determine if an amplified stethoscope is available, but it does not assure the learner that a device will be provided. The learner may volunteer to share specific information about a disability, but it is inappropriate for the educator to require documentation on the severity of the disability (Choice D).
Reference: Billings & Halstead (2020), pp. 62–83

24. B. Using case studies that incorporate ethical principles in decision making
Rationale: Given the nature of the nursing profession, the nurse educator needs to be concerned with ethics as an important area to emphasize and should provide opportunities for learners to apply the principles of ethical behavior. The most effective activity would be using case studies that incorporate ethical principles in decision making (Choice B). Acting as an ethical role model (Choice A) is important and will assist in developing ethical behaviors but is not the most effective method in the application of these behaviors. Providing a safe environment in which learners can discuss ethical principles (Choice C) is another important foundational consideration when addressing this content but does not specifically allow for the application of ethical behavior. Using learner discussion groups to talk about personal experiences involving ethics (Choice D) is helpful in applying principles of ethical behavior but does not provide a scenario for which ethical decision making can be dissected and discussed; therefore it is not the best activity to apply principles of ethical behavior. Additionally, discussing personal issues among a group presents an issue related to violation of privacy.
Reference: Cannon & Boswell (2016), pp. 96–97

25. D. Pursue mentors who align with career goals.
Rationale: Nurse educators should carefully reflect on their career development needs and seek out mentors who have the background to help them achieve their career goals (Choice

D). Experienced mentors (Choice A) are a consideration, but is not the only area of consideration when seeking mentors. Mentors from the nursing field (Choice B) may be of benefit; however, nurse educators can also benefit from having mentors outside of the nursing field. It is not required to have a mentor from a different institution (Choice C).
Reference: Billings & Halstead (2020), pp. 7–8

26. D. Support for achieving learning is adequate and accessible.
Rationale: When evaluating learner services, the nurse educator should consider and assess whether adequate and accessible support for learning is provided (Choice D). Ensuring guidance for financial aid is only one service available to learners (Choice A). Ensuring transcript evaluation processes are accurate and timely (Choice B) and ensuring learners receive an adequate orientation to the program (Choice C) are also important considerations. However, these options are less specific to the role of the nurse educator and not directly associated with learning support.
Reference: Billings & Halstead (2020), p. 549

27. A. Manageable workload
Rationale: Nurse educators need a manageable workload (Choice A) to support continuous productivity in teaching, service, and scholarship. Even as nurse educators become accustomed to their role, a manageable workload is essential to functioning in a challenging and demanding environment. If one becomes overwhelmed due to an unmanageable workload, productivity will inevitably suffer. Ongoing self-evaluation (Choice B) is very helpful in directing ways to improve teaching, service, and scholarship, but it is not the most important factor. Administrative support (Choice C) is important in retaining nurse educators but does not specifically support continuous productivity on a daily basis. Teaching relevance and competence (Choice D) is important in functioning in the nurse educator role in general but, again, it does not specifically support continuous productivity in the role.
Reference: Halstead (2019), pp. 126–128

28. C. Sharing teaching innovations in a public forum
Rationale: The Scholarship of Teaching is critically important as part of fostering the science of nursing education. One of the issues today is that too few nurse educators share their work so others can benefit from it. The nurse educator can fulfill the role obligation to disseminate scholarly work by sharing teaching innovations in a public forum (Choice C). Engaging in interprofessional activities (Choice A) is an important step to foster collaboration in health care professionals, but it is not specific to dissemination of scholarly work. Working as an advisor on a doctoral committee and serving as a manuscript reviewer (Choices B and D) are critical to the development of future nurse scientists, but they also are not specific to dissemination of scholarly work related to the role of the nurse educator.
Reference: Oermann et al. (2022), p. 398

29. D. Teaching and Application
Rationale: The assistant professor rank is usually held by nurse educators without many years of experience and is therefore a time to seek opportunities to develop as a teacher (Scholarship of Teaching). Growing as a professional while developing teaching expertise is also an important beginning role of the nurse educator (Choice D). The Scholarship of Discovery relates to developing and conducting research, which occur more at higher educator ranks such as associate or full professor (Choices A and C). The Scholarship of Integration provides opportunities for educators to collaborate with members of the interprofessional faculty team in a spirit of inquiry (Choices B and C).
Reference: Billings & Halstead (2020), pp. 539–540

30. B. Scholarship is an expectation of all faculty regardless of experience.
Rationale: All nurse educators are considered scholars, and most institutions have expectations for scholarship for faculty at all levels of nursing education regardless of experience (Choice B).

Scholarship is required for faculty appointed on the tenure track (Choice A) but is also required of faculty on other tracks. Although teaching is a focus for novice nurse educators, they are still expected to engage in scholarship as well (Choice C). Often, research-intensive institutions require faculty to have scholarship productivity (Choice D); however, teaching-intensive institutions likely have scholarship expectations as well.
Reference: Oermann et al. (2022), pp. 398–400

31. C. Serving on a nursing program progression committee

Rationale: Service responsibilities are often a requirement of nurse educators as academic faculty. Professional service typically includes leadership in professional organizations, committee work, and community service. Working on a nursing program progression committee (Choice D) is an example of service that nurse educators can use to satisfy their service requirements. Substituting as a guest lecturer in a nursing class (Choice A) and meeting with learner advisees on an ongoing basis (Choice C) are aligned with teaching responsibilities. Presenting at a local nursing education conference (Choice B) is an example of scholarship engagement.
Reference: Oermann et al. (2022), pp. 398–400

32. C. It involves inquiry about teaching and learning.

Rationale: Broadly conceptualized, the Scholarship of Teaching in nursing education involves inquiry about teaching and learning (Choice C). Research describes the Scholarship of Discovery (Choice A), and Choice B reflects the Scholarship of Integration. Service-learning activities are an example of the Scholarship of Application (Choice D).
Reference: Oermann et al. (2022), pp. 398–400

33. B. Networking at professional nursing conferences

Rationale: Networking with other professionals with similar interests, such as at professional nursing conferences (Choice B), is an important aspect of socialization to the role of nurse educator. This activity provides opportunities for conversation, discourse, and relationship building that connect the educator to the profession. Obtaining a terminal degree (Choice A) and becoming certified in a specialty area in nursing (Choice B) are activities that promote the Scholarship of Teaching, but they do not necessarily promote role socialization. Maintaining a portfolio documenting teaching quality (Choice D) is a way to demonstrate role effectiveness and scholarship productivity.
Reference: Oermann et al. (2022), pp. 398–400

34. B. The need for professional development changes as experience is gained in the role.

Rationale: In pursuing professional development opportunities, the nurse educator should recognize that career enhancement changes as experience is gained in the role (Choice B). Nurse educators should select opportunities that are aligned with career goals and trajectory (Choice A). These choices can be discussed with a mentor, but they do not necessarily need to be approved. Professional development activities should be targeted and directed, aimed at increasing effectiveness in the uniqueness of their educator role, not broad and varied (Choice C). Most nursing programs allocate monies in the operational budget for professional development. When those funds are depleted, foundations, grants, or other sources often support nursing professional development opportunities such that the educator does not need to pay for them (Choice D).
Reference: Oermann et al. (2022), p. 27

35. A. Provides advice and support for the educator

Rationale: The role of the faculty mentor is to offer advice and support for the nurse educator at any point in the educator's career (Choice A). The mentor does not evaluate the educator's performance, report the educator's progress in the role, or take on any of the educator's workload (Choices B, C, and D).
Reference: Billings & Halstead (2020), pp. 7–8

36. D. "I will need permission from the learner before I can discuss the learner's grades with you."
Rationale: Family Educational Rights and Privacy Act (FERPA) laws protect learners' rights by preventing access to the learners' school records without their permission. Therefore no one, including the learner's parents, is allowed to know anything about the learner's grades or progress without learner permission (Choice D). Choices A, B, and C do not indicate the need for learner permission.
Reference: Billings & Halstead (2020), pp. 278–279

37. A. Conducting research on the impact of COVID-19 infection on the quality of life of nursing home residents
Rationale: Boyer's Scholarship of Discovery focuses on conducting and disseminating the result of research, such as described in Choice A. Choice D is an example of the Scholarship of Application and demonstrates professional development. Choices B and C are not examples of scholarship but rather are active learning strategies for adult learners.
Reference: Oermann et al. (2022), pp. 398–400

38. D. Scholarship of Integration
Rationale: The Scholarship of Integration is demonstrated in the spirit of inquiry through interprofessional research. The study in the test question describes the nurse educator's research with a social worker, which meets this definition (Choice D). The other areas of scholarship do not involve interprofessional colleagues (Choices A, B, and C).
Reference: Billings & Halstead (2020), p. 540

39. C. Planning a service-learning experience
Rationale: The Scholarship of Application is demonstrated through the educator's activities in professional service and practice. Choice C is an example of professional service. Choice A represents the Scholarship of Discovery, Choice B is an example of the Scholarship of Teaching, and Choice D is an example of the Scholarship of Integration.
Reference: Billings & Halstead (2020), p. 539

40. D. Accepting the chair position for an institutional committee
Rationale: Functioning as a committee chair for a department or at an institution level is an example of educator socialization into the academic role as a leader. Socialization indicates that the educator is recognized has having the knowledge, skills, attitudes, and abilities (KSAs) needed for the academic role (Choice D). Joining an organization and reading journals are responsibilities of any professional nurse and not specific to academic nurse educators (Choices A and B). Choice C is part of the educator role but does not indicate that the individual has the KSAs needed for full role socialization.
Reference: Halstead (2019), pp. 124–126

41. B. Notifying learners of academic changes in a clear and timely manner
Rationale: Nurse educators should always notify learners of any changes in the curriculum, course syllabus, or policies in an effective, clear, and timely manner to be fair (Choice B). This communication can be verbal, written, and/or electronic. Adding points to a test may or may not be fair, depending on the statistical analysis of test results (Choice A). Allowing learners to leave early is a violation of the learning contract between the learners and the institution (Choice C). Developing policies is not necessarily an example of fairness but instead is an expectation that learners are expected to follow (Choice D).
Reference: Billings & Halstead (2020), p. 42

42. A. Conduct a needs assessment.
Rationale: A needs assessment (Choice A) is the most important process for collecting and analyzing information for curriculum development. This information is used to make decisions about

the need for initiating new programs or revising existing programs and their continued need. External (and internal) frame factors (Choice B) are considered in a needs assessment. External frame factors are those that influence curriculum in the environment outside the program or institution, such as health care needs of the populace, regulations, and accreditation. Internal frame factors, such as resources within the institution, the organizational structure within the school, and faculty or learners, influence curriculum from within the program and institution. Population demographics (Choice C) are useful information when developing or revising curricula and also would be considered in the needs assessment, but they are only one aspect of the needs assessment. Input from community stakeholders (Choice D) is also an aspect of needs assessment and would be considered an external frame factor for curriculum development.
Reference: DeBoor (2023), pp. 330–337

43. A. Predictions for future nursing workforce needs
Rationale: When designing curriculum for a new nursing program, the nurse educator would conduct a needs assessment. A needs assessment involves considering factors that are outside of the nursing program that inform decisions about curricula, while also considering factors that are within the program that affect the design. Predictions for future nursing workforce needs (Choice A) is a factor that needs to be considered initially. Mission, vision, philosophy, and goals of the school (Choice B); resources within the nursing program and institution (Choice C); and organizational structure of the parent academic institution (Choice D) are other factors to be considered once the broader understanding of nursing workforce needs is determined.
Reference: DeBoor (2023), pp. 330–337

44. B. Faculty beliefs and values
Rationale: A philosophy statement is one of the components of the curriculum and is a statement that embraces faculty beliefs and values (Choice B). It is used to inform curriculum development and decision making. Additional components include the mission, vision, and theoretical framework. The mission statement describes the overarching goals for the work being done (Choice C). The vision statement describes the broad vision for the program (Choice A). The theoretical framework serves as the guiding framework for program development (Choice D).
Reference: DeBoor (2023), pp. 34–35

45. D. Level course outcomes sequentially to align with program learning outcomes.
Rationale: The nurse educator, in developing curriculum for a new nursing program, should level outcomes that sequentially lead to end-of-program outcomes (Choice D). Creating weekly lesson outcomes that are tied to course outcomes (Choice A) and aligning course assignments and grading criteria with course outcomes (Choice B) are helpful and important strategies in aligning course content but are not specific to developing course or program outcomes. Crosswalking course outcomes with guiding bodies in nursing education (Choice C) may assist in curriculum development, but it does not specifically formulate course or program learning outcomes.
Reference: DeBoor (2023), p. 128

46. D. Ensures essential knowledge and skills are integrated into the curriculum
Rationale: The process of concept analysis or mapping is important for ensuring that essential knowledge and skills are integrated into the curriculum (Choice D). Conducting a needs assessment assists in projecting future needs of health care and educational consumers (Choice A), in determining needed resources for implementation of planned activities (Choice B), and in examining relationships between curricular concepts and stakeholder needs (Choice C).
Reference: DeBoor (2023), pp. 47–48

47. D. Psychomotor
Rationale: Organizing course and program outcomes in a methodical fashion is important to ensure alignment and consistency in the nursing curriculum, such as by using Bloom's taxonomy

to develop outcomes. Bloom's taxonomy categorizes domains of learning into the affective, cognitive, behavioral, and psychomotor domains. Vital sign measurement, or any nursing skill or concept, can be assessed differently to address each of the domains. The skill of accurately measuring vital signs addresses the psychomotor domain (Choice D). The affective domain (Choice A) would be addressed by assessing learners' attitudes and beliefs surrounding vital sign measurement. The cognitive domain (Choice B) would be addressed by assessing their understanding of the pathophysiology of vital sign changes with certain conditions. The behavioral domain (Choice C) would be addressed by observing the learner's behaviors and interactions while performing the skill.
Reference: DeBoor (2023), p. 128

48. **B.** Graduation rates
Rationale: Program effectiveness is best measured by summative evaluation strategies at the end of or after the program, such as licensure or certification exam pass rates, employment rates, and graduation rates (Choice B). Summative evaluation strategies involve looking at the "final product." Course evaluations (Choice A), learner course surveys (Choice C), and learner course exam scores (Choice D) are examples of formative evaluation strategies because they are not obtained at the end of the program.
Reference: DeBoor (2023), pp. 254–255

49. **A.** The state nurse practice act
Rationale: Each state regulates higher education and approves programs based on specific requirements. The nursing practice act (Choice A) provides guidance for each state and defines the role of the nurse through each state's regulations. Educational and programmatic requirements may include accreditation standards (Choice B), but these standards do not serve as a reference source for scope of practice for the state. Each state regulates licensure requirements, and there is no national licensure requirement (Choice C). The institution's mission statement (Choice D) does not provide regulatory guidance.
Reference: DeBoor (2023), pp. 278–279

50. **B.** Failure to seek accreditation will result in ineligibility for federal monies.
Rationale: Program approval by accreditation is a necessary and important process to ensure program quality. Accreditation in the United States is voluntary (Choice A); however, failure to seek program accreditation will result in ineligibility for federal monies (Choice B) or ineligibility for development funds and other financial support. State regulatory bodies, not accreditation bodies, provide oversight of licensure requirements (Choice C), which is done after graduation from the program. Learner transfer credits from nonaccredited institutions typically are not recognized (Choice D).
Reference: DeBoor (2023), pp. 275–277

51. **D.** To determine the extent to which the program meets expected outcomes
Rationale: The purpose of systematic program evaluation is to determine the extent to which all activities for the program meet the established goals or outcomes (Choice D). Ensuring a process for formal complaints (Choice A) and defining programmatic policies and procedures (Choice D) are responsibilities of the faculty and administrators within the school, but they are not specifically related to systematic program evaluation. Ensuring national standards are met and quality is maintained (Choice C) is a requirement set forth by accrediting agencies.
Reference: Billings & Halstead (2020), p. 514

52. **D.** Advisory group meeting minutes
Rationale: A number of data sources, both external and internal, can be used for assessment as part of the program evaluation plan. Advisory groups (Choice D) are an example of an external support for a nursing program. Other external data and support sources include administrators,

agencies such as state boards of nursing and nursing accreditation bodies, alumni, clinical agency staff, faculty, learners, and the institution in which the nursing program is housed. Course evaluation survey results (Choice A), standardized examination results (Choice B), and learner engagement survey reports (Choice C) are examples of sources of data that come from internal processes within the program. Other sources of data that come from internal processes used for nursing program assessment and evaluation may include examinations, focus groups, institutional records or reports, interviews, projects, papers, assignments, or other surveys.
Reference: Oermann (2017), p. 61

53. B. Ensuring concepts and content in the curriculum are complete and relevant
Rationale: The faculty role in curriculum design focuses on ensuring concepts and content in the curriculum are complete and relevant (Choice B). Confirming physical space is available for planned learning activities (Choice A) is usually done by staff supporting the program. Determining instructional resources are adequate to achieve learning outcomes (Choice C) is often considered a fiscal resource decision and is ultimately determined by administration of the program. Obtaining clinical experiences that are varied and appropriately sequenced (Choice D) may be done by a faculty member or another staff person whose role is dedicated to obtaining and maintaining clinical placements.
Reference: Iwasiw et al. (2020), pp. 430–431

54. D. Determining whether strategies effectively facilitated achievement of learning outcomes
Rationale: The primary consideration when evaluating the effectiveness of teaching and learning strategies is determining whether strategies effectively helped learners achieve desired learning outcomes (Choice D). Ascertaining if learners were satisfied with strategies used (Choice A), judging whether content complexity increased with strategies used (Choice B), and assessing if strategies used were designed in accordance with best practice (Choice C) are less important considerations in the evaluation process.
Reference: Oermann (2017), p. 23

55. A. The ability for learners to meet learning outcomes in the clinical site
Rationale: All of the choices should be taken into consideration when selecting clinical sites for learner experience. However, the primary or most important element is that each site allows learners the opportunity to meet clinical learning outcomes (Choice A). Depending on the clinical site, learners may have the opportunity to perform complex skills (Choice B). Patient census should be adequate to allow learners the ability to meet outcomes, but this is not the primary consideration (Choice D). Ideally, the clinical educator would have experience in the agency, but this is not a requirement (Choice C).
Reference: Billings & Halstead (2020), pp. 328–329

56. C. "It is not part of the nurse educator's academic role to develop curriculum."
Rationale: All of these statements are correct about barriers to curriculum development with the exception of Choice C. The National League for Nursing (NLN) competencies for the academic nurse educator include the responsibility of educators to participate in curriculum development and revision. Therefore mentors need to follow up with educators who state this work is not within their role. Many faculty are inexperienced with curriculum development (Choice A) and feel they need assistance from a consultant (Choice D). Others feel they have insufficient time to complete such a large task (Choice B) due to other obligations for scholarship, service, and leadership.
Reference: Halstead (2019), pp. 91–102

57. B. Clinical partners
Rationale: Stakeholders are individuals and groups who have a vested interest in the nursing program. Internal stakeholders are those within the institution, such as learners, faculty, and

nursing administration (Choices A, C, and D). External stakeholders are individuals and groups who are outside the institution, such as partners in clinical agencies. Therefore Choice B is the correct response.
Reference: Billings & Halstead (2020), p. 148

58. D. Assessing standardized patients

Rationale: Simulation is a process in which health care is imitated in a safe environment for learners. High-fidelity simulation has a high degree of reality and allows learners to learn and make mistakes without fear of harming the "patient." Using high-fidelity mannequins and human beings are the best examples of high-fidelity simulation. Standardized patients are people who play a role in the clinical scenario, often with a predetermined script of what to say and do. Therefore Choice D is the correct response to this question. Task trainers (Choice A) and static mannequins (Choice C) are examples of low-fidelity simulation due to their lower degree of imitating reality. Unfolding case studies describe simulated clinical situations but have no hands-on component. Some experts classify unfolding cases as low-fidelity simulation (Choice B).
Reference: Billings & Halstead (2020), p. 503

59. C. Cognitive

Rationale: The three domains of learning for nursing practice are psychomotor (developing technical clinical skills), cognitive (acquiring nursing knowledge and thinking skills), and affective (exploring and developing professional values, attitudes, and beliefs). The course objective in the question requires the learner to analyze knowledge to make a comparison, which requires thinking. Therefore the course objective measures learning in the cognitive domain (Choice C). The objective does not measure psychomotor or affective learning (Choices A and D). Performance is not one of the three learning domains (Choice B).
Reference: Oermann & Gaberson (2021), pp. 15–19

60. A. Remembering

Rationale: The objective requires the learner to recall (identify) social determinants of health for a population and reflects the lowest level on the cognitive taxonomy, known as remembering (Choice A). This recall does not require understanding (Choice B) or complex thinking at an applying or analyzing level (Choice D).
Reference: Oermann & Gaberson (2021), pp. 15–16

61. A. Ensure the nursing department philosophy is congruent with the institution's philosophy and values.

Rationale: A nursing program or department philosophy is a statement of the faculty's values and beliefs about nursing and nursing education and serves as the foundation of program curriculum. The nursing department functions as part of the educational institution and its culture. Therefore it is essential that the nursing and institutional philosophy, goals, and values align or are congruent (Choice A). There is no purpose for conducting a literature search or surveying learners because the department philosophy represents the faculty's beliefs (Choices B and D). The philosophy should represent a collective consensus among faculty rather than include each faculty's opinion (Choice C).
Reference: Billings & Halstead (2020), pp. 135–146

62. D. Creating

Rationale: The creating taxonomic level of the cognitive learning domain requires that the learner combine information to develop a new product. The course objective states that the learner will develop a teaching plan that would be specific to the new birth parent. Therefore the correct response to this question is Choice D. The other cognitive taxonomy levels require less complex thinking (Choices A, B, and C).
Reference: Oermann & Gaberson (2021), pp. 15–16

63. D. Increased focus on diversity and health equity issues

Rationale: A major current societal trend is increased awareness of and focus on diversity, inclusivity, and health equity. This issue has affected every facet of life, including educational programs. Therefore Choice D is the correct response. U.S. immigration has increased rather than decreased (Choice B). Changes in licensure and certification examinations could also influence curriculum revision, but they are not societal or health care trends (Choice A). Most social media platforms are used for communication and sharing personal information and should not be used for sharing patient or professional nursing content, which would be a breach of privacy and confidentiality (Choice C).

Reference: Billings & Halstead (2020), pp. 57–58

64. B. It reflects the program's philosophy and allows students to meet course outcomes.

Rationale: Nursing faculty should develop specific courses based on their expertise rather than involve the entire nursing faculty (Choice D). Not all courses would be provided in a hybrid format or address current trends in nursing and health care, depending on subject content (Choices A and C). However, all courses should reflect the philosophy of the nursing program and be designed to allow all learners to meet the course outcomes.

Reference: Billings & Halstead (2020), pp. 181–201

65. C. Analyze the possible reasons for the pass rate decline to develop an action plan.

Rationale: Certification exam pass rate is an outcome that reflects the effectiveness of a program as part of the program's systematic plan for evaluation. The expected level of passing licensure and certification exams is often established by nursing accrediting bodies. If a group does not meet the established benchmark, the faculty need to examine possible causes for the low pass rate and develop an action plan to help improve it (Choice C). Continuing to monitor the pass rates without an action plan is not appropriate for continuous quality improvement (Choice D). The expected outcome should not be changed to meet the actual pass rate, as that would lower the standard for the program (Choice A). The faculty may also want to determine if the certification exam underwent any major changes, but that is not the most important action (Choice B).

Reference: Billings & Halstead (2020), pp. 551–552

66. B. To make learners aware of how learning activities align with course objectives

Rationale: Lesson plans are part of course design by faculty and delineate learning outcomes, learning activities, assignments, and evaluation methods to measure achievement of learning. Although lesson plans can help educators organize their modules or classes, they do not have to be shared with learners (Choices A and C). The primary purpose for sharing with learners is to help them recognize how assignments, class/online activities, and evaluation methods help to meet course learning outcomes and objectives (Choice B). Regulatory and accrediting bodies usually do not mandate lesson plans, but they may recommend that faculty develop them if they are not part of course design (Choice D).

Reference: Billings & Halstead (2020), pp. 183–184

67. D. Empower learners and graduates to become leaders in nursing.

Rationale: Nurse educators can effect change in the nursing profession through their own personal contributions. As educators, they are uniquely positioned, however, to effect change by empowering learners and graduates to become leaders in nursing (Choice D). Serving as a faculty advisor to a group of learners (Choice A) is part of the role of the nurse educator and is a good opportunity to mentor learners; however, it does not specifically create a downstream effect. Obtaining grant funding to support leadership initiatives (Choice B) provides resources for this initiative but also does not necessarily create a downstream effect. Attending a leadership academy to improve leadership skills (Choice C) personally develops the nurse educator's skills in this area but is not targeted at promoting change.

Reference: Halstead (2019), p. 107

68. B. Leadership skills

Rationale: Leadership skills (Choice B) are integral in advancing the nursing profession. Nurse educators have the responsibility of fostering leadership skills in their learners as a concerted effort in advancing nursing. Critical thinking (Choice A), technology fluency (Choice C), and communication strategies (Choice D) are important aspects of the nursing role, such as in providing safe and effective patient care, but do not necessarily advance the profession of nursing.
Reference: Halstead (2019), pp. 115–117

69. A. Social and political forces

Rationale: Social and political forces (Choice A) are factors in academia that need to be considered because they influence the direction of professional nursing education. Nurse leaders and faculty need to have an understanding of these forces so the curriculum can be responsive and serve to prepare learners to function effectively after graduation. Technologic resources (Choice B), teaching best practice guidelines (Choice C), and learner characteristics and preferences (Choice D) are important considerations in determining curricular and course content and are effective teaching and learning strategies. These factors do not influence the direction of professional nursing education but rather support it.
Reference: Billings & Halstead (2020), p. 84

70. A. Create instructional strategies that support equity.

Rationale: The nurse leader can model teaching for cultural competence by recommending fellow educators create instructional strategies that support equity (Choice A). Encouraging learners to participate in professional groups (Choice C) can foster the development of cultural competence, but this is not a teaching method to address this skill. The nurse educator does not necessarily need to engage in scholarly work focused on culturally competent care (Choice C) to teach for cultural competence. Threading cultural competence content throughout the curriculum (Choice D) is a strategy that can be used to ensure this content is adequately addressed in the curriculum, but it does not refer to the teaching or learning facilitation of cultural competence.
Reference: Billings & Halstead (2020), p. 306

71. C. Share teaching innovations with other educators.

Rationale: Scholarship is essential to nursing education. Without scholarship, educational practices cannot develop further. The nurse educator can share innovations with other educators (Choice C) as a means of engaging in scholarship to make contributions to the body of knowledge in nursing education. Conducting original clinical research (Choice A) is also scholarship but does not contribute to nursing education science. Obtaining certification in a specialty area (Choice B) supports teaching and practice but does not contribute to the science of nursing education. Seeking grant funding to support scholarly work (Choice D) is also a desirable scholarship endeavor but is not specific to the body of knowledge in nursing education.
Reference: Oermann et al. (2022), pp. 398–400

72. D. Time and resources to establish a firm scholarship foundation

Rationale: Novice nurse educators need to be provided with adequate time and resources to lay a firm foundation in developing their scholarship programs (Choice D). Establishing a clear direction early on will result in higher productivity. Clinical competence in the assigned teaching area (Choice A) and training on working with diverse learner populations (Choice C) will help novice nurse educators to be more proficient in their teaching role. Continuing education focused on nursing leadership (Choice C) would be helpful in growing in their role, but it is not specific to developing a successful scholarship program.
Reference: Cannon & Boswell (2016), pp. 306–307

73. A. Create a diversity, equity, and inclusion committee.

Rationale: Diversity within the learning community is important and allows for strengths and limitations of all learners to be supported by educators and others in the group. Diversity

contributes to equipping future work forces to handle the complexity and the challenges in health care. When an institution is interested in expanding a particular effort or has specific strategic goals, a mechanism that is useful in promoting this effort is to create a committee to move the work forward. A diversity, equity, and inclusion committee (Choice A) would be accountable for producing results. Threading diversity, equity, and inclusion content in the curriculum (Choice B) and obtaining affiliation agreements with clinical sites offering diverse experiences (Choice C) are curricular changes that support learning, but they are not institution-level mechanisms to address this change. Engaging learners in scholarship focused on diversity, equity, and inclusion (Choice D) is another way to support learning in this area, but it does not broadly disseminate the work at the institutional level.
Reference: Cannon & Boswell (2016), pp. 308–310

74. B. Becoming a scholar in a leadership academy
Rationale: Nurse educators are charged with maintaining competence and expertise in their role while also developing leadership skills in nursing education. There are many continuing education activities available, such as attending a nursing leadership conference (Choice A), taking a graduate-level nursing leadership course (Choice C), and reading journal articles about nursing leadership styles (Choice D). The most helpful activity would be becoming a scholar in a leadership academy (Choice B), as this activity is designed to provide a structured, mentored experience and involves application of leadership skills in nursing education.
Reference: Cannon & Boswell (2016), pp. 303–304

75. B. Engage in the spirit of inquiry.
Rationale: A nursing scholar is one who has a persistent spirit of inquiry or curiosity that informs practice and education. Therefore Choice B is the correct response. Developing expertise in clinical practice and using active teaching-learning strategies are part of the nurse educator's responsibility but do not demonstrate scholarship (Choices A and C). Conducting literature searches is part of conducting research but does not demonstrate scholarship as a separate activity (Choice D).
Reference: Oermann et al. (2022), p. 398

76. C. Publishing the effectiveness of an innovative teaching strategy
Rationale: Nurse educators who demonstrate the Scholarship of Teaching show evidence of effective teaching and dissemination of knowledge gained through that teaching. Publishing the effectiveness of an innovative teaching-learning strategy meets this description (Choice C) and is therefore the correct response. Conducting interprofessional research demonstrates the Scholarship of Integration (Choice A). Serving on a nursing education committee is an example of the Scholarship of Application. Developing an unfolding case study does not demonstrate nurse educator scholarship (Choice B).
Reference: Billings & Halstead (2020), p. 539

77. A. Using evidence-based approaches to teaching-learning
Rationale: Scholarly teaching implies that the educator would use best practices based on current evidence when approaching the teaching-learning process; therefore Choice A is the correct response. Active learning, respecting diverse learning styles, and maintaining high learner satisfaction are good teaching practices, but are not necessarily evidence based (Choices B, C, and D).
Reference: Oermann et al. (2022), 398–400

78. C. Teaching
Rationale: Depending on the type of educational institution, nurse educators may or may not be required to conduct research or service (Choices A and B). All educators should be good teachers and leaders (Choice D). However, the primary role of all educators, regardless of the type of program, is teaching (Choice C).
Reference: Billings & Halstead (2020), pp. 4–8

79. D. Ensure protection of research participants
Rationale: The purpose of an IRB is to ensure ethical conduct and to ensure protection of subjects when disseminating findings from any research project (Choice D). The other choices are not within the purview of the IRB (Choices A, B, and C).
Reference: DeBoor (2023), p. 99

80. A. Obtaining certification in nursing education
Rationale: Joining a professional organization is not the same as influencing its work or accepting a leadership position. Therefore Choice B is not the correct response. Teaching an online course and submitting a manuscript are typical educator activities and do not best demonstrate leadership (Choices C and D). However, taking the certification in nursing education recognizes the special knowledge and expertise needed to be competent as an academic nurse educator. Therefore Choice A is the best answer.
Reference: Billings & Halstead (2020), pp. 4–8

81. B. Creating a vision for the department
Rationale: Formal leaders in education who are part of nursing administration are responsible for providing direction for the nursing department by creating and implementing a vision; therefore Choice B is the correct response. The leader may also participate in the other choices (A, C, and D), but these activities are not the most important quality for department success.
Reference: Halstead (2019), pp. 107–116

82. D. Ensuring the group is ready for the change
Rationale: The role of a change agent, who may be from within or outside the organization, is to facilitate the desired change, starting with evaluating if the group is ready to change (Choice D). The change agent does not decide on the need for change (Choice C) or plan and implement the change for the faculty (Choices A and B).
Reference: Iwasiw et al. (2020), pp. 134–147

83. C. Integrate nursing leadership competencies throughout the curriculum.
Rationale: Developing a case study on nursing leadership and assigning learners to partner with a nursing leader are one-time activities that would help them learn about leadership skills (Choices B and D). However, integrating multiple leadership competencies throughout the curriculum provides a more effective method for promoting leadership skills for learners, making Choice C correct. Choice A is an assessment method and not a learning activity.
Reference: Oermann et al. (2022), pp. 79–80

84. C. Collaborating with interprofessional faculty to develop a new course
Rationale: Nurse educators can demonstrate leadership at the program, department, and/or institutional level. Collaborating with faculty from other disciplines to develop a new course demonstrates leadership to meet learner needs and is therefore the correct response (Choice C). The other choices are department or program activities (Choices A, B, and D).
Reference: Halstead (2019), pp. 119–129

85. B. Ensuring cultural sensitivity and inclusivity
Rationale: At times, planning a change on a department or organizational level requires an external expert consultant. However, this action is an option and not a requirement (Choice A). Including faculty, staff, and learner input may be needed for some institutional changes, but they are not always required (Choices C and D). Every institutional change does require cultural awareness and sensitivity to ensure its success (Choice B) to foster and maintain a positive organizational climate.
Reference: Halstead (2019), pp. 112–115

86. A. Transformational
Rationale: The administrator using a participative leadership style would involve all faculty, which promotes faculty morale. However, the decision-making process is very slow and communication can be noneffective. This style does not help retain faculty (Choice B). As a transactional leader, the administrator sets specific achievable goals for the team, and team motivation and productivity may increase. Faculty satisfaction and retention are not necessarily improved with this type of leadership (Choice C). Authoritative leadership allows leaders to make decisions and can cause faculty rebellion (Choice D). Transformational leaders role model their vision and empower faculty to motivate them. The result is usually increased faculty satisfaction and retention; thus Choice A is the correct response.
Reference: Iwasiw et al. (2020), p. 222

87. A. Unfreezing
Rationale: The first phase of the change process using Lewin's theory is unfreezing, which is needed when faculty do not want to change or do not support the change. Therefore Choice A is the correct response. Choices B and C are not phases in Lewin's mode, and refreezing occurs after the change is made to ensure it will continue (Choice D).
Reference: Iwasiw et al. (2020), pp. 90–92

88. B. Serve on a professional organization's legislative committee.
Rationale: The nurse educator needs to role model political advocacy for learners. Although all of these choices demonstrate ways to learn about this attribute (Choices A, C, and D), serving on a legislative committee shows commitment by the educator to political advocacy (Choice B).
Reference: Halstead (2019), pp. 117–120

89. D. Learners meet the program learning outcomes and graduate.
Rationale: The purpose of evaluation during the admissions process is to ascertain whether learners have achieved their potential and have acquired the knowledge, skills, and abilities set forth in learning activities, courses, and curricula (Choice D). Self-directed learning may be a learning style preference, but it is not an evaluation measure related to the admissions process (Choice A). Learners that require little direction may be admitted to the program; however, feedback and collaboration are a best practice in nursing and should be encouraged. These factors are also not an evaluation measure related to the admissions process (Choice A). In general, learners should not be expected to meet clinical outcomes without feedback from their instructors (Choice B), and this does not provide evidence of an effective admissions policy. Learners admitted to the program exceeding minimum grade requirements (Choice C) is only one measure of academic success, and the expectation would be that learners meet—not necessarily exceed—the requirements.
Reference: Billings & Halstead (2020), pp. 451, 475–476

90. C. Provides information on effectiveness of teaching and learning methods
Rationale: Nurse educators need to evaluate their courses and whether learners are achieving course outcomes. Primarily, this activity allows nurse educators to gather information on the effectiveness of teaching and learning methods (Choice C) and make necessary modifications to improve the methods used. Course evaluations may produce data for program evaluation and accreditation (Choice A), may provide insight into whether additional resources are needed (Choice B), and may also uncover personal opportunities for improvement for the nurse educator (Choice D).
Reference: Oermann (2017), p. 23

91. D. Require learners to describe conflict resolution strategies to promote teamwork among staff in an acute care setting.
Rationale: The emphasis in the cognitive domain of learning is on knowledge attainment. Therefore requiring learners to describe conflict resolution strategies to promote teamwork

among staff in an acute care setting (Choice D) assesses learning in the cognitive domain. Demonstrating safe sterile technique in the insertion of an indwelling urinary catheter (Choice A) and gathering needed supplies to correctly change a peripheral intravenous line dressing (Choice B) assess the psychomotor domains of learning. Asking learners to justify the application of cultural competence skills when conducting health assessments (Choice C) assesses the affective domain of learning.
Reference: Billings & Halstead (2020), pp. 188–189

92. C. Determine the learners' ability to prepare intravenous medications before administration.
Rationale: The emphasis of the psychomotor domain is on developing manual or physical competencies. Nursing skills are usually the focus of psychomotor learning. Determining the learner's ability to safely prepare a patient's intravenous medications before administration (Choice C) is a method the novice nurse educator can use to assess learning in the psychomotor domain. Observing communication between learners and their assigned patients (Choice A) assesses the affective domain. Reviewing learners' assessment findings documented in the medical record for accuracy (Choice B) and assessing the learners' knowledge of their patients' medication before administration (Choice D) assess the cognitive domain.
Reference: Billings & Halstead (2020), pp. 190–191

93. A. Evaluate a learner's written reflection on clinical experiences with a dying patient.
Rationale: The emphasis of the affective domain is on attitudes, beliefs, values, feelings, and emotions. Evaluating learners' written reflection on clinical experiences (Choice A) assesses their attitudes and beliefs related to the clinical experiences. Reviewing a learner's competency checklist before doing a dressing change (Choice B) assesses the psychomotor domain. Critiquing a learner's clinical assignment submission and offering feedback for improvement (Choice C) and asking the learner to describe the significance of laboratory results for a patient with chronic kidney disease (Choice D) evaluate the cognitive domain.
Reference: Billings & Halstead (2020), pp. 189–190

94. D. To determine if learners met expected outcomes
Rationale: Assessment and evaluation are critical in nursing education to obtain important information about learning, to evaluate competencies and learner progression in meeting expected outcomes, and to enable decision making about needed improvements (Choice D). Learner engagement and learner satisfaction (Choices A and B) may be improved using evidenced-based assessment and evaluation practices in nursing education; however, decision making is the primary purpose. Data generated from these practices may be used to satisfy regulatory requirements (Choice C), with the primary purpose being to enable programmatic decision making for improvements.
Reference: Oermann & Gaberson (2021), p. 3

95. B. Relate the rubric criteria to the learning objectives of the course.
Rationale: When developing a rubric to be used for evaluation of written assignments, the rubric criteria should be related to the learning outcomes of the course (Choice B) to ensure alignment of the assignment and expected performance. Specifying the number of drafts to be submitted with due dates (Choice A) and providing a template for learners to use when developing the assignment (Choice C) is helpful supplemental information that will likely improve the quality of the work submitted by learners, but do not relate to developing the rubric for evaluation purposes. Reviewing assignment guidelines with learners before they begin working on it (Choice D) may also be helpful to the learners and will likely improve their work, but it is also not related to the development of the rubric itself.
Reference: Oermann & Gaberson (2021), pp. 166–168

96. B. Provides a way of evaluating learning outcome achievement
Rationale: The most common use of tests is to assign grades and, in this way, to primarily serve as a way of evaluating learning outcomes (Choice B). Tests provide summative evaluation of

learning, which can then be used to determine grades. Test performance does not give direct insight into learner clinical performance ability (Choice A); depending on the learner, test performance may be aligned with clinical performance, or it can be the opposite. Test performance may indirectly assist the nurse educator in determining teaching effectiveness (Choice C) and indirectly allow for interpretation of projected learner performance on the final course examination (Choice D); however, its primary purpose is to evaluate learning outcome achievement.
Reference: Billings & Halstead (2020), pp. 25, 474–475

97. C. The scores of a group of individuals being evaluated form the basis for comparison.
Rationale: Norm-referenced interpretation of tests refers to interpreting data in terms of group norms. The scores of a group form the basis of comparison (Choice C). On the other hand, in criterion-referenced test interpretation, scores are judged against preestablished criteria (Choice A), it typically involves evaluation of competency-based learning models (Choice B), and there is an emphasis on mastery and potential for all learners to achieve competence (Choice D).
Reference: Billings & Halstead (2020), pp. 445–446

98. A. It reflects whether learners have met predetermined learning outcomes.
Rationale: Criterion-referenced test interpretations are judged against preestablished criteria; in this case the criteria are learning outcomes (Choice A). Norm-referenced interpretation allows for interpretation of groups of learners in terms of norms, or national performance (Choice B). There is the ability to make comparisons within the learner group and outside the group (Choice C). In this method of interpretation there will always be learners who achieve the highest-level scores and those who achieve the lowest-level scores (Choice D), but the criteria are preestablished and not based on those scores.
Reference: Billings & Halstead (2020), p. 446

99. D. Determine the learning outcomes to be measured.
Rationale: The purpose of developing a test blueprint is to ensure the test measures what it intends to measure and serves its intended purpose. The first step in developing a test blueprint is to determine the learning outcomes to be measured (Choice D). The second step is to determine the instructional content to be evaluated (Choice C) followed by deciding on the weight to be assigned to each area (Choice A). The type and number of items (Choice B) should be determined last.
Reference: Billings & Halstead (2020), p. 476

100. D. The reliability of test scores increases as the length of the test increases.
Rationale: Test length is an important factor that should be guided by the purpose of the test, abilities of the learners, item formats being used, amount of testing time available, and desired reliability of test scores. In general, the reliability of test scores increases as the length of the assessment increases (Choice D). Validity (not reliability) improves by having other educators review the test (Choice A). Test validity also depends on adequate content coverage of the test (Choice B). Validity (not reliability) can also be addressed by having varying item types on the test (Choice C).
Reference: Oermann & Gaberson (2021), pp. 49–50

101. B. Unit exams
Rationale: The nurse educator uses collaborative testing, which is an assessment method where small groups or pairs of learners work together during unit exams (Choice B). This method involves the learners taking the same test twice, once individually and then again collaboratively. Clinical case studies (Choice A), simulation experiences (Choice C), or scholarly papers (Choice D) may serve as the basis or be a component of a formative assessment but do not incorporate collaborative testing.
Reference: Oermann & Gaberson (2021), pp. 192–194

102. A. Educator bias

Rationale: Observation is a common strategy used to evaluate learner performance in the clinical setting. There are threats to the reliability and validity of observation as an evaluation strategy because of the nurse educator's values, attitudes, and biases (Choice A). The educator needs to be aware of biases and take steps to be as fair and consistent as possible in evaluating learner performance. The clinical setting (Choice B), patient diagnosis (Choice C), and learner attitude (Choice D) are considered as part of the evaluation but usually do not have an impact on the evaluation process.

Reference: Oermann & Gaberson (2021), pp. 269–270

103. C. Beginning self-assessment with the first clinical course

Rationale: Self-assessment is an evaluation approach that can be used as a part of evaluation of learner performance in the clinical setting. Ideally, self-assessment begins with the first clinical course in a program (Choice C). If started at the end of the program (Choice A), there is less opportunity to identify strengths and areas of improvement. Self-assessment is often included as part of the clinical rather than theory grade (Choice B). Self-assessment is conducted before or at the same time as the educator's evaluation of the learner's clinical performance (Choice D).

Reference: Oermann & Gaberson (2021), pp. 290–291

104. D. The exam demonstrates internal consistency.

Rationale: Test reliability refers to the degree to which a test measures or evaluates learning consistently over time (Choice D). A KR-20 of 0.73 is considered acceptable reliability and therefore is not unreliable (Choice A). Test validity refers to the exam measuring intended concepts (Choice B). If validity or reliability is violated, certain items on the exam likely require revision (Choice C); however, in this example, reliability is acceptable.

Reference: Oermann & Gaberson (2021), p. 246

105. A. 68% of learners who took the test got this item correct.

Rationale: A p level for a test item indicates the percentage of learners who got the item correct expressed as a decimal. The p level in this item is 0.68, which when converted to a percentage (move the decimal point two digits to the right) means that 68% of the learners who took the test got the item correct. Therefore Choice A is the correct response. The p level represents the item difficulty, not discrimination (Choice B) or reliability (Choice C). Choice D is not the answer, as explained.

Reference: Oermann & Gaberson (2021), pp. 232–233

106. B. Choices B and C

Rationale: For a four-choice multiple-choice test item, one choice is correct and the others are incorrect. The incorrect choices are called distractors. For most items, the nurse educator would want more test takers to select the correct response more often than selecting one of the distractors. For the sample item in this question, only 5 of 39 learners selected the correct response. However, 16 learners selected B—three times more learners selected this choice. Therefore if using this difficult item in the future, at a minimum, the educator should possibly revise the answer, Choice C, and the distractor that most test takers selected, that is, Choice B (making Choice B the correct response). If the educator desires, all of the choices could be revisited, but the priority would be B and C. Choices A and D in the question do not include Choice C in the sample test item.

Reference: Oermann & Gaberson (2021), pp. 232–233

107. D. This test item discriminated well between high and low scorers.

Rationale: The point biserial (PBS) coefficient is the appropriate measure of discrimination for multiple-choice items (Choice A). The desired PBS for a multiple-choice test item is a high value, preferably above 0.20, but greater than 0.10 is marginally acceptable. The PBS for the sample item is 0.39 because it is the PBS associated with the correct response, or Choice B. This high

PBS demonstrates that the high scorers on the test selected the correct response much more than the lower scorers. The PBS values for the distractors are very low or negative, which shows that the lower scorers selected these choices much more than the higher scores. Therefore the sample test item discriminated very well between high and low scorers (Choice D), and the item does not need to be nullified (Choice C). PBS is a measure of item discrimination, not difficulty (Choice B).
Reference: Oermann & Gaberson (2021), pp. 234–235

108. C. This test question should be nullified because it poorly discriminated.
Rationale: In this sample item the PBS for the correct choice (and thus for the item) is very low, at 0.05. One of the distractors had a very high PBS, showing that high scorers selected that choice. Because the sample item negatively or poorly discriminates, the item should be nullified (Choice C). Nullification means that all choices of the item are accepted as correct because the item was poorly written, causing unacceptable discrimination. Choices A, B, and D are therefore incorrect.
Reference: Oermann & Gaberson (2021), pp. 234–235

109. B. Course grade of B
Rationale: The learner earned 122 + 27 + 25 + 16 = 190 points. To determine the percentage of points the learner obtained, divide 190 by the total possible course points of 225: 190/225 = 84.44%, which falls within the range for a course grade of a B (83%–91%). Therefore the answer to the test item is Choice B. This means that the Choices A, C, and D are not correct grades.
Reference: Oermann & Gaberson (2021), pp. 338–339

110. A. To establish content-related evidence of measurement validity
Rationale: The most important component of a test blueprint is learning outcomes, also called course objectives. Identifying these objectives helps the educator ensure that the test items will measure what was intended to be measured. This purpose is called content-related evidence of measurement validity, content-related validity, or merely content validity (Choice A). If learners have access to the blueprint, they may find it helpful to study for the test, but that is not the primary purpose of the blueprint (Choice C). A test blueprint does not indicate or ensure any type of reliability (Choices B and D).
Reference: Oermann & Gaberson (2021), p. 56

111. B. Interrater reliability
Rationale: A clinical evaluation tool is used by multiple nurse educators in a course. Each educator uses this tool to evaluate the clinical performance of a small group of learners. Therefore it is important that the educators use the tool in the same way. Establishing interrater reliability is needed to ensure fair and accurate evaluations (Choice B). The other types of reliability are not applicable for this type of tool (Choices A, C, and D).
Reference: Oermann & Gaberson (2021), p. 293

112. C. One-minute paper
Rationale: Capstone assignments and final examinations are used as summative assessments (Choices B and D). The portfolio is also usually used for summative assessment (Choice A). However, the one-minute paper is intended to assess what learners have gained as a result of an ongoing learning experience. If content has not been learned as evidenced by the one-minute paper, there is an opportunity to remediate or provide additional teaching (Choice C).
Reference: Oermann & Gaberson (2021), pp. 9–10

113. D. Observation of learner's performance
Rationale: Choices A and B are written clinical assignments that supplement clinical performance, but they are not the best way to assess clinical competence. Direct observation of the learner by the educator is the best way to assess clinical competence and performance (Choice

D). Weekly progress notes are a written record of how learners performed and are part of the formative assessment (Choice C).
Reference: Oermann et al. (2022), p. 309

114. C. "I gave the preceptors our clinical evaluation tool so they can complete it for each learner."
Rationale: The statement in Choice C needs follow-up by the mentor because it is incorrect. Nurse educators are responsible for evaluating learner performance in any clinical model because they have the expertise to do this. Preceptors are not educators, but they can provide feedback on the learner's progress. The other statements are correct in that it is also the responsibility of the educator to orient, monitor, and mentor selected preceptors (Choices A and B). The educator should also ask preceptors and learners about how effectiveness of the preceptorship experience by completing an evaluation that can be trended and analyzed by course faculty (Choice D).
Reference: Billings & Halstead (2020), p. 346

115. B. Comprehensive final examination
Rationale: Formative assessment occurs during a learning experience to provide learners with the opportunity to improve. Unit examinations, quizzes, and the muddiest point are formative assessment methods (Choices A, C, and D). The comprehensive final exam is given at the end of the course and tests content from the entire course as a summative evaluation, making Choice B correct.
Reference: Oermann & Gaberson (2021), pp. 9–10

116. A. The test item is likely too easy.
Rationale: A p level of 0.97 means that 97% of the learners who answered the item on the test got the correct answer. Ninety-seven percent is almost the entire class, making the test item likely too easy (Choice A). Therefore the item is not too difficult (Choice B). The p level is about test item difficulty and not about discrimination (Choices C and D).
Reference: Oermann & Gaberson (2021), pp. 232–233

117. D. The feedback should be frequent, timely, and constructive.
Rationale: Learners need frequent, timely, and constructive feedback about their performance and progress during a course (Choice D), not once or twice (Choices B and C). Frequent feedback allows learners the opportunity to improve in any area in which they are not meeting course expectations. Feedback should not be recorded unless the learner has permission from the nurse educator (Choice A).
Reference: Billings & Halstead (2020), pp. 338–340

118. B. Use a validated instrument for assessing learning style.
Rationale: Obtaining information about learners and their learning style preferences is a very helpful measure in the facilitation of learning. Nurse educators interested in assessing learning style preferences for their learners can begin this process by using a validated instrument (Choice B). Determining learning style based on age of learners (Choice A) and deciphering learning style based on current learner study habits (Choice C) are not helpful in providing information about learning style. In fact, the study habits should be based on the learning style preferences once determined. The nurse educator developing and administering a survey asking about learning preferences (Choice D) is not the best method to assess learning style because the survey has not been validated; many validated instruments can be used to do this.
Reference: Billings & Halstead (2020), pp. 30–31

119. A. Practicing listening to heart sounds in the skills laboratory
Rationale: Kinesthetic learners prefer hands-on experiential learning, such as performing physical assessment skills like practicing listening to heart sounds (Choice A). Listening to a recorded slide presentation would appeal best to auditory learners (Choice B); watching a video would be

preferred by visual learners (Choice C). The read-write learner would prefer taking notes on class reading (Choice D).
Reference: Billings & Halstead (2020), pp. 29–30

120.   **C.** Faculty development focused on online instruction
Rationale: Distance education systems are constantly undergoing rapid change and are becoming a mainstay in the delivery of education. Use of distance learning technology requires significant planning and time for development in addition to support for the nurse educators. To enable nurse educators to provide distance-accessible programs that meet the educational needs of learners enrolled in online courses, faculty development opportunities focused on online instruction (Choice C) need to be available. Online course management software (Choice A), information technology support for learners (Choice B), and communication platforms for collaboration with learners (Choice D) are all necessary resources for quality distance education, but they do not specifically assist the nurse educators in providing quality distance education as much as faculty development opportunities do.
Reference: Billings & Halstead (2020), pp. 392–395

121.   **C.** Tend to be self-directed, flexible, and technology adept
Rationale: The nurse educator is charged with supporting educational environments in which generational diversity is accepted. Doing so aids in creating better learning opportunities. Understanding the common characteristics of each generation will assist the nurse educator in responding effectively to each generation's learning needs. Generation X learners tend to be self-directed, flexible, and technology adept (Choice C). Millennials, or Generation Y learners, are accustomed to structure and very little free time (Choice A) and are often optimistic, team-oriented, and rule following (Choice B). Generation Z learners absorb information instantaneously and lose interest quickly (Choice D).
Reference: Billings & Halstead (2020), pp. 18–20

122.   **D.** Audience response systems
Rationale: Nurse educators continue to face the arrival of new technologies that affect teaching and learning. Educators need to remain apprised of the new educational technology capabilities that can be integrated into course requirements as a way of responding to learning needs. To promote engagement during class activities, the educator could use audience response systems (Choice D), which are systems that gather learner responses to a question asked during class and display the results for everyone to see. Having this information available provides the educator with the opportunity to address gaps or deficits in learning in real time. Electronic books (Choice A) are available for learners and can be used on a number of different devices. Although these may be convenient for the learner, they do not directly support engagement during class activities. Podcasting or live captures (Choice B) are compressed audio files or recorded lectures that provide ways for educators to make class recordings available for asynchronous viewing. Although these may also be helpful in facilitating learning, they do not promote learner engagement during class activities. Drug reference manuals (Choice C) are invaluable resources for the learner and can be used on a number of different devices and to provide needed information quickly and easily. These resources are particularly helpful in the clinical setting but also do not directly promote learner engagement during class activities.
Reference: Billings & Halstead (2020), pp. 375–387

123.   **A.** Using a virtual simulator in a flipped classroom
Rationale: Nurse educators have learned of the importance of creating and implementing teaching methodologies in the classroom that replace inactive traditional classroom learning. Simulation is one way to do this and, in particular, using a virtual simulator in a flipped classroom (Choice A) is one way the nurse educator can incorporate simulation as an active learning strategy in the classroom setting. Employing Socratic questioning (Choice B) and dividing learners into groups

to construct a concept map (Choice C) are both active learning strategies but do not specifically relate to facilitating learning using simulation. Assigning a classroom debate on ethics (Choice D) is an active learning strategy, not a simulation activity.
Reference: Billings & Halstead (2020), pp. 358–359

124. D. Clinical judgment and critical thinking

Rationale: Evidence supports the use of the clinical simulation process and, in particular, debriefing within that process, as a way of promoting clinical judgment and critical thinking skills (Choice D). Debriefing allows for direct interaction in the clinical scenario, allowing for critical thinking and decision making and clinical judgment opportunities. Time management (Choice A) may indirectly be developed through repeated use of clinical simulation, but it is not specific to the debriefing aspect. Clinical skills and techniques (Choice B) and a broadened nursing knowledge base (Choice C) are not direct outcomes of debriefing during simulation.
Reference: Cannon & Boswell (2016), pp. 223–226

125. B. Case studies

Rationale: Learning opportunities to develop critical thinking and clinical judgment in the classroom are very important to learners in nursing courses and programs. Inactive teaching and learning strategies are not useful in promoting critical thinking and the abilities needed for the nurse. Case studies (Choice B) are a teaching and learning strategy that can be used to promote the development of critical thinking. Other strategies include role-playing and problem-based learning. Lecture (Choice A), assigned reading (Choice C), and written assignments (Choice D) are inactive or passive learning strategies and therefore are not the best methods to promote the development of critical thinking.
Reference: Cannon & Boswell (2016), p. 163

126. B. Group projects

Rationale: Practical use of adult learning theory may include the following learning strategies: group collaboration projects (Choice B), self-study activities, self-directed learning, self-paced learning modules, service learning, case-based learning, observation, and case studies. Concept mapping (Choice A) and peer-to-peer teaching (Choice C) align best with social learning theory. Creating drug cards aligns best with cognitive learning theory (Choice D).
Reference: Billings & Halstead (2020), p. 251

127. D. Clinical simulation

Rationale: Experiential learning theory, often called "learning by doing," involves concrete experiences, reflection, abstract conceptualization, and active experimentation. Clinical simulation (Choice D) is a teaching and learning strategy that allows the learner to accomplish this and is reflective of experiential learning. Brief lectures (Choice A), practice questions (Choice B), and clinical care plans (Choice C) are teaching and learning strategies that do not address aspects of the experiential learning theory as clinical simulation does; in particular, active experimentation is not supported by these strategies.
Reference: Billings & Halstead (2020), p. 252

128. D. Understanding the needs of learners

Rationale: Clinical education often does not offer opportunities for learners to engage in more complex aspects of nursing practice for a variety of reasons. Nurse educators are charged with improving clinical education. Synergy between learners and facilitators of learning, such as the clinical instructors understanding the needs of learners (Choice D), is key to a positive clinical learning experience, and often nurse educators need to advocate for learning in the clinical setting. Although clinical site availability (Choice A), learner confidence and self-efficacy (Choice B), and having an adequate number of patient assignments (Choice C) are also important factors

in clinical learning, they are not the most important or key factors in promoting a positive clinical experience. This starts with having an environment that promotes learning.
Reference: Halstead (2019), pp. 24–27

129. **B.** Generational differences
Rationale: Considering previous life experiences in learning needs is an important part of facilitating learning. The nurse educator should begin by considering generational differences as a starting point (Choice B) because these differences are often common to generational cohorts and can create a disconnect between learners and educators if not considered. From here, considering individual characteristics such as military status (Choice A), previous work experiences (Choice C), and racial and ethnic background (Choice D) are effective ways to individualize the teaching and learning process.
Reference: Billings & Halstead (2020), pp. 16–18

130. **A.** Mentorship
Rationale: Academic success initiatives are needed for both learners and faculty to promote retention. Mentorship (Choice A) is one of the best methods to increase retention of diverse learners. Mentoring helps provide role modeling opportunities for learners and educators and addresses both academic and nonacademic needs for learners. Academic support (Choice B) and English-language programs (Choice D) are helpful resources for diverse learners, but these resources do not address the nonacademic needs and are not typically resources available to educators. Leadership development (Choice C) is important for both learners and educators and may offer support in varying ways; mentorship, however, is more directed and individualized and therefore is the best method to promote retention.
Reference: Billings & Halstead (2020), pp. 25–26

131. **C.** Clinical competence in nursing practice
Rationale: The priority for clinical teaching is competence in teaching and competence in nursing practice (Choice C) to ensure patient safety. Leadership and management skills (Choice A), effective communication skills (Choice B), and ability to collaborate with others (Choice D) are helpful skills in clinical teaching, but they are not as important as clinical competence.
Reference: Billings & Halstead (2020), pp. 340–341

132. **A.** Using class time to clarify and illustrate concepts
Rationale: Promoting a supportive and engaging learning environment is essential to integrating teaching-learning strategies aimed at developing critical thinking in the classroom environment. Using class time to clarify and illustrate concepts (Choice A), ideally done after the learners review information on their own outside of class, is a strategy that is effective in achieving this. Coordinating guest lecturers on specialty topic areas (Choice B), placing additional resources on the course learning management system (Choice C), and asking the learners to take detailed notes during lecture (Choice D) are not active learning strategies and therefore do not assist in developing critical thinking in the classroom.
Reference: Cannon & Boswell (2016), pp. 161–163

133. **C.** Using learning activities that incorporate research utilization
Rationale: Research utilization (Choice C) is an effective way to promote critical thinking in clinical learning. It allows learners to understand and interpret evidence and translate it into practice. Assigning discussion board assignments focusing on clinical reflection (Choice A), requiring learners to complete clinical care plans before the clinical day (Choice B), and ensuring learners understand pathophysiology concepts for disease processes encountered in the clinical setting (Choice D) may also assist with promoting critical thinking in the clinical setting, but they are not the best approaches. The nurse educator would need to use additional methods to assess critical thinking.
Reference: Cannon & Boswell (2016), pp. 226–229

134. C. Ensure opportunities for collaboration.

Rationale: The nurse educator should use a variety of strategies to promote a culture of caring in the learning environment. Ensuring opportunities for collaboration and creativity, such as by pairing peers to work together on an assignment (Choice C), is an effective strategy. Minimizing communication between peers (Choice A) does not promote a caring learning environment because peer learner relationships are an important aspect of creating this climate. Emphasizing socialization to the nursing role by encouraging learners to interact with nursing staff (Choice B) is important, but it does not specifically contribute to promoting a culture of caring in learning. Presenting caring theory content in postconference (Choice D) will likely support learning but is not a specific strategy to promote a culture of caring in the clinical environment.

Reference: Billings & Halstead (2020), pp. 286–288

135. D. Piloting the technology

Rationale: Active learning is an important teaching strategy for learners in nursing. Audience response systems are a technologic advancement that promote interaction in learning. The nurse educator should pilot the technology first (Choice D) to determine any problems or glitches. Using the technology to assess learning (Choice A) should not be done until the technology has been piloted. Next, surveying learners on their perception of the system (Choice C) would be helpful, and then the nurse educator could make decisions about integrating the technology into all planned lessons (Choice B) based on the overall experience.

Reference: Billings & Halstead (2020), pp. 286–288

136. A. Developing clinical decision-making abilities

Rationale: Clinical education provides a foundation for learners in nursing and provides an avenue for application of learned information to practice. The nurse educator should prioritize the development of decision-making abilities (Choice A) among learners in a clinical setting, as this is what will be required of them as new nurses. Often, there is an incorrectly placed emphasis on observing learners performing nursing skills (Choice B) as the priority outcome in clinical learning; although this is important, there should be a greater emphasis on decision-making abilities. Offering equitable clinical assignments among learners (Choice C) is not feasible given the dynamic nature of health care and the varying needs of patients cared for in this setting. In addition, the nurse educator can use a variety of patient assignments to meet clinical outcomes. The clinical environment is a strategic setting to provide guidance for socialization into the profession (Choice D), but once again, the emphasis should be on developing decision-making abilities.

Reference: Cannon & Boswell (2016), pp. 226–230

137. B. Strong clinical practice partnerships

Rationale: Clinical education is critical to learning in nursing programs. Nurse educators should seek continued improvement of clinical experiences. Strong clinical practice partnerships (Choice B) are foundational to supporting the quality of clinical learning. Having good relationships with clinical partners provides the nurse educator with the tools and resources needed to support learning. Qualified clinical nurse educators (Choice A) and validated clinical learning evaluation tools (Choice C) are also integral to learning, but without a strong clinical practice partnership, these resources would not assist in improving clinical experiences for learners. Integration of high-fidelity simulation in clinical learning (Choice D) is an excellent addition to augment clinical learning, but it is not foundational and cannot be the only method to achieve clinical learning outcomes.

Reference: Halstead (2019), pp. 24–27

138. C. Ability to critically appraise the literature

Rationale: Integration of evidence-based teaching strategies has become an expectation in nursing education. As evidence is becoming available in the literature, the ability to critically appraise the literature (Choice C) is critical to the successful integration of evidence-based teaching

strategies. This will allow nurse educators to know what the strategies are and will provide them with information about how to successfully use recommendations from the literature. Public speaking proficiency (Choice A) is not a necessary skill to do this; however, often, decisions are made based on individuals who are most vocal. Educators should be mindful and aware of this potential barrier to integration of evidence in teaching. A willingness to take on complex tasks (Choice B) is helpful; however, not all strategies integrated will be overly complex. Understanding of high-level statistical analyses (Choice D) is not a necessary skill in this endeavor.
Reference: Cannon & Boswell (2016), pp. 19–21

139. D. Low-fidelity simulation
Rationale: Educational technology allows nurse educators to achieve learning outcomes more deliberately and efficiently. Low-fidelity simulation (Choice D) includes using case studies and role-playing. Static mannequins (Choice A) are meant to allow learners to practice specific skills, but on their own they are not as useful as low-fidelity simulation in accommodating these strategies. App-based practice questions (Choice B) are helpful in promoting knowledge application, but they are not as useful as integrating case studies and role-playing. Electronic information resources (Choice C) may be accessed as part of a scenario that uses a case study and role-playing, but they are not the most helpful technology in doing so.
Reference: Cannon & Boswell (2016), pp. 217–218

140. D. College degree
Rationale: Choices A, B, and C are intrinsic motivational factors for learning because they are internal qualities within individuals. Earning a college degree is an extrinsic motivational factor for learning because it is not an internal individual characteristic, making Choice D correct.
Reference: Billings & Halstead (2020), pp. 27–28

141. A. Audio recording of breath sounds
Rationale: The auditory learner enjoys hearing information and would prefer the audio recording of breath sounds (Choice A). Attending a lecture would also appeal to the auditory learner (Choice D) but that is not the most appropriate teaching-learning activity. Listening to breath sounds on a patient would be appropriate for the kinesthetic learner (Choice B). Interpreting breath sounds (Choice C) requires analysis in the cognitive learning domain and could be appropriate for many types of learners.
Reference: Billings & Halstead (2020), pp. 29–30

142. B. It fosters student engagement in the learning process.
Rationale: Active learning strategies promote learner engagement, which facilitates understanding and possible application of knowledge (Choice B). Although some active learning strategies can be practiced in groups, this is not a requirement (Choice C). Active learning can occur individually, in pairs, and/or in larger groups. Planning and implementing active learning strategies often take more time and are more challenging for educators (Choice A). Using active learning is not a primary principle of adult learning; some adults prefer more traditional passive strategies such as lecture (Choice D).
Reference: Billings & Halstead (2020), p. 187

143. C. Select a later time to talk with staff about how they perceive the learners' experiences.
Rationale: In this situation, approaching the staff nurses at this time may cause them to become defensive and is not the best action (Choice A). However, the comments should not be ignored or reported to nursing administration (Choices A and D). The best approach is to get feedback from staff at a later time about how the clinical experience with learners is going, which is important in going forward in this experience and for planning future experiences, making Choice C correct.
Reference: Oermann et al. (2022), p. 213

144. B. Provide alternative hands-on clinical experiences in the campus simulation laboratory.
Rationale: The clinical hours must be made up and should be made up with equivalent experiences such as simulation (Choice B). Clinical paper assignments do not replace hands-on care of patients (Choice C). Students are obligated to fulfill clinical practice hour requirements as soon as possible (Choice A). Learning in other environments does not substitute for clinical practice (Choice D).
Reference: Oermann et al. (2022), pp. 171–175

145. D. "When do you need to start the IV so I can be available to help you?"
Rationale: The most important quality of a clinical nurse educator is clinical competence and expertise (Choice D). Therefore the educator would agree to find the time, assist with the procedure, and supervise the learner who wants to start a peripheral IV line. Performing a skill on an actual patient is a better learning experience than practicing the skill in the lab (Choice C). It is not the responsibility of the staff nurses to take time from their work to supervise the learner (Choices A and B).
Reference: Billings & Halstead (2020), pp. 187–188

146. A. Ask staff nurses for help with selecting patient assignments for learners.
Rationale: Involving staff nurses in the clinical experience would likely help with relationship building, especially if the educator asked for their assistance to help build their self-concept. Therefore Choice A is the correct response. Based on accountability, learners should always communicate first with staff nurses regarding any patient changes or other information (Choice B). Attending a staff meeting would benefit the educator but would not necessarily help build a strong relationship (Choice C). Offering a staff development session would also not necessarily help strengthen educator–staff relationships (Choice D).
Reference: Billings & Halstead (2020), p. 333

147. B. Patience
Rationale: Although clinical competence is the most important clinical nurse educator attribute, it does not guarantee that the educator knows how to facilitate learning and decrease learner anxiety (Choice A). Confidence and respect are also important attributes of the educator in a clinical setting, but they do not necessarily mean that the educator can facilitate learning and decrease learner anxiety (Choices C and D). However, patience is needed when trying to teach learners in the clinical setting because they are often slower than practicing nurses when completing any task or skill. Additionally, being patient often helps to decrease anxiety, especially for learners who lack confidence or are having difficulty providing care, making Choice B correct.
Reference: Oermann et al. (2022), pp. 209–213

148. C. Games
Rationale: Games like *Jeopardy!* are the most appropriate way to engage learners in active learning to help them acquire, retain, and retrieve knowledge (Choice C). Case studies (Choice A), concept maps (Choice B), and discussion forums (Choice D) stimulate and develop critical thinking and clinical reasoning using retrieved knowledge and are therefore not the correct response.
Reference: Billings & Halstead (2020), p. 294

149. C. Using a just culture approach
Rationale: A just culture approach does not blame an individual for an error or near-miss, which helps the learner feel safe and motivated in the learning environment. This type of approach is best for learners and health care professionals who face challenges every day (Choice C). Providing feedback to correct learner errors (Choice A) can be very intimidating if the feedback is not constructive. Learners often enjoy pairing with staff nurses (Choice D) because they obtain insight into current nursing practice from the staff's perspectives. However, this method may or

may not motivate learners. Presenting patient cases in postconference (Choice B) can facilitate learning but does not necessarily motivate learners.

Reference: Oermann et al. (2022), p. 226

150. D. Learners prepare for class by completing learning activities.

Rationale: Using a flipped classroom approach requires learners to prepare in advance before class by completing reading and written learning activities (Choice D). Learners do not usually conduct a literature search before class (Choice A); readiness testing is associated with team-based learning (Choice B), and group presentations may be part of any type of classroom or online approach (Choice C).

Reference: Billings & Halstead (2020), p. 292

References for Answers and Rationales

American Association of Colleges and Universities (AACU). (2008). *High impact educational practices.* https://www.aacu.org/node/4084.

Bastable, S. (2016). *Essentials of patient education.* Burlington, MA: Jones & Bartlett Learning.

Billings, D. M., & Halstead, J. A. (2020). *Teaching in nursing: A guide for faculty* (6th ed.). St. Louis: Elsevier.

Bradshaw, M. J., Hultquist, B. L., & Hagler, D. (2021). *Innovative teaching strategies in nursing and related health professions.* Burlington, MA: Jones & Bartlett Learning.

Cadet, M. J. (2021). Examining the learning characteristics of nursing students: A literature review. *Journal of Nursing Education, 60*(4), 209–215.

Cannon, S., & Boswell, C. (2016). *Evidence-based teaching in nursing: A foundation for educators* (2nd ed.). Burlington, MA: Jones & Bartlett Learning.

Christenbery, T. (2014). The curriculum vitae: Gateway to academia. *Nurse Educator, 39*(6), 267–268.

Christensen, L. S., & Simmons, L. E. (2020). *The scope of practice for academic nurse educators and academic clinical nurse educators.* Washington, DC: National League for Nursing.

CITI Program. (n.d.). *Get to know CITI Program.* https://about.citiprogram.org/get-to-know-citi-program/.

DeBoor, S. S. (2023). *Keating's curriculum development and evaluation in nursing education* (5th ed.). New York: Springer Publishing.

Grady, C. (2015). Institutional review boards: Purpose and challenges. *Chest, 148*(5), 1148–1155. https://doi.org/10.1378/chest.15-0706.

Halstead, J. (2019). *NLN core competencies for nurse educators: A decade of influence.* Washington, DC: National League for Nursing-Wolters Kluwer.

He, Y., & Hutson, B. (2016). Appreciative assessment in academic advising. *Review of Higher Education, 39*(2), 213–240.

Ignatavicius, D. (2019). *Teaching and learning in a concept-based nursing curriculum: A how-to best practice approach.* Burlington, MA: Jones & Bartlett Learning.

International Institute for Management Development (IMD). (Updated May 2021). *The 5 leadership styles you can use.* https://www.imd.org/imd-reflections/reflection-page/leadership-styles/.

Iwasiw, C. L., Andrusyszyn, M., & Goldenberg, D. (2020). *Curriculum development in nursing education* (4th ed.). Burlington, MA: Jones & Bartlett Learning.

Lafayette. (2021). *The three types of IRB review.* https://irb.lafayette.edu/the-three-types-of-irb-review/.

Marzinsky, A., & Smith-Miller, C. (2019). *Nurse research and the institutional review board.* American Nurse. https://www.myamericannurse.com/nurse-research-and-the-institutional-review-board/.

McDonald, M. (2018). *The nurse educator's guide to assessing learning outcomes.* Burlington, MA: Jones & Bartlett Learning.

Metzger, M., Dowling, T., Guinn, J., & Wilson, D. (2020). Inclusivity in baccalaureate nursing education: A scoping study. *Journal of Professional Nursing, 36*, 5–14.

National League for Nursing (NLN). (2006). Position-statement: Mentoring of nurse faculty. *Nursing Education Perspectives, 27*(2), 110–113.

National League for Nursing (NLN). (2016). NLN releases a vision for advancing the science of nursing education: The NLN nursing education research priorities (2016–2019). *Nursing Education Perspectives, 37*(4), 236.

National League for Nursing (NLN). (2019). *Certification in nursing education.* http://www.nln.org/Certification-for-Nurse-Educators.

National League for Nursing (NLN). (2020). *NLN fair testing guidelines for nursing education.* www.nln.org/fairtestingguidelines.

Oermann, M. H. (2017). *A systematic approach to assessment and evaluation of nursing programs.* Philadelphia: Wolters Kluwer.

Oermann, M., & Gaberson, K. (2021). *Evaluation and testing in nursing education* (6th ed.). New York: Springer Publishing.

Oermann, M. H., DeGagne, J. C., & Phillips, B. C. (2022). *Teaching in nursing and role of the educator* (3rd ed.). New York: Springer Publishing.

Stevens, D. D., & Levi, A. J. (2012). *Introduction to rubrics: An assessment tool to save grading time, convey effective feedback, and promote student learning.* Sterling, VA: Stylus.

University of Buffalo. (n.d.). *High quality learning outcomes.* http://www.buffalo.edu/ubcei/enhance/designing/learning-outcomes/high-quality-learning-outcomes.html.

University of Minnesota Libraries. (2010). *Organizational behaviors.* https://open.lib.umn.edu/organizationalbehavior/chapter/15-5-creating-culture-change/.

U.S. Department of Health and Human Services (USDHHS). (n.d.). *Healthy People 2020: Social determinants of health.* https://health.gov/healthypeople/objectives-and-data/social-determinants-health.

Vajoczki, S., Savage, P., Martin, L., Borin, P., & Kustra, E. (2011). Good teachers, scholarly teachers and teachers engaged in the scholarship of teaching and learning: A case study from McMaster University, Hamilton, Canada. *The Canadian Journal for the Scholarship of Teaching and Learning, 2*(1). https://doi.org/10.5206/CJSOTL-RCACEA.2011.1.2. article 2.

Walker, D., Altmiller, G., Hromadik, L., Barkell, N., Barker, N., Boyd, T., et al. (2020). Nursing students' perception of just culture in nursing programs. *Nurse Educator, 45*(3), 133–138.

Weir, S., Dickman, M., & Fuqua, D. (2005). Preferences for academic advising styles. *NACADA Journal, 25*(1), 74–80.

Index

NOTE: Page numbers followed by *b* indicate boxes, *f* indicate illustrations, and *t* indicate tables.

Notes

Notes

Notes

Notes

Notes